Essential Medical Ophthalmology

A Problem-oriented Approach

The ˮ   Book

To Ali, Harry and Oliver

Acquisitions editor: Melanie Tait
Development editor: Zoë Youd
Production controller: Chris Jarvis
Desk editor: Jane Campbell
Cover designer: Alan Studholme

Essential Medical Ophthalmology:
A Problem-oriented Approach

JOHN D. FERRIS FRCOphth

Consultant Ophthalmologist
Gloucestershire Eye Unit, Cheltenham

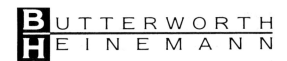

OXFORD AUCKLAND BOSTON JOHANNESBURG MELBOURNE NEW DELHI

Butterworth-Heinemann
Linacre House, Jordan Hill, Oxford OX2 8DP
225 Wildwood Avenue, Woburn, MA 01801-2041
A division of Reed Educational and Professional Publishing Ltd

A member of the Reed Elsevier plc group

First published 2001

Reed Educational and Professional Publishing Ltd 2001

British Library Cataloguing in Publication Data
Ferris, John
    Essential medical ophthalmology: a problem oriented approach
    1. Ocular manifestations of general diseases
    I. Title
    617.7

Library of Congress Cataloguing in Publication Data
A catalogue record for this book is available from the Library of Congress

ISBN 0 7506 4937 2

Typeset by David Gregson Associates, Beccles, Suffolk
Printed and bound in Italy

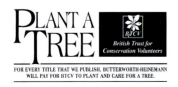

WW 100

Contents

Preface

There have been many books that have aimed to cover the ocular manifestations of systemic disease, most of which are in a photo-atlas format with numerous illustrations and a relatively truncated text. The aim of this book is to highlight ocular conditions associated with common systemic diseases, with a particular emphasis on the medical management of the underlying systemic disorders.

Each section involves the recognition and interpretation of physical signs, radiological imaging or laboratory investigations. It would be impossible to have an exhaustive discussion of each condition in the accompanying text, and therefore many conditions such as diabetes mellitus, Graves' disease and multiple sclerosis feature in two or more sections. The aim of the 'question and answer' format is to assess the readers' knowledge of the natural history and manifestations of the disease and to explore common diagnostic and management problems relevant to the clinic and examination setting. The questions are designed in such a way as to promote tangential thinking and to emphasise the common ground shared by ophthalmolo-gists and physicians in the management of these patients.

In order to facilitate an evidence-based approach to clinical practice, the results of many clinical trials and their influence on current clinical practice are discussed in detail. A recommended reading list consisting of these landmark papers and in-depth review articles is included after many questions. I hope this format will be more conducive to stimulating further reading than a lengthy bibliography.

Over the last decade there has been an increasing trend towards subspecialisation in both ophthalmology and medicine. Although there have been benefits for both clinicians and patients as a result of these changes, the price that has been paid is a narrowing of our medical perspective. There is a need for ophthalmologists and physicians to be aware of the ocular and systemic manifestations of the diseases they are treating, and also the effect their treatments have on the management of the patient as a whole. I hope this book will go some way to heightening this awareness in both ophthalmologists and physicians alike.

Acknowledgements

There have been many people who have helped me during the course of writing this book. I would like to thank Mr Declan Flanagan FRCS FRCOphth, Mr Nicholas Sarkies MRCP FRCS FRCOphth, Dr Wendy Marshman FRACO and Mr Eric Barnes MRCP FRCOphth for reviewing sections of the manuscript. I would especially like to thank Dr Paul Siklos FRCP whose advice regarding the format and medical content of the book was invaluable.

Many colleagues have generously allowed me to use clinical photographs, radiological images and electrodiagnostic recordings from their personal collections. In this regard I would like to thank Mr Jack Kanski MD FRCS FRCOphth, Mr Tony Moore MA FRCS FRCOphth, Mr Tony Vivian FRCOphth, Mr Martin Snead MD FRCOphth, Dr Paul Meyer MD MRCP FRCS FRCOphth, Dr Brian Hazelman FRCP, Dr Owen Edwards FRCP, Dr Carlos Parvesio MD FRCS FRCOphth, Dr Keith Bradshaw PhD and Mr Ken Nischal FRCOphth.

I would also like to thank Dr Fiona Rowe for her help with the illustrations in the visual field and ocular motility sections and Dr Les Culank for providing the biochemical investigations.

Finally, I would like to acknowledge the invaluable help I received from Katherine Haslam in the Medical Photography Department of Addenbooke's Hospital, Cambridge. I am not only indebted to Katherine for her skill as photographer, but also for her abundant patience and good humour as we compiled the illustrations for this book.

Section 1

Fundi

1.1

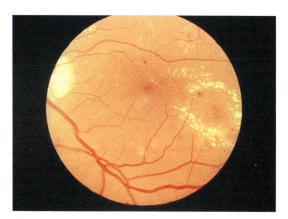

Fig. 1.1a

Q: *Describe this fundal appearance. What is the diagnosis? (see Fig. 1.1a)*

A: There are numerous microaneurysms with associated areas of circinate exudate and intra-retinal haemorrhages scattered throughout the posterior pole. There are no cotton wool spots or areas of venous beading, this can therefore be classified as background diabetic retinopathy. The discrete areas of circinate exudate are indicative of a focal diabetic maculopathy.

Q: *What are the pathological features of this microvasculopathy?*

A: Diabetic microvasculopathy arises as a result of a number of changes in the retinal circulation:

(1) Loss of microvascular intramural pericytes.
(2) Microaneurysm formation, which may in part be linked to pericyte loss.
(3) Thickening of microvascular basement membranes.
(4) Endothelial cell dysfunction results in a breakdown of the blood–retinal barrier.
(5) Capillary and arteriolar closure, possible causes for which can be divided into three categories:

(a) Intraluminal factors such as erythrocyte aggregation, elevated plasma fibrinogen, increased platelet adhesiveness and aggregation may all promote thrombosis within small retinal vessels.
(b) Intramural factors; basement membrane changes coupled with endothelial abnormalities may result in luminal narrowing and haemodynamic alterations.
(c) Extramural factors in the form of increased interstitial fluid in the retina have been proposed as a factor in capillary closure.

(6) Retinal hyperperfusion secondary to a loss of retinal autoregulation causes shearing damage to capillaries. Conditions such as moderate carotid artery stenosis and raised intraocular pressure, which reduce retinal hyperperfusion, tend to protect from advancing retinopathy. Conversely, hypertension, hyperglycaemia and pregnancy, which exacerbate hyperperfusion, worsen diabetic retinopathy.

Q: *How should this condition be treated?*

A: Focal diabetic retinopathy that threatens the fovea, as this large temporal circinate exudate does, should be treated promptly with argon laser directed at the leaking microaneurysms. Close follow-up in the ophthalmology clinic is essential to monitor the resolution of the exudates and to check for any progression of the retinopathy.

Q: *Describe the fundal appearance of this 65-year-old non-insulin-dependent diabetic woman. What would you expect her visual acuity to be? (see Fig. 1.1b)*

A: There are a number of scattered microaneurysms, intraretinal haemorrhages and subtle changes in the retinal pigment epithelium

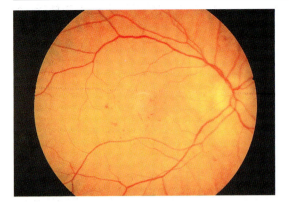
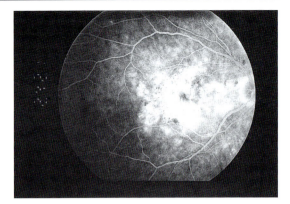

Fig. 1.1b

(RPE), but there is very little in the way of exudate. At a casual glance this would appear to be an example of mild background diabetic retinopathy; however, what this two-dimensional view does not reveal is the marked retinal thickening which may be difficult to detect with direct ophthalmoscopy. This picture is characteristic of diffuse diabetic macular oedema, the extent of which may be confirmed by fluorescein angiography. This demonstrates extensive extravasation of fluorescein (white) from the incompetent retinal capillaries in the late venous phase of the angiogram. The visual acuity in this eye was 6/24.

Q: *How would you manage this patient?*

A: The Early Treatment Diabetic Retinopathy Study (EDTRS) demonstrated that eyes with clinically significant macular oedema benefited from focal argon laser photocoagulation. This was defined as follows:

(1) Retinal thickening at or within 500 µm of the centre of the macula.
(2) Hard exudate at or within 500 µm of the centre of the macula associated with thickening of adjacent retina.
(3) A zone(s) of retinal thickening 1 disc area or larger, any part of which is within one disc diameter of the centre of the macula. This is assessed using lens biomicroscopy and/or stereophotographs. Treatment was found to increase the chance of visual improvement, decrease the frequency of persistent macular oedema and reduce the risk of visual loss. However, despite treatment, 12% of patients with central diabetic macular oedema lost 15 or more letters over a 3-year period (Fig. 1.1c). The prognosis

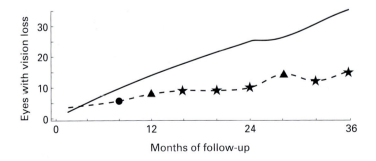

Fig. 1.1c – – – immediate photocoagulation;
——— deferral of photocoagulation unless high risk characteristics develop

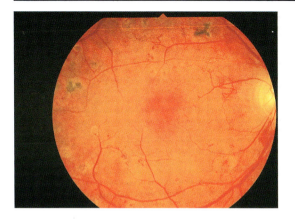
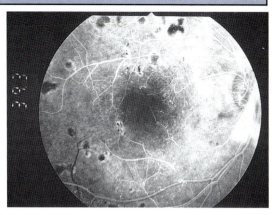

Fig. 1.1d

was particularly poor in those eyes with an initial visual acuity of 6/18 or less.

Treatment is normally in the form of a grid laser treatment, with applications of concentric 100 μm burns increasing to 200 μm with increasing eccentricity from the fovea. The papillomacular bundle is usually avoided, at least in initial treatments. It is also essential to ensure that any hypertension is adequately treated, as no amount of laser treatment will compensate for the deleterious effect of uncontrolled hypertension and a leaking capillary bed. The best visual results occur when the initial (pre-treatment) visual acuity is 6/24 or better.

Q: *Describe the fundal and fluorescein appearances of this 32-year-old man with insulin-dependent diabetes. What would you expect the visual acuity to be? (see Fig. 1.1d)*

A: There are a number of intraretinal haemorrhages, microaneurysms and laser scars visible in an otherwise relatively featureless posterior pole. However, closer inspection reveals an intraretinal microvascular abnormality (IRMA) along the superotemporal arcade and some early venous irregularities. The most striking feature of the mid-venous phase angiogram is the grossly enlarged foveal avascular zone (the foveal avascular zone is normally < 500 μm in diameter, i.e. 1/3 of a disc diameter). These appearances are typical of an

ischaemic maculopathy, which has reduced the visual acuity to 6/36.

Q: *How would you manage this patient and what is the visual prognosis?*

A: Ischaemic maculopathy has a variable visual prognosis, with surprisingly little effect on visual acuity until the foveal avascular zone is 1000 μm in diameter. In eyes with arteriolar as well as capillary closure the visual prognosis is uniformly poor. There is no role for focal laser treatment, unless the angiogram demonstrates that it is associated with a significant degree of macular oedema (ischaemic and oedematous maculopathy frequently coexist). It is invariably associated with more global fundal ischaemia and these patients are at risk of developing proliferative retinopathy if they have not done so already. They should therefore be followed up 3-monthly in the eye clinic and every effort should be made to improve their diabetic control. The UK Prospective Diabetes Study Group was the first study to prove that tight control of hypertension in patients with type 2 diabetes reduces the risk of clinical complications of diabetic eye disease. In this study a 10 mmHg fall in systolic blood pressure and a 5 mmHg fall in diastolic blood pressure was associated with a 47% reduction in the risk of doubling the visual angle at 9 years. There is evidence that hypertension is the major risk factor in the development of ischaemic maculopathy and as such should be treated aggressively.

The two cases above are good examples of how potentially sight-threatening maculopathy may be misdiagnosed as 'background' diabetic retinopathy by the unsuspecting physician. As it may be difficult to fully assess the diabetic fundus by direct ophthalmoscopy, any patient with apparently 'mild diabetic retinopathy' and unexplained visual loss (which is not improved using a pinhole) should be referred promptly for an ophthalmological opinion. Physicians and ophthalmologists alike should be mindful of the fact that 'background' diabetic retinopathy, in the form of maculopathy, is the most common cause of blind registration in diabetic patients.

Recommended reading

Bresnick, G. H. (1994) Nonproliferative diabetic retinopathy. In *Retina*, 2nd edn (S. J. Ryan, ed.), pp. 1277–1318. Mosby-Year Book, St Louis, MO.

The Early Treatment of Diabetic Retinopathy Study Research Group (1985) Photocoagulation for diabetic macular edema. *Arch. Ophthalmol.*, **103**, 1796–1806.

UK Prospective Diabetes Study Group (1998) Tight blood pressure control and the risk of macrovascular and microvacsular complications in type 2 diabetes: UKPDS 38. *Br. Med. J.*, **317**, 703–713.

1.2

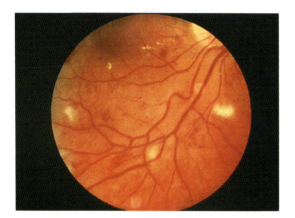

Fig. 1.2a

Q: *Describe the fundal appearance of this 30-year-old diabetic woman. What stage of retinopathy is this? (see Fig. 1.2a)*

A: There are deep intraretinal and superficial nerve fibre layer haemorrhages. Four cotton wool spots (note that the term cotton wool spot refers to a focal nerve fibre layer infarct; some medical textbooks still refer to these lesions as 'soft exudates' as they are neither soft nor exudates this terminology should no longer be used), an IRMA and a degree of venous beading are also present. These latter changes are indicative of preproliferative retinopathy.

Q: *What percentage of such eyes will progress to proliferative retinopathy?*

A: These eyes will demonstrate a marked degree of ischaemia on fluorescein angiography and 50% of them will progress to proliferative retinopathy over a period of 15 months. These patients should therefore be reviewed at least 4-monthly by an ophthalmologist.

Q: *What simple 'investigations' may be performed in the clinic to assess the risk of progression to proliferative retinopathy and other end-organ damage?*

A:

(1) Urinalysis to check for proteinuria – although conventional 'stix' testing will not detect microalbuminuria it is a useful screening test of renal function. The presence of proteinuria detectable on routine urinalysis is indicative of albumin excretion >300 mg/24 h and signifies established nephropathy. These patients are at high risk of developing proliferative retinopathy.
(2) Blood pressure – hypertension is a risk factor for both macrovascular and microvascular disease, early detection and aggressive treatment may prevent or at least delay the onset of end-organ damage.

Q: *What are the indications for performing panretinal argon laser photocoagulation at this preproliferative stage?*

A: One of the issues addressed by the Early Treatment of Diabetes Retinopathy Study was whether patients with preproliferative retinopathy would benefit from early panretinal photocoagulation (PRP). They concluded that for eyes with mild to moderate preproliferative changes, e.g. numerous cotton wool spots, scattered IRMA and moderate venous beading PRP was not indicated. However, in eyes which were deemed as being at high risk of developing proliferative changes, e.g. those with extensive venous calibre irregularities, numerous deep intraretinal haemorrhages and large areas of capillary closure on angiography, then prophylactic PRP could be justified. A patient's previous attendance record and the quality of their diabetic control may well influence the ophthalmologist's scheduling of PRP.

Q: *How does pregnancy influence the development and progression of diabetic retinopathy? How would you manage this patient if she was in the first trimester of pregnancy?*

A: It is essential for ophthalmologists, physicians and obstetricians to be aware of the effect of pregnancy on diabetic retinopathy and the effect of diabetic retinopathy on pregnancy. It is now well established that diabetic retinopathy worsens during pregnancy, although the mechanism by which progression occurs is still a subject of debate. The following factors have been implicated in the progression of retinopathy during pregnancy:

(1) Metabolic control – The Diabetes in Early Pregnancy (DIEP) study clearly showed that those women with the greatest reduction in HbA_{1C} over the first 14 weeks of pregnancy were at an increased risk of progression of retinopathy. These patients also had the largest improvement in diabetic control in early pregnancy. It was impossible to determine whether this or the poor baseline control was the most important risk factor for progression.

(2) Duration of diabetes – this is probably not as important as the baseline severity of retinopathy. However, there is a close correlation between duration of diabetes and the stage of retinopathy. There is evidence to suggest that progression to proliferative retinopathy is more common in women with more than a 15-year history of diabetes.

(3) Baseline severity of retinopathy – approximately 12% of women with no retinopathy at the start of pregnancy will develop minor background changes by term, these usually regress in the postpartum period. The DIEP study showed that only 6.3% of women with minimal baseline retinopathy developed proliferative disease during pregnancy. This increased to 29% if patients had moderate retinopathy at baseline. The severity of retinopathy has also been shown to adversely affect outcome in pregnancy.

Proliferative retinopathy at baseline is associated with the development of pregnancy-induced hypertension, congenital malformations and/or foetal death.

(4) Hypertension is a risk factor for the progression of diabetic retinopathy and this adverse effect on retinopathy is even more marked during pregnancy.

Despite the risks of imposing strict glycaemic control it is also recognised that normalisation of blood sugar is the most important factor for the successful outcome of pregnancy in diabetes. The following is a protocol for the management of the expectant mother with diabetes:

(1) Strict glycaemic control aiming for an HbA_{1C} of 8% should ideally be instigated prior to conception or as early as possible in the pregnancy.

(2) Patients with minimal background retinopathy can be safely monitored on a 3-monthly basis. Patients with more marked background changes should have a fundal examination at each obstetric visit, if there is any evidence of progression 2-weekly follow-up is advisable.

(3) Patients with preproliferative retinopathy (such as the above patient) should be reviewed on a monthly basis or more frequently if previous glycaemic control has been poor and a rapid improvement in glycaemic control is anticipated.

(4) Treatment of proliferative retinopathy prior to conception reduces the risk of visual loss during pregnancy. If proliferative disease is detected during pregnancy prompt laser treatment sufficient to promote regression is indicated. Under no circumstances should laser treatment be delayed for 1–2 weeks, if adequate treatment is not possible because of patient discomfort, retrobulbar anaesthesia or a short general anaesthetic should be considered.

Recommended reading

Best, R. M. and Chakravarthy, U. (1997) Diabetic retinopathy in pregnancy [Review]. *Br. J. Ophthalmol.*, **81**, 249–251.

Early Treatment of Diabetic Retinopathy Study Research Group (1991) Early Photocoagulation for diabetic retinopathy. ETDRS report # 9. *Ophthalmology*, **98** (Suppl.), 766–785.

1.3

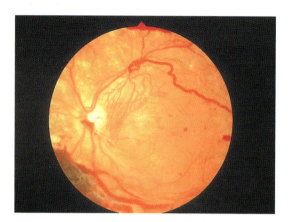

Fig. 1.3a

Q: *Describe the fundal appearance of this 25-year-old woman with diabetes. What stage of retinopathy is this? (see Fig. 1.3a)*

A: The fundus photograph shows marked neovascularisation superotemporal, inferior and adjacent to the disc. The inferior new vessels have bled resulting in a localised subhyaloid haemorrhage. There are gross venous calibre irregularities and evidence of previous laser treatment. This is the typical appearance of proliferative diabetic retinopathy.

Q: *What distinguishes new vessels from IRMAs?*

A: Both true neovascularisation and IRMA are responses of the retinal circulation to increasing ischaemia. IRMA as their name would suggest are intraretinal vessels (and hence appear flat on ophthalmoscopy or biomicroscopy) that represent 'shunt vessels' between the retinal arterioles and venules, although some observers view them as areas of intraretinal neovascularisation. The endothelium of IRMA possesses tight junctions, therefore they do not leak fluorescein. Neovascularisation arises from retinal venules, endothelial buds under the influence of vasoproliferative factors sprout fronds of new vessels, which grow in a characteristic 'carriage

wheel' pattern between the internal limiting membrane of the retina and the posterior hyaloid. New vessels may arise anywhere in the retina but are most commonly found within 45° of the optic disc. One of their unique features is that they extend across both arterial and venous branches of the underlying retinal vascular network. As neovascularisation progresses connective tissue composed of fibrocytes and glial cells may be associated with the vessels. If there is a partial detachment of the posterior hyaloid membrane the vessels may appear elevated. As the neovascular endothelium lacks tight junctions they will leak fluorescein, resulting in the characteristic hyperfluorescence seen with angiography.

Q: *What is the visual prognosis for eyes with proliferative retinopathy. What is the evidence that PRP is of benefit?*

A: The first study to conclusively prove the benefits of PRP was the Diabetic Retinopathy Study (DRS). This was a large multicentre trial published in 1978 that demonstrated an overall reduction in the rate of severe visual loss from 15.9% in untreated groups to 6.4% in those receiving PRP, a reduction of 60%. The trial also highlighted groups of patients who were at especially high risk of developing severe visual loss (visual acuity of <5/200) over a 2-year period (Table 1.1).

The cumulative rates of severe visual loss for eyes classified by presence of proliferative retinopathy (PDR) and high-risk characteristics (HRC), in baseline DRS fundal photographs, are illustrated in Fig. 1.3b.

Q: *What is the rationale behind PRP for proliferative retinopathy? How should treatment be monitored and what are the potential side effects?*

A: The exact method by which argon laser photocoagulation produces regression of

Table 1.1

Group	Treated	Untreated
NVD (mild) with vitreous haemorrhage	43%	25.6%
NVD (moderate to severe) without vitreous haemorrhage	8.5%	26.2%
NVD (moderate to severe) with vitreous haemorrhage	20.1%	36.9%
NVD (moderate to severe) without vitreous haemorrhage	7.2%	29.7%

proliferative retinopathy is not fully understood, possible explanations include:

(1) Destruction of ischaemic retina, which is postulated to be producing vasoproliferative factors.
(2) Improved oxygenation of the overlying inner retina by destruction of the highly metabolically active photoreceptors, so allowing oxygen from the choriocapillaris to permeate to these superficial layers.
(3) Retinal pigment epithelial cells may produce a new vessel inhibiting factor, the release of which may be stimulated by photocoagulation injury.

In most cases of proliferative retinopathy a minimum of 1000–1500 burns should be applied as an initial treatment. The patient should then be reviewed within 1 month for further photocoagulation of the peripheral retina. Although there is not a fixed number of burns that will insure regression of new vessels, after 2500–3000 burns most ophthamologists would monitor the eye for signs of regression prior to applying further laser treatment.

Signs of regression include:

(1) A return to normal venous calibre is often the first sign of regressing retinopathy.
(2) Disappearance of the new vessels (this may never occur in some eyes).
(3) The development of closed loops at the end of neovascular fronds.
(4) Fibrotic changes around the new vessels.

When these changes are observed no further PRP is required. However, even inactive new vessels may bleed in the event of a posterior vitreous detachment, resulting in a subhyaloid or intragel haemorrhage. If there are no signs of regression after an initial PRP, fill-in treatment should be carried out until regression is achieved, or until vitreous haemorrhage precludes further treatment. Figure 1.3c is the

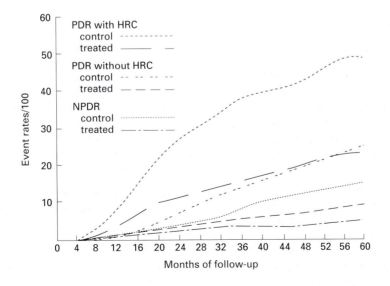

Fig. 1.3b

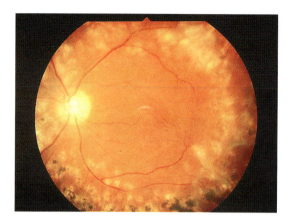

Fig. 1.3c

fundal appearance of the eye in Fig. 1.3a after adequate PRP.

Fully informed consent outlining the side effects of PRP is mandatory prior to treatment. Potential side effects include decreased night vision, colour vision and peripheral vision. The latter may be severe enough to preclude the patient from holding a driving licence. Occasionally one or more lines of best corrected visual acuity may be lost, this is often the result of an exacerbation of pre-existing macular oedema; grid laser treatment should therefore be performed prior to PRP in all such patients.

Q: *What is the evidence that tighter diabetic control retards the development or progression of diabetic retinopathy? (see Fig. 1.3c)*

A: All ophthalmologists and physicians should be familiar with the Diabetes Control and Complications Trial (DCCT). This multicentre trial recruited approximately 1400 insulin-dependent diabetics who either had no retinopathy at presentation (the primary-prevention cohort) or mild retinopathy (the secondary-intervention cohort). All patients were randomised into two groups and followed up for a mean of 6.5 years:

(1) Those who were maintained on an intensive insulin regime aimed at achieving an HbA_{1C} of 6.5%. The average blood glucose

in this cohort during the trial period was 8.6 mmol/l.

(2) Those who were maintained on a standard b.d. insulin regime. The mean HbA_{1C} in this group was 9.2% and the mean blood glucose 12.8 mmol/l.

The main parameters that the trial looked at were retinopathy, nephropathy and neuropathy.

Intensive therapy reduced the adjusted mean risk for the development of retinopathy by 76% and slowed the progression of retinopathy by 54%. The incidence of severe preproliferative and proliferative retinopathy was reduced by 47%. In the two cohorts combined intensive treatment reduced the occurrence of microalbuminuria by 39%, albuminuria by 54% and clinical neuropathy by 60%. However, these impressive results were achieved at the expense of a 2- to 3-fold increase in the frequency of severe hypoglycaemic episodes.

The UK Prospective Diabetes Study Group reported the results of strict glycaemic control with sulphonylureas or insulin in patients with type 2 diabetes. This study recruited 3867 newly diagnosed patients with type 2 diabetes and randomised them to intensive or conventional glycaemic control. Over 10 years the HbA_{1C} was 7.0% in the intensive group and 7.9% in the conventional group. Progression of retinopathy was reduced by 21% and albuminuria by 34% in the intensively treated cohort. The fact that the HbA_{1C} only differed by 0.9% between the two cohorts in this study (versus 1.9% in the DCCT) may explain the less dramatic reduction in microvascular disease.

Recommended reading

The Diabetic Retinopathy Study Research Group (1978) Photocoagulation treatment of proliferative diabetic retinopathy: the second report of Diabetic Retinopathy Study findings. *Ophthalmology*, **85**, 82–106.
The Diabetic Retinopathy Study Research Group (1981) Photocoagulation treatment of proliferative diabetic retinopathy: clinical application of

Diabetic Retinopathy Study (DRS) findings, DRS report 8. *Ophthalmology*, **88**, 583–600.

The Diabetes Control and Complications Trial Research Group (1993) The effect of intensive treatment of diabetes on the development of long-term complications in insulin-dependent diabetes mellitus. *N. Engl. J. Med.*, **329**, 977–986.

The UK Prospective Diabetes Study Group (1998) Intensive blood glucose control with sulphonylureas or insulin compared with conventional treatment and risks of complications in patients with type 2 diabetes (UKPDS 33). *Lancet*, **352**, 837–853.

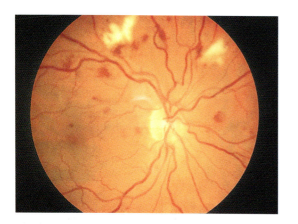

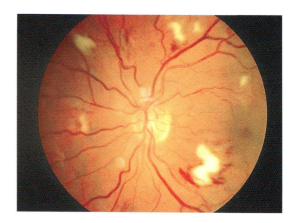

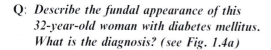

Fig. 1.4a

Q: *Describe the fundal appearance of this 32-year-old woman with diabetes mellitus. What is the diagnosis? (see Fig. 1.4a)*

A: The most striking fundal features are the numerous cotton wool spots and scattered nerve fibre layer and intraretinal haemorrhages. There are no microaneurysms, retinal exudates nor evidence of venous beading, thus ruling out the diagnosis of diabetic retinopathy. These fundal changes are in fact secondary to the relatively recent onset of hypertension, this explains the absence of arteriovenous crossing changes and signs of arteriosclerosis.

Q: *What are the cardinal features of a hypertensive retinopathy?*

A: The degree of retinopathy will be dependent on the duration and the severity of the hypertension. When examining the fundi of a hypertensive patient the following features should be sought:

(1) Changes in the arterioles:
 (a) Generalised narrowing.
 (b) Generalised sclerosis (i.e. 'copper and silver wiring').
 (c) Focal constriction.
 (d) Tortuosity.
(2) Arteriovenous crossing changes:
 (a) Arteriovenous nipping or apparent compression of the vein (Gunn's sign).
 (b) A deflection in the course of the vein (Salus' sign).
(3) Retinal haemorrhages:
 (a) These are usually flame shaped nerve fibre layer haemorrhages.
 (b) Occasionally deep intraretinal haemorrhages may occur (this is in marked contrast to diabetic retinopathy where deep intraretinal haemorrhages predominate).
(4) Cotton wool spots. These represent infarction of the nerve fibre layer. They are white greyish lesions, that have feathery edges and are a transient phenomenon. They may be confused with focal intraretinal periarteriolar transudates (FIPTs), a term coined by Hayreh to describe pinpoint to pinhead size, round or oval, dull white transudates. FIPTs are one of the earliest and most common lesions in hypertensive retinopathy. These lesions, like nerve fibre

layer infarcts, are transient. Although unlike cotton wool spots they are thought to be specific to malignant arterial hypertension.

(5) Exudates. Exudates usually accumulate in the posterior pole where they may produce a 'macular star'. These residues tend to have a relatively low fat content and appear grey or silver, this is in contrast to the waxy exudates seen in diabetic retinopathy.

(6) Disc swelling. There may be a significant degree of inter-observer variability when it comes to assessing the optic disc in cases of hypertensive retinopathy, thus rendering disc swelling an unreliable physical sign. Recent studies have shown that disc swelling does not adversely influence the prognosis in patients who already have bilateral retinal haemorrhages and exudates, when effective treatment is instigated. Some authors have therefore suggested, that papilloedema should no longer be regarded as a necessary feature of malignant hypertension.

Q: *What is the pathogenesis of optic disc swelling in severe hypertension? What are the risks to vision of rapidly reducing the blood pressure in such patients?*

A: There is considerable debate as to what is the cause of disc swelling in severe hypertension.

(1) The raised intracranial pressure (ICP) theory. Historically disc swelling was thought to be secondary to raised ICP. Numerous studies have shown a close correlation between the increased CSF pressure and the diastolic blood pressure in patients with optic disc oedema. Others have proposed a direct relationship between the occurrence of optic disc oedema and the CSF pressure.

(2) *The ischaemic theory*. As the optic nerve head is supplied primarily by the posterior ciliary and not the retinal circulation, hypertensive optic neuropathy should not be considered to be part of the hypertensive retinopathy spectrum. The development of hypertensive optic neuropathy is, however, linked with hypertensive choroidopathy. It has been suggested that vasoconstriction of the choroidal vascular bed, perhaps associated with failure of autoregulation in the optic nerve head (failure of cerebral autoregulation is the primary cause of hypertensive encephalopathy), produces optic nerve head ischaemia, stasis in axoplasmic flow proximal to the ischaemic site and axonal swelling at the optic disc. Animal studies have confirmed that disc swelling is present in the absence of a raised CSF pressure.

The severity of this anterior ischaemic optic neuropathy is extremely variable but it is well documented that sudden lowering of the blood pressure may inflict a further ischaemic insult on an already compromised optic nerve head. This may result in bilateral infarction of the optic nerve head.

Q: *If asked to examine this patient what features of the systemic examination would be of relevance?*

A: Approximately 90% of hypertension can be labelled as essential. The remaining 10% is in the main secondary to endocrinological disease, renal disease or cardiovascular disorders. Bearing this in mind your examination should include the following to ascertain both the aetiology of the hypertension and also its possible sequelae.

(1) General inspection. Look for evidence of endocrine dysfunction (e.g. acromegaly and Cushing's syndrome) and of neurofibromatosis.

(2) Cardiovascular examination:
 (a) Radio-femoral delay signalling coarctation of the aorta.
 (b) Left ventricular heave secondary to hypertrophy of the left ventricle.
 (c) Carotid bruits and peripheral pulses for evidence of more generalised vascular disease.
 (d) Measure the blood pressure.

(3) Abdominal examination:
  (a) Palpate the abdomen for polycystic kidneys.
  (b) Abdominal bruits of renal artery stenosis.
(4) Urinalysis. Check for glucosuria, proteinuria and haematuria.

Q: *What are the ocular side effects of anti-hypertensive/arrhythmic medications?*

A:

(1) Disturbance of colour vision, especially the yellow discoloration of images (xanthopsia), may be caused by a number of medications. Digoxin is the most common culprit, the visual problem is dose related and occurs when the serum digoxin level is >2 µg/l. Digoxin may also cause scotomas. Thiazide duiretics may occasionally produce xanthopsia.
(2) Corneal verticilata are commonly seen with amioderone therapy, but very rarely do they cause any visual symptoms.
(3) Treatment of hypertension especially in the elderly may cause periods of relative hypotension when the patient is supine. In patients with glaucoma in whom the optic nerve head circulation is compromised, these periods of nocturnal hypotension may lead to further ganglion cell drop-out with resultant visual field loss.
(4) Cortical infarction in the watershed zone between the middle and posterior cerebral circulations has been reported with nifedipine therapy.
(5) Quinidine may cause a quinine-like optic neuritis.

Q: *What is the threshold for the treatment of hypertension? What is the appropriate target blood pressure?*

A: The WHO/International Society of Hypertension 1999 guidelines use a systolic blood pressure criterion of >140 mmHg or a diastolic blood pressure of >90 mmHg for a definition of hypertension. The decision as to which patients should be treated is based on cardiovascular

risk factor assessment, which takes into account factors such as diabetes, smoking, family history and raised serum cholesterol. Hypertension has long been implicated as a major risk factor for coronary and cerebrovascular disease. However, despite treatment there is often a higher incidence of cardiovascular complications in patients with hypertension than in normotensive individuals. The Hypertension Optimal Treatment randomised trial has recently addressed the issue of what constitutes optimal blood pressure control.

The trial recruited 18 790 patients aged 50–80 years with hypertension and a diastolic blood pressure between 100 and 115 mmHg. They were randomised into three groups with target diastolic blood pressures of ≤90, ≤85 and ≤80 mmHg. Felodipine was the baseline therapy and other agents were then added according to a set protocol. The lowest incidence of major cardiovascular events occurred at a mean diastolic blood pressure of 82.6 mmHg and the lowest risk of cardiovascular mortality occurred at 86.5 mmHg. Further reduction below these blood pressures was found to be safe, thus casting doubt on the historical concept of a J-shaped mortality curve in hypertension. In diabetic patients there was a 51% reduction in major cardiovascular events in the <80 mmHg target group.

Recommended reading

Hansson, L., Zanchetti, A., Carruthers, S. G., Dahlof, B., Elmfeldt, D., Julius, S., *et al.* (1998) Effects of intensive blood-pressure lowering and low-dose aspirin in patients with hypertension: principle results of the Hypertension Optimal Treatment (HOT) randomised trial. HOT Study Group. *Lancet*, **351**, 1755–1762.

McGregor, E., Isles, C. G., Jay, J. L., Lever, A. F. and Murray, G. D. (1986) Retinal changes in malignant hypertension. *Br. Med. J.*, **292**, 233–234.

Tso, M. O. M. and Jampol, L. M. (1982) Pathophysiology of hypertensive retinopathy. *Ophthalmology*, **89**, 1132–1145.

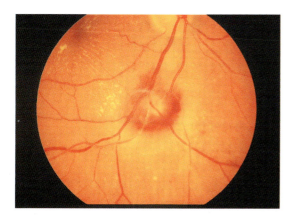
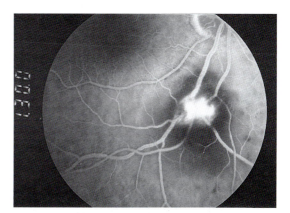

Fig. 1.5a

Q: *This 75-year-old lady presented with a sudden loss of vision in her left eye. What is the diagnosis? What is the natural history of this condition? (see Fig. 1.5a)*

A: This is a retinal macroaneurysm that has burst resulting in intraretinal haemorrhage and exudate in the vicinity of the macroaneurysm, and more distal exudate in a macular star distribution. These lesions are most commonly seen in elderly (70 years plus) hypertensive women. They occur in the first three orders of arteriolar bifurcation or at an arteriovenous crossing.

The natural history of this condition is variable, in many cases retinal macroaneurysms remain asymptomatic and are an incidental finding on ophthalmoscopy. Other sequelae include:

(1) Thrombosis and spontaneous involution.
(2) Exudative changes which may threaten the macula.
(3) Subretinal, intraretinal and subhyaloid haemorrhage.

Q: *How would you manage this condition?*

A: In cases where exudate from a leaking aneurysm is involving or threatening, the macula laser photocoagulation is indicated. Fluorescein angiography will identify the site of the aneurysm and laser treatment should be performed circumferentially. The exudate and intraretinal haemorrhage will then resolve slowly over 4–8 weeks. Occasionally haemorrhage from a ruptured macroaneurysm will result in a large subhyaloid haemorrhage. If this occurs in the superior fundus the subhyaloid haemorrhage may obscure the fovea, as illustrated in Fig. 1.5b (note the fluid level). In these cases the posterior hyaloid membrane,

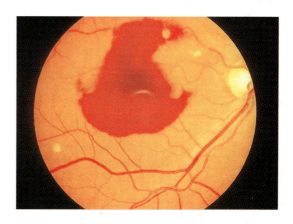

Fig. 1.5b

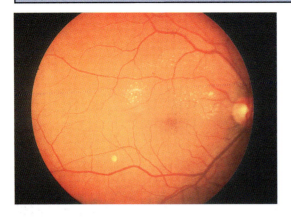

which is containing the haemorrhage can be disrupted with YAG laser allowing the blood to disperse into the vitreous (Fig. 1.5c; this photograph was taken 4 months after YAG laser treatment).

Fig. 1.5c

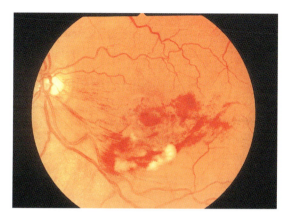 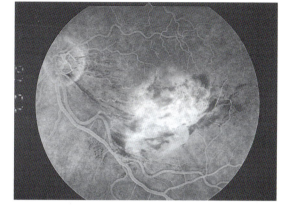

Fig. 1.6a

Q: *This 64-year-old man presented with sudden loss of vision in his left eye. What is the diagnosis? How would you manage this condition? (see Fig. 1.6a)*

A: There are extensive intraretinal/preretinal haemorrhages and cotton wool spots in the inferotemporal quadrant of the fundus extending to the fovea. This is an inferior branch retinal vein occlusion (BRVO). The early-venous frame of the fluorescein angiogram shows there is little in the way of capillary closure, indicating this is a non-ischaemic BRVO. As the venous occlusion is relatively recent there is no evidence of collateral vessel formation.

A full medical and ophthalmic history should be taken. Investigations should be confined to blood pressure measurement and a full blood count. A coagulation profile may be indicated if there is a suggestion of a hypercoagulable state.

Fluorescein angiography will define the degree of capillary closure and hence the risk of neovascularisation. It will also illustrate the extent to which the perifoveal vasculature is involved and the degree of macular oedema. However, if there are extensive retinal haemor-

rhages fluorescein angiography should be deferred for 3–6 months.

Q: *What is the natural history of BRVOs? What is the role of laser photocoagulation in the management of BRVO?*

A: The visual prognosis in BRVO is generally good, with 33–50% of eyes regaining a visual acuity of 6/12 or better. Visual loss may be secondary to macular oedema, non-clearing macular haemorrhage or macular ischaemia. The prognosis for visual recovery is less certain when there is macular oedema associated with non-perfusion, but even in this situation improvement can occur up to one year after BRVO.

Approximately 50% of large BRVOs (involving a quadrant or more) will induce >5 disc diameters of capillary non-perfusion; 40% of these eyes will go on to develop retinal neovascularisation (Fig. 1.6b). Vitreous haemorrhage will occur in 60% of eyes with retinal neovascularisation. Iris neovascularisation is a rare complication of BRVO.

BRVO is usually unilateral, with bilateral involvement being reported in 10% of patients.

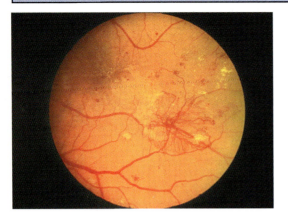

Fig. 1.6b

The two principal indications for argon (bluegreen) laser photocoagulation in patients with BRVO are persistent cystoid macular oedema and retinal neovascularisation. The guidelines for laser photocoagulation based on the Branch Vein Occlusion Study data are as follows:

(1) No laser treatment should be considered for 3–6 months as spontaneous improvement is common.
(2) If the vision is 6/12 or worse and fluorescein angiography demonstrates cystoid macular oedema, but no non-perfusion (Fig. 1.6c), grid macular photocoagulation is indicated.
(3) If there is >5 disc diameters of capillary closure the patient should be followed up at

4-monthly intervals. If neovascularisation develops this should be treated with photocoagulation to that quadrant. This study did not recommend prophylactic laser treatment.

Grid photocoagulation will on average improve the vision from 6/24 to 6/12, whilst scatter treatment reduces the risk of vitreous haemorrhage from 60% to 30% in eyes with established neovascularisation.

Q: *What conditions other than BRVO may cause dilation and leakage of the perifoveal capillary bed?*

A: There are a number of other conditions which may mimic the capillary dilation and leakage seen after BRVO, they include:

(1) *Idiopathic parafoveal capillary telangiectasis (see Fig. 1.6d).* In unilateral cases telangiectatic changes are usually confined to one clock hour at the temporal edge of the foveal avascular zone. The retinal vascular abnormalities and associated oedema are often subtle and are best illustrated by fluorescein angiography. Although bilateral cases may be associated with more extensive involvement of the foveal vasculature, hard exudates remain uncommon. Patients are typically men aged 50–70. The visual acuity is rarely <6/9 and photocoagulation is not recommended because of the lack of

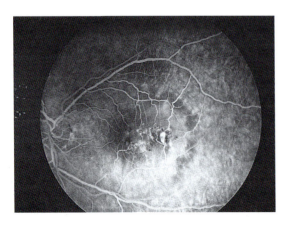
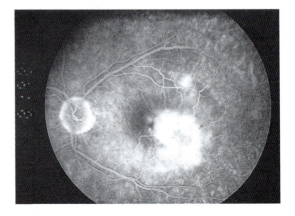

Fig. 1.6c

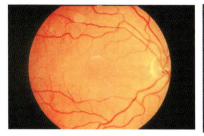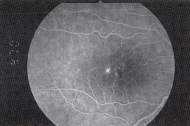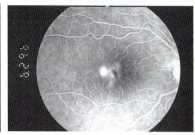

Fig. 1.6d

leakage (in most cases) and the proximity to the fovea.

(2) *Radiation retinopathy (see Fig. 1.6e)*. The earliest changes are capillary dilation, telangiectasis, microaneurysm formation and capillary closure. This occlusive angiopathy may also be associated with cotton wool spots, retinal oedema, neovascularisation and vitreous haemorrhage. As in the above case, the extent of the retinal vascular changes are clearly defined by fluorescein angiography. Radiation retinopathy is usually progressive, although spontaneous improvement has been reported. The incidence of retinopathy is dependent upon both the total dose and the daily fraction size. What constitutes a safe dose of radiation is still a contentious area, but most studies report that doses need to be in excess of 30–35 Gy of cephalic radiation to induce radiation retinopathy. However,

it should be noted that diabetic patients and those receiving certain chemotherapeutic drugs may develop radiation retinopathy at much lower doses.

(3) *Coats' disease (see Fig. 1.6f)*. This is an idiopathic condition characterised by telangiectatic and aneurysmal vessels with intraretinal and subretinal exudates. It is unilateral in 80% of cases and has a 3:1 male to female ratio. The less common adult form of Coats' typically presents with visual loss secondary to parafoveal retinal exudates. The associated telangiectatic changes may be very subtle and are often only detected on angiography. In all cases of unexplained retinal telangiectasis the examiner should make a thorough inspection of the temporal retinal periphery. The discovery of more extensive vascular anomalies and subretinal exudate can confirm the diagnosis of Coats' disease.

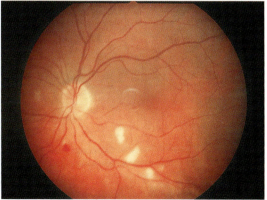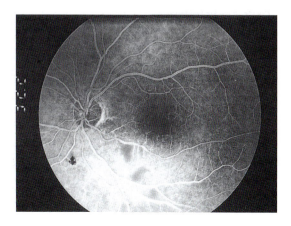

Fig. 1.6e

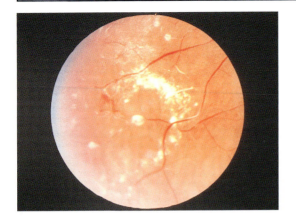 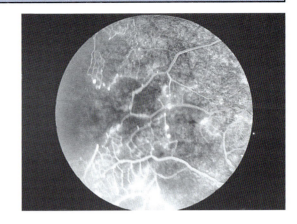

Fig. 1.6f

Recommended reading

Branch Vein Occlusion Study Group (1984) Argon laser photocoagulation for macular edema in branch vein occlusion. *Am. J. Ophthalmol.*, **98**, 271–282.

Branch Vein Occlusion Study Group (1986) Argon laser scatter photocoagulation for prevention of neovascularisation and vitreous hemorrhage in branch vein occlusion. *Arch. Ophthalmol.*, **104**, 34–41.

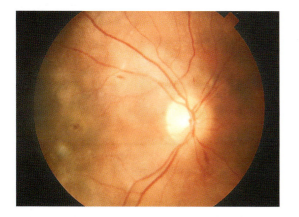 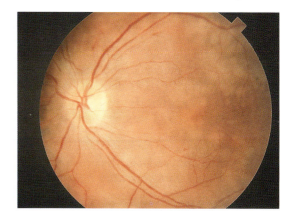

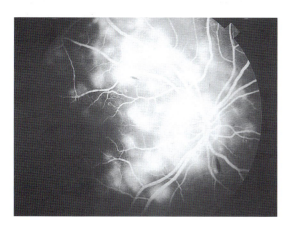 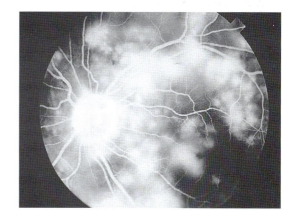

Fig. 1.7a

Q: *Describe these fundal photographs. What is the differential diagnosis? (see Fig. 1.7a)*

A: These fundus photographs and fluorescein angiogram frames illustrate multifocal exudative retinal detachments and underlying greyish choroidal infarcts. The differential diagnosis for this condition should include the following:

(1) Hypertensive retinopathy.
(2) Acute renal failure.
(3) Choroiditis, e.g. Harada's disease.
(4) Posterior scleritis.

The underlying aetiology of this condition was an acute hypertensive crisis, the absence of arteriolar changes such as narrowing and sclerosis, plus the relative lack of haemorrhages suggest that the hypertension was of recent onset.

Q: *What underlying condition would you suspect in a 25-year-old female who presents with blurred vision, 'blindspots' and this fundal picture?*

A: This fundal appearance is characteristically produced by a sudden and marked increase in blood pressure, such as that associated with pre-eclampsia. Pre-eclampsia may occur as early as the 20th week of pregnancy and in some cases the patient may be 'unaware' that she is in fact pregnant. In the UK 10–15% of primigravid women will develop some form of hypertension. The 6% who develop hypertension after the 20th week of pregnancy fall into the category of pregnancy-induced hypertension (PIH). Severe PIH is defined as a blood pressure >160/110 mmHg with proteinuria and develops in 2% of women with PIH.

Q: *What are the acute pathophysiological fundal changes in this condition? What is the relationship with hypertensive retinopathy?*

A: Hypertensive choroidopathy is caused by fibrinoid necrosis of the choroidal arteries and arterioles. These occlusive changes in the choroidal vascular bed result in marked ischaemia of the overlying RPE. The RPE lesions can be subdivided into initial acute focal lesions (due to focal infarction), known as Elschnig's spots, and progressive degenerative changes, which develop later in the macular and peripheral regions of the fundus. The serous retinal detachments are less common manifestations. They are usually confined to the posterior pole and arise as a result of RPE decompensation and a breakdown of the inner blood–retinal barrier.

Hypertensive choroidopathy and retinopathy are two independent manifestations of renovascular hypertension.

Q: *If this woman was 33 weeks pregnant how should she be managed? What is the visual prognosis?*

A: The blood pressure should be measured and urinalysis performed to detect any proteinuria. If these are suggestive of pre-eclampsia urgent referral to an obstetrician is indicated. Unfortunately despite prompt and aggressive treatment of the hypertension (usually with hydralazine) the visual prognosis for the above fundal picture is often poor as there is usually some degree of retinal pigment epithelial impairment, even after resolution of the serous detachments. Some authors have reported an improved visual prognosis following haemodialysis in patients presenting with this fundal picture as a result of acute renal failure with or without hypertension.

Recommended reading

Hayreh, S. S., Servais, G. E. and Virdi, P. S. (1986) Fundal lesions in malignant hypertension. VI. Hypertensive choroidopathy. *Ophthalmology*, **93**, 1383–1400.

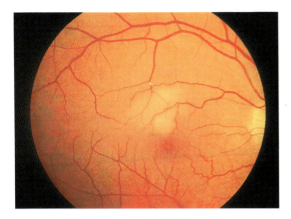

Fig. 1.8

Q: *This patient presented with a sudden loss of vision predominantly affecting the inferior aspect of the central visual field. What is the diagnosis? If you were asked to examine this patient what features of the systemic examination would be of particular relevance? (see Fig. 1.8)*

A: The acute pathology is a small superior macular artery occlusion. The cholesterol embolus is clearly visible, as is the pale ischaemic retinal infarct.

The systemic examination should include the following:

(1) Cardiovascular examination:
    (a) Arrhythmias, e.g. atrial fibrillation.
    (b) Hypertension.
    (c) Thoracotomy scars and cardiac murmurs indicative of valvular heart disease.
    (d) Carotid bruits (bearing in mind that the absence of a bruit does not rule out carotid stenosis and the presence of a bruit is not always indicative of significant stenosis).
    (e) Splinter nail fold and tarsal conjunctival haemorrhages.

(2) A full neurological examination to look for any neurological sequelae of embolic disease.

Q: *What is the most common source of cholesterol emboli? What other emboli may become lodged in the retinal circulation?*

A: Cholesterol emboli are one of the most common causes of amaurosis fugax and invariably arise from atheromatous plaques at the carotid artery bifurcation. Calcific emboli usually originate from diseased mitral or aortic valves and tend to result in branch or central retinal artery occlusions rather than simply causing amaurotic episodes. Fibrin-platelet emboli arising from areas of carotid atheroma may also cause symptomatic compromise of the retinal circulation. Other rarer forms of emboli include talc emboli in intravenous drug users. Attacks of amaurosis fugax may be single or multiple and in most patients, without retinal infarction, the prognosis for visual recovery is good.

Q: *What non-embolic conditions may cause amaurosis fugax?*

A: A number of non-embolic disorders can abruptly reduce perfusion to one eye resulting in amaurosis fugax.

(1) Vasculitides:
    (a) Giant cell arteritis.
    (b) Systemic lupus erythematosus (SLE).
    (c) Polyateritis nodosa.
(2) Low perfusion pressure:
    (a) Postural hypotension.
    (b) Intracranial hypertension.
    (c) Glaucoma.
    (d) Multiple occlusions of extracranial cerebral arteries.
(3) High resistance to retinal perfusion:
    (a) Migraine.
    (b) Malignant hypertension.

(c) Thrombophilic tendencies, e.g. protein C or S, Factor V Leiden deficiency, elevated erythrocyte sedimentation rate (ESR).

(d) Vasospasm (this is very much a diagnosis of exclusion).

This list emphasises that amaurosis fugax may be the presenting sign of a host of potentially severe conditions. Clinicians should therefore not automatically assume that amaurosis fugax is secondary to a retinal embolus.

Q: *What non-invasive investigations may be helpful in the management of a patient with amaurosis fugax and/or a visible retinal embolus?*

A: Having said that most cholesterol emboli arise from atheromatous plaques in the region of the carotid bifurcation it would still be prudent to perform an ECG and a echocardiogram to rule out arrhythmias, valvular disease and ventricular aneurysms. When it comes to assessing the internal carotid arteries a number of non-invasive tests are available.

(1) Duplex scanning. This technique combines the benefits of Doppler ultrasound and B scanning to provide a sensitive test for carotid artery stenosis (95% detection rate of stenoses >50% with a false-negative rate of <5%). Duplex scanning will also provide some information on the presence of ulceration of the atheromatous plaque and associated thrombus formation. With the advent of colour Doppler technology transverse studies of the vessels are possible, as is the ability to distinguish between a complete stenosis and a very narrowed lumen (the 'string' sign). Duplex scanning has been shown to be just as accurate in predicting the degree and nature of carotid occlusive disease as digital subtraction angiography.

(2) Magnetic resonance angiography (MRA). This technique is unique in that it provides information about the extra- and intracerebral carotid circulation, and the brain parenchyma in one examination. Results

compare favourably with angiography although there is a tendency to overestimate the degree of stenosis because of turbulence induced dephasing beyond the stenosis. Reversal of flow from the proximal internal carotid artery into the common carotid artery during diastole may show up as a false narrowing of the proximal internal carotid artery and severe stenoses may be misdiagnosed as complete occlusions. MRA is a non-invasive procedure, therefore there is no risk of stroke or arterial injury and no contrast agents or ionising radiation are used. An additional 10–15 min is all that is required for MRA to be added to conventional parenchymal studies.

Clinicians should be aware that the presence of a visible retinal embolus has a relatively low correlation with the detection of haemodynamically significant (>60%) carotid artery stenosis, in the setting of acute retinal artery occlusion. The presence of an embolus should not therefore influence their decision to perform carotid Doppler ultrasonography in patients with acute retinal arterial occlusion.

Q: *What are the pros and cons of performing angiography on patients suspected of having cerebrovascular disease?*

A: The advantages of angiography over the non-invasive techniques described above are that it may define the character of some atheromatous plaques more accurately, it is a better discriminator between severe narrowing and complete occlusion, and it provides additional information about the intracerebral circulation. However, angiography is not a risk-free procedure; in patients with suspected cerebrovascular disease the incidence of subjective neurological complaints or objective neurological findings within 24 h of angiography is 4.2% and the incidence of permanent neurological sequelae is 0.63%. The complication rate can be minimised by using soft catheters, non-ionic contrast medium and by keeping patients well hydrated. Although angiography may now be performed as an outpatient, it is still considerably more expensive than duplex scanning and is not suitable for serial examinations.

Q: *What is the annual incidence of stroke in patients with amaurosis fugax? What is the main cause of death in these patients?*

A: The annual stroke rate in untreated patients with amaurosis fugax is thought to be approximately 2%. The stroke rate in patients with hemispheric transient ischaemic attacks (TIAs) is 10% in the first year, 8% in the second year and 5% each year thereafter. Untreated patients with amaurosis fugax, retinal infarcts and monocular TIAs have an equal prevalence of atherosclerosis, a 30% 5-year expectancy of myocardial infarction and an 18% mortality rate during the same interval. Ischaemic heart disease and not cerebrovascular disease is the most common cause of death in this group of patients.

Recommended reading

Arruga, J. and Saunders, M. (1982) Ophthalmic findings in 70 patients with evidence of retinal embolism. *Ophthalmology*, **89**, 1333–1347.

Gautier, J.-C. (1993) Amaurosis fugax [Editorial]. *N. Engl. J. Med.*, **329**, 426–428.

Sharma, S., Brown, G. C., Pater, J. L. and Cruess, A. F. (1998) Does a visible retinal embolus increase the likelihood of hemodynamically significant carotid artery stenosis in patients with acute retinal arterial occlusion? *Arch. Ophthalmol.*, **116**, 1602–1606.

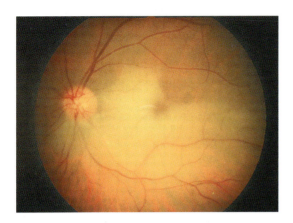

Fig. 1.9

Q: *What is the diagnosis and what is the likely visual acuity? (see Fig. 1.9)*

A: This is an inferior branch retinal artery occlusion. The retina along the inferior arcade is pale and oedematous, the presence of a cherry-red spot indicates foveal involvement and the visual acuity was reduced to counting fingers. Although there are no emboli visible in the retinal circulation the most likely aetiology is still embolic.

Q: *What advice would you give this patient regarding carotid endarterectomy surgery if duplex scanning revealed an ipsilateral stenosis of 80% and he was already taking 300 mg aspirin daily?*

A: The initial treatment for all patients with retinal or hemispheric TIAs is the commencement of antiplatelet therapy with aspirin, as well as treatment of coexisting hyperlipidaemia, hypertension and diabetes. The role of carotid endarterectomy has been investigated in several large randomised trials over recent years.

(1) The North American Symptomatic Carotid Endarterectomy Trial was conducted in 50 centres and recruited 659 patients with a recent hemispheric or retinal TIA, or a recent non-disabling stroke, who had an ipsilateral 70–99% carotid artery stenosis. Patients were randomised into two groups, those who received medical therapy alone and those who in addition to antiplatelet therapy underwent carotid endarterectomy. The cumulative 2-year risk of ipsilateral stroke in the medical group was 26% and in the surgical group was 9% (the relative benefit increased with increasing degrees of stenosis). The cumulative rates of a fatal ipsilateral stroke over the same period were 13% in the medical group and 2.5% in the surgical group. The perioperative fatality was 0.6% and perioperative rate of major stroke or death was 2.1%.

(2) The MRC European Carotid Surgery Trial recruited over 2500 patients with a similar history of TIAs who were randomised into a medical group and a joint medical and surgical group. For patients with severe stenosis (70–99%) the risks of surgery were significantly outweighed by its later benefits. Although 7.5% had a stroke or died within 30 days of surgery, during the next three years the risks of ipsilateral ischaemic stroke were an extra 2.8% for surgery-allocated and 16.8% for control patients. A 6-fold reduction. At 3 years the total risk of surgical death, surgical stroke, ipsilateral ischaemic stroke or any other stroke was 12.3% for surgery and 21.9% for controls.

It would therefore be reasonable to advise this patient that carotid endarterectomy offers better long-term protection from ipsilateral stroke than medical therapy alone, with the proviso that the surgeon has a perioperative mortality of <2% and there are no operative risk factors.

Q: *What would be your advice to the same patient if the degree of stenosis was 60%?*

A: There is no evidence from any of the above trials that the rate of ipsilateral stroke in patients with symptomatic stenoses between 50–75%, who are on antiplatelet therapy, is reduced further by carotid endarterectomy.

Q: *What advice would you give to an asymptomatic patient who is found to have a unilateral 85% carotid artery stenosis?*

A: The question of whether carotid endarterectomy provides an additional benefit to medical therapy in patients with asymptomatic carotid stenosis has been addressed in two large multicentre trials.

(1) The CASANOVA Study (Carotid Artery Stenosis with Asymptomatic Narrowing: Operation Versus Aspirin) randomised 410 asymptomatic patients with 50–90% internal carotid stenoses into two groups. Group A was a surgical group where patients with unilateral or bilateral stenosis had unilateral or bilateral surgery respectively. In group B, patients with unilateral stenosis did not have surgery but those with bilateral disease had surgery on the more affected side. All patients were treated with aspirin 300 mg and dipyridamole 75 mg t.d.s. The minimum follow-up was 3 years and end points were ischaemic neurological deficits exceeding 24 h or death due to surgery or stroke. Complications of angiography and surgery were 6.9%, when these were included in the statistical analysis there was no significant difference in the number of neurological incidents or deaths between the two groups.

(2) The Veterans Affairs Cooperative Study Group enrolled 444 patients who had asymptomatic stenoses of >50%. They were randomised into surgery and aspirin, and aspirin alone groups. The mean follow-up was 4 years. The incidences of ipsilateral neurological events and ipsilateral stroke were 8 and 4.7% in the surgical group and 20.6 and 9.4% in the medical group. However, there were no significant differences between the groups for stroke and death combined. The conclusion that seems to have been drawn from both of these studies is that in asymptomatic patients with stenoses <90% carotid endarterectomy should only be performed as part of a controlled clinical trial.

Recommended reading

European Carotid Surgery Trialists' Collaborative Group (1991) MRC European Carotid Surgery Trial: interim results for symptomatic patients with severe (70–99%) or with mild (0–29%) carotid stenosis. *Lancet*, **337**, 1235–1243.

North American Carotid Endarterectomy Trial Collaborators (1991) Beneficial effect of carotid endarterectomy in symptomatic patients with high-grade carotid stenosis. *N. Engl. J. Med.*, **325**, 445–453.

The CASANOVA Study Group (1991) Carotid surgery versus medical therapy in asymptomatic carotid stenosis. *Stroke*, **22**, 1229–1235.

The Veterans Affairs Cooperative Study Group (1993) Efficacy of carotid endarterectomy for asymptomatic carotid stenosis. *N. Engl. J. Med.*, **328**, 221–227.

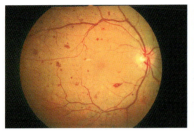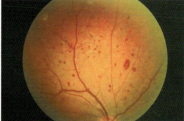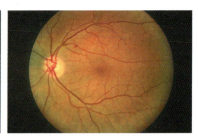

Fig. 1.10a

Q: *Describe the fundi of this 75-year-old woman. What is the differential diagnosis? (see Fig. 1.10a)*

A: There is evidence of mild hypertensive retinopathy in the left fundus. In the right eye there are intraretinal and some preretinal haemorrhages scattered along the vascular arcades extending to the mid-peripheral fundus. There is no evidence of arteriovenous changes, cotton wool spots, exudates nor disc swelling. The other findings of note are subtle disc neovascularisation and arterial narrowing. Although diabetic retinopathy may be asymmetrical it would be very unusual to find disc neovascularisation in one eye with no evidence of any retinopathy in the fellow eye. The same can be said for hypertensive retinopathy, although it should be noted that neovascularisation is never a feature of purely hypertensive retinopathy.

The differential diagnosis should therefore include:

(1) Ocular ischaemic syndrome.
(2) Non-ischaemic central retinal vein occlusion (CRVO).

The lack of disc swelling makes a CRVO unlikely. In patients with severe carotid artery obstruction there will be decreased central retinal artery perfusion pressure, this may be confirmed by observing central retinal artery pulsation when gentle digital pressure is applied to the globe.

Q: *What is the aetiology of the ocular ischaemic syndrome? How do patients with ocular ischaemic syndrome present?*

A: The ocular ischaemic syndrome, or venous stasis retinopathy as it was originally termed, is secondary to severe carotid artery obstruction (stenosis >90%). Most patients present in their 50s or 60s, there is 2:1 male preponderance and bilateral involvement is found in approximately 20% of cases. Presenting symptoms are typically visual loss or pain, which may be related to changes in illumination. The visual loss, which is present in 90% at presentation, is usually gradual occurring over a period of weeks or months. The degree of visual loss is variable, approximately one-third of eyes will have acuities of 6/6 to 6/12, one-third will range from 6/18 to 3/60 and one-third will be severely affected with acuities of counting fingers to light perception. The pain described by 40% of patients is centred over the eye or brow and may radiate to the temple. It is secondary to a combination of globe ischaemia and neovascular glaucoma. The latter complicates one-third of eyes with the ocular ischaemic syndrome.

Q: What are the characteristic angiographic features of this condition?

A:

(1) A prolonged arm-to-choroid circulation time has been described. However, these measurements can be difficult to interpret as they may be influenced by other variables such as the speed of injection.
(2) Choroidal filling is normally complete within 5 s of the appearance of dye in the choroidal circulation. Patchy choroidal filling of >5 s duration is found in 60% of affected eyes.
(3) Increased retinal arteriovenous transit times are found in 95% of affected eyes. This is measured from the initial appearance of dye within the retinal arteries of the temporal arcade until the corresponding veins are completely filled. It is <11 s in normal subjects.
(4) Staining of retinal vessels in the late stages of the angiogram, which affects the arteries more than the veins, is seen in 80% of cases. In CRVOs venous staining is prominent, but the arteries generally do not stain. The ocular ischaemic syndrome is also the only condition in which the retinal arteries are dilated.
(5) Leakage from disc neovascularisation will be present in 40% of affected eyes and 25% of these eyes will have associated retinal new vessels.
(6) Retinal capillary closure in the mid-periphery is a sign of increasing ischaemia. The latter two features are demonstrated in Fig. 1.10b.

Q: *What are the late complications of this condition and how may they be prevented?*

A: Treatment is aimed at preventing severe visual loss and neovascular glaucoma. PRP

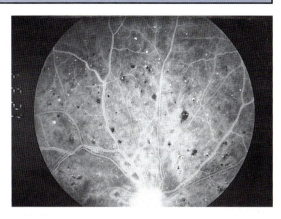

Fig. 1.10b

for cases of rubeosis where the angle is still open may be effective. However, the regression of iris neovascularisation is less marked than that seen in diabetic eyes or in those with a CRVO.

Although the data on the role of carotid endarterectomy is sparse (and controversial), stabilisation or improved vision has been reported in 25% of eyes following surgery. A potential ocular side effect of carotid endarterectomy in patients with closed angles but normal preoperative intraocular pressures is that improved ciliary body perfusion increases aqueous production and may cause a marked rise in intraocular pressure. Despite the above treatment modalities an initial visual acuity of counting fingers or less, or the presence of rubeosis iridis are very poor visual prognostic signs.

Recommended reading

Raman, M., Gregory-Evans, K. (2000) Management of ocular ischaemic syndrome. *Br. J. Ophthalmol.*, **84**, 1428–1431.

1.11

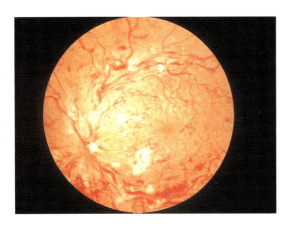

Fig. 1.11a

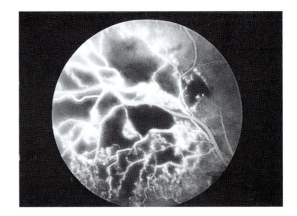

Fig. 1.11b

Q: *This 75-year-old hypertensive man noted a sudden deterioration in the vision of his left eye. What is the diagnosis? (see Fig. 1.11a)*

A: This is the typical appearance of a CRVO. There are four quadrant intraretinal and preretinal haemorrhages, numerous cotton wool spots, venous dilatation, and optic nerve head swelling. Following diabetic retinopathy, central or branch retinal vein occlusions are the most common retinal vascular disorders.

Q: *What features of the ocular examination and fluorescein angiography may point to the development of rubeosis and neovascular glaucoma?*

A: The most serious complication of CRVO is the development of rubeosis and subsequently neovascular glaucoma. It is notoriously difficult to predict which patients with CRVOs will develop rubeosis, but bad prognostic signs include:

(1) A visual acuity of hand movements or less that does not improve with time.
(2) A relative afferent pupillary defect.
(3) Multiple deep intraretinal haemorrhages and cotton wool spots.

(4) Greater than 10 disc areas of capillary closure on fluorescein angiography is probably the most reliable indicator of an ischaemic CRVO. Although retinal haemorrhages often mask the posterior pole preventing an accurate assessment of the capillary circulation in this area, it is often possible to demonstrate capillary closure in the mid-peripheral fundus in patients with an ischaemic CRVO (Fig. 1.11b).

Electrophysiological investigations including the ERG and the EOG have also been used to differentiate ischaemic from non-ischaemic CRVOs.

Q: *What are the major risk factors for the development of a CRVO in the elderly patient?*

A: Most large CRVO series report that 50% or more occur in patients over 65 years of age and that 50–70% of cases are associated with one or more of the following.

(1) Hypertension.
(2) Cardiovascular disease.
(3) Diabetes mellitus.

Other less common risk factors in the elderly are glaucoma and hyperviscosity syndromes.

Q: *How should patients with ischaemic CRVOs be managed?*

A: The Central Vein Occlusion Study Group has published their results of early PRP in CRVO. The primary outcome of this study was the development of two clock hours of iris neovascularisation or any angle neovascularisation (TC-INV/ANV). In the early treatment group 20% of eyes developed TC-INV/ANV, compared with 35% in the untreated group. This difference was not statistically significant when baseline variables were accounted for. Neovascular glaucoma developed in 4% of eyes in both patient groups. The most important factor in predicting the development of neovascularisation was the amount of capillary closure. The risk in eyes with 10–29 disc areas of closure was 16% and this increased to 52% in eyes with more than 75 disc areas of non-perfusion. The study recommended that in patients with an ischaemic CRVO prophylactic PRP is not beneficial and these patients should be reviewed monthly with careful examination of the undilated pupil and of the angle. PRP should be performed only if TC-INV/ANV develops and monthly follow-up should be continued until there is evidence of regression of the neovascularisation.

These recommendations have been criticised as being impractical when dealing with busy outpatient clinics and patients who may not attend for regular follow-up. Despite these recommendations many ophthalmologists continue to perform prophylactic PRP for ischaemic CRVOs.

Q: *What is the likelihood of developing a venous occlusion in the fellow eye following a non-ischaemic CRVO? How long should such patients be kept under review?*

A: The risk of a patient with a non-ischaemic CRVO developing a similar venous occlusion in their fellow eye is 6.6% at 2 years and 7.7% at 4 years. In patients over 65 years the probability of developing a contralateral retinal venous occlusion of any type (branch, hemiretinal or ischaemic CRVO) is 13 and 18% after 2 and 4 years respectively. Patients with non-ischaemic CRVOs should be followed up for 18 months as approximately 18% of non-ischaemic CRVOs in patients over 65 years of age will convert to ischaemic CRVOs over this period. The probability of conversion from a non-ischaemic to an ischaemic CRVO is only 8% in younger patients.

Recommended reading

Hayreh, S. S., Zimmerman, M. B. and Podhagsky, P. (1994) Incidence of various types of retinal vein occlusion and their recurrence and demographic characteristics. *Am. J. Ophthalmol.*, **117**, 429–441.

The Central Vein Occlusion Study (1993) Baseline and early natural history report. *Arch. Ophthalmol.*, **111**, 1087–1095.

The Central Vein Occlusion Study Group Report (1995) A randomised clinical trial of early panretinal photocoagulation for ischaemic central vein occlusion. *Ophthalmology*, **102**, 1434–1444.

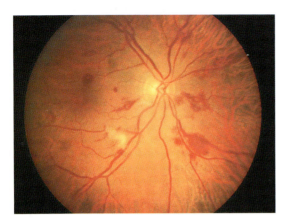 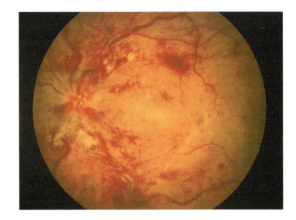

Fig. 1.12a

Q: *Describe the fundal appearances of this 35-year-old man. What is the differential diagnosis? (see Fig. 1.12a)*

A: In the left eye there are extensive retinal and preretinal haemorrhages in all quadrants, scattered cotton wool spots, and marked disc swelling. There are scattered retinal and preretinal haemorrhages in all four quadrants of the right eye, a single cotton wool spot but no disc swelling. The differential diagnosis should include:

(1) CRVOs.
(2) Grade IV hypertensive retinopathy.
(3) Valsalva or Purtscher's retinopathy.

The patient was in fact normotensive and there was no history of a crushing chest/abdominal injury to suggest a valsalva retinopathy; the diagnosis is one of bilateral (established and incipient) CRVOs.

Q: *What features of his history and examination may be of relevance in determining the aetiology of these venous occlusions?*

A: The majority of young adults with CRVOs are otherwise healthy with no other systemic or ocular disease. However, the following have all been associated with retinal venous occlusions in patients under 45 years of age:

(1) Cardiovascular disease:
    (a) Hypertension.
    (b) Diabetes mellitus.
    (c) Hyperlipidaemia.
    (d) Mitral valve prolapse.
    (e) Carotid artery disease.
(2) Medications:
    (a) Oral contraceptives.
    (b) Diuretics.
    (c) Sympathomimetics.
(3) Collagen vascular diseases.
(4) Haematological disorders:
    (a) Coagulopathies.
    (b) Leukaemia.
    (c) Hyperviscosity syndromes.
(5) Acquired immunodeficiency syndrome.

The above patient did in fact have acute myeloid leukaemia.

Q: *How would you investigate abnormalities in the coagulation or fibrinolytic system in a young patient with a CRVO?*

A: It is imperative to take a detailed family history in all young patients with an unexplained thrombotic episode. A careful history of previous thrombo-embolic episodes in the patient, their siblings, parents and children should be taken. A history of recurrent miscarriages may also be relevant. A negative family history does not rule out the possibility of inherited thrombophilia as these defects have a low penetrance and spontaneous mutations can occur. Screening tests should include:

(1) Antiphospholipid antibody tests:
   (a) Platelet count.
   (b) Partial thromboplastin.
   (c) Lupus anticoagulant.
   (d) VDRL (Venereal Disease Research Laboratories) test and anticardiolipin antibodies. The presence of anticardiolipin antibodies is the most frequently reported haematological abnormality in patients with retinal vascular occlusions. In the majority of cases there is an underlying disease or the antibodies are drug induced, but it is not uncommon to find raised titres in apparently normal individuals.
(2) Factor V Leiden mutation leads to a relative resistance of coagulation factor V to breakdown by activated protein C. Estimates of the prevalence of this mutation vary, but approximately 5% of the white population are thought to be carriers. Activated protein C resistance has been found in 12% of patients with CRVO.
(3) Antithrombin III is the major inhibitor of activated coagulation factors including thrombin, factor IXa and Xa. Glycosaminoglycans produced by endothelial cells act as high-affinity binding sites for antithrombin III and deficiencies in either of these can induce a thrombotic state. The prevalence of antithrombin III deficiency in young patients with venous thrombosis ranges from 2 to 5%. Antithrombin III levels should be determined by functioning assays, either coagulation or amidolytic.

(4) Protein C is a vitamin K-dependent serine protease that is a potent inhibitor of coagulation factors Va and VIIIa. The deficiency is inherited as an autosomal dominant trait and clinically affected individuals are heterozygous with a protein C concentration of about 50% normal. The prevalence of protein C deficiency in young patients with venous thrombosis is reported as 6–8%. Functional rather than immunological assays are the investigation of choice. Protein S and phospholipid are cofactors in the inactivation of factors Va and VIIIa by activated protein C.
(5) Protein S is only active in its free form (40%) the remainder is bound to C4b-binding protein. Like protein C deficiency, inheritance is autosomal dominant. The prevalence in young patients with thrombotic episodes is 5–8%. Functional protein S activity can now be measured using the snake venom-derived protein C activator.

Q: *How does the natural history and visual prognosis of a CRVO in a young patient differ from that seen in a patient over 65 years of age?*

A: Large CRVO series have reported that 8–19% of CRVOs occur in individuals under 50 years of age. Unlike CRVO in patients over 65 years the visual acuity tends to be less profoundly affected. A slow spontaneous resolution over a 3–6 month period is reported as typical, although approximately one in five will have significant, permanent visual loss. The improved visual prognosis is secondary to the higher proportion of non-ischaemic CRVOs in younger patients. Visual acuities of 6/12 or better have been reported in 34–47% of non-ischaemic CRVOs. The figure for ischaemic CRVOs is 7–14%.

The colour photograph and fluorescein angiogram of this patient's left eye (Fig. 1.12b) were taken 3 months after presentation. There is no evidence of capillary closure nor of macular oedema and the visual acuity was 6/9.

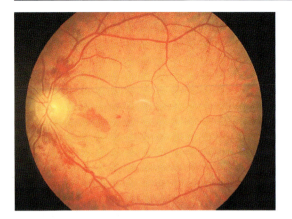 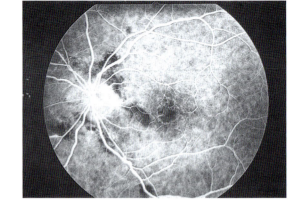

Fig. 1.12b

Recommended reading

Fong, A. C. O. and Schatz, H. (1993) Central retinal vein occlusion in young adults. *Surv. Ophthalmol.*, **37**, 393–417.

Vine, A. K. and Samama, M. M. (1993) The role of abnormalities in the anticoagulant and fibrinolytic systems in retinal vascular occlusions. *Surv. Ophthalmol.*, **37**, 283–292.

Williamson, T. H. (1997) Central retinal vein occlusion: what's the story? [Perspective]. *Br. J. Ophthalmol.*, **81**, 698–704.

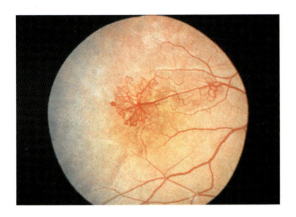

Fig. 1.13a

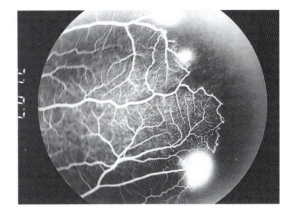

Fig. 1.13b

Q: *Describe the peripheral fundus of this 26-year-old West Indian woman. What is the most likely diagnosis? What are the other characteristic fundal abnormalities associated with this condition?*
(see Fig. 1.13a)

A: There is an area of neovascularisation in the retinal periphery in which the vessels have a 'sea-fan' configuration. The retinal vasculature appears to be absent peripheral to these areas of neovascularisation. The most common aetiology of such lesions in young Afro-Caribbean patients is sickle cell retinopathy. The features of sickle cell retinopathy have been classified by Goldberg and are as follows:

Stage I   Background non-proliferative fundal changes including salmon patch intraretinal haemorrhages (secondary to occlusion, infarction and blow-out of retinal arterioles), black sunburst lesions caused by subretinal haemorrhage, iridescent spots and occluded peripheral vessels.

Stage II   Arteriolar-venular anastomoses connecting arterioles to medium-sized veins in the equatorial retina.

Stage III   Proliferative sickle retinopathy (PSR) illustrated above. The sea-fans are initially flat but may with time grow into the vitreous and circumferentially.

Stage IV   Vitreous haemorrhage.

Stage V   Retinal detachment. These are usually tractional but some may have a rhegmatogenous component.

The fluorescein frame in Fig. 1.13b demonstrates arteriolar-venular anastomoses, hyperfluorescence associated with neovascularisation and complete peripheral capillary closure.

Q: *What form of sickle cell haemoglobinopathy is this patient likely to have?*

A: From the physician's point of view the most serious form of sickle cell is sickle cell disease Hb SS, which affects 0.4–0.2% of black Americans. However, the most severe retinopathy is found in SC disease, which affects 0.1% of black Americans. Several explanations have been put forward to account for this. The most plausible of which is that with haemoglobin SS ischaemia secondary to sickling cells in the precapillary arterioles progresses rapidly to infarction, whereas with haemoglobin SC the progression is slower allowing the areas of neovascularisation to develop.

Q: *What features of the systemic examination may help distinguish between patients with sickle cell disease and sickle cell trait?*

A: Patients with sickle cell trait are usually asymptomatic and will not suffer any adverse sequelae unless they become anoxic. Features indicative of sickle cell disease include:

(1) Painful swellings of the fingers and toes in young patients.
(2) Abdominal findings:
   (a) Hepatosplenomegaly.
   (b) Splenectomy and/or cholecystectomy scars.
(3) Anaemia or mild jaundice.
(4) Chronic leg ulcers due to ischaemia.
(5) Evidence of osteomyelitis, or aseptic necrosis (particularly of the femoral heads).

Q: *At what age do patients develop PSR and what is the natural history of these areas of neovascularisation?*

A: Workers at the Medical Research Council laboratories in Jamaica have undertaken extensive natural history studies of sickle cell retinopathy. In a study of almost 400 children aged 5–13 years peripheral retinal vessel closure was present in 50% of SS and SC genotypes at age 6 years, and 90% of children by age 12 years. In SS disease complete closure was associated with lower total haemoglobin and foetal haemoglobin levels, and lower weight. Whereas in SC disease the risk factors were a high mean cell volume and low platelet count.

In a cohort of almost 800 sickle cell disease and 500 sickle cell trait patients the prevalence of PSR was 17% in the SS group and 70% in the SC group. Bilateral disease developed in 49% of SS patients with PSR and in 70% of SC patients with PSR, although simultaneous development was rare. In SC disease the risk of developing PSR was highest between 15 and 24 years in males, between 20 and 39

years in females, and in SS disease between 25 and 39 years in both sexes.

Regarding the natural history of PSR, peripheral arterial occlusions lead to remodelling of the retinal vasculature with the formation of arteriovenous anastomoses. Preretinal 'sea-fan' neovascularisation arises from these anastomoses at the edge of the ischaemic retina. The MRC group have studied the influence of genotype on the natural history of untreated PSR and found that spontaneous regression occurred in 40% of SS patients, and in 20% of SC patients.

Q: *What is the incidence of significant visual loss in sickle cell disease?*

A: Natural history studies have shown that visual acuity loss of $\leq 6/18$ attributable to sickle cell retinopathy occurs in 10% of untreated eyes over a 7-year period. In 90% of cases the visual loss arose as a direct consequence of PSR, i.e. vitreous haemorrhage, tractional retinal detachment or epiretinal membranes. The prevalence of visual loss in eyes with PSR was 34% over the same period, half of these eyes had a best corrected visual acuity of $< 6/60$. Only 2% of eyes without PSR had significantly reduced acuities, the most common cause for which was angioid streaks with disciform degeneration.

Q: *What is the role of photocoagulation in the management of PSR?*

A: The first attempts at treating PSR utilised the xenon arc and later the argon laser to photocoagulate the sea-fan feeder vessels. However, although this treatment was effective in producing regression of the sea-fans there was a high incidence of iatrogenic chorioretinal neovascularisation. This often converted to choriovitreal neovascularisation with associated vitreous haemorrhage and tractional retinal detachment. The current treatment of choice is scatter argon laser photocoagulation around areas of PSR, avoiding the sea-fans and their feeder vessels. The moderate benefit of treatment has been proven in the only randomised prospective clinical trial of photocoagulation in

Table 1.2

	Treated	Untreated
Complete closure of new vessels	30%	23%
Partial closure of new vessels	50%	24%
Recurrent new vessels or new vessels in previously normal retina	34%	41%
Significant visual loss*	3%	8%
Vitreous haemorrhage (of any degree)	11%	19%

* Significant visual loss was defined as a loss of three or more Snellen lines from baseline, on two visits at least two months apart

PSR. The average length of follow-up was 42 months, the results of this trial are summarised in Table 1.2.

Although complications were unlikely to occur in eyes with <30° of PSR the authors still recommended treating these patients.

Q: *If this patient required a vitrectomy for a tractional retinal detachment what preoperative, perioperative and postoperative measures would be advisable to minimise the risk of sickle cell related complications?*

A: A thorough preoperative work-up is essential if systemic and ocular complications of sickle cell disease are to be prevented.

(1) Exchange transfusion is recommended if electrophoresis indicates <50% haemoglobin A and the haematocrit is <35%. The purpose of such a transfusion is to reduce the risk of the following complications:
  (a) Anterior segment ischaemia.

(b) Optic nerve infarction and macular capillary occlusion, which may occur at intraocular pressures as low as 25 mmHg.
(c) Sickle cell crisis. Prior to exchange transfusion the potential risks of transfusion and the benefits outlined above should be discussed fully with the patient.

(2) Intraoperative measures:
  (a) The risk of anterior segment ischaemia is reduced by avoiding transection or unnecessary traction on the rectus muscles, careful placement of cryotherapy avoiding the long posterior ciliary arteries, and minimising the use of phenylephrine for pupillary dilation.
  (b) Maintaining a lowered intraocular pressure using a carbonic anhydrase inhibitor or intravenous mannitol and by drainage of subretinal fluid prior to scleral buckling wherever possible.

(3) The general principles of keeping the sickle cell patient well hydrated, oxygenated and adequately analgesed postoperatively are essential if late complications are to be prevented.

Recommended reading

Farber, M. D., Jampol, L. M., Fox, P., Moriarty, B. J., Acheson, R. W., Rabb, M. F. and Sergeant, G. R. (1991) A randomised clinical trial of scatter photocoagulation of proliferative sickle cell retinopathy. *Arch. Ophthalmol.*, **109**, 363–367.

Jampol, L. M., Ebroon, D. A. and Goldbaum, M. H. (1994) Peripheral proliferative retinopathies: an update on angiogenesis, etiologies and management. *Surv. Ophthalmol.*, **38**, 519–540.

1.14

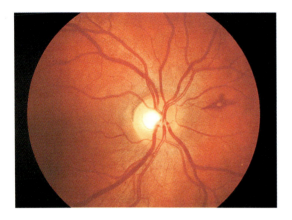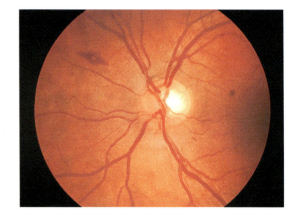

Fig. 1.14a

Q: *Describe these fundal photographs. What are the causes of these retinal haemorrhages? (see Fig. 1.14a)*

A: These white centred retinal haemorrhages are Roth spots. Roth spots are features of the following conditions:

(1) Acute leukaemias.
(2) Severe anaemia.
(3) Bacterial endocarditis.

Q: *This patient was suspected of having bacterial endocarditis. What features of the systemic examination would support this diagnosis?*

A:

(1) Cardiac findings:
  (a) Murmurs are present in 90% of patients with endocarditis. The development of a new murmur or change in the character of an existing murmur are warning signs.
  (b) Signs of cardiac failure in 50% of cases.
(2) Vascular lesions:
  (a) Petechial or mucosal haemorrhages.
  (b) Nailfold splinter haemorrhages.
  (c) Flat erythematous macules on thenar and hypothenar eminences (Janeway lesions).
(3) Anaemia.
(4) Splenomegaly.
(5) Focal neurological signs secondary to cerebral emboli occur in 20% of patients with endocarditis.

Q: *What are the appropriate investigations in cases of suspected infective endocarditis?*

A: A comprehensive work-up for a case of suspected infective endocarditis should include the following investigations:

(1) Full blood count – findings may include:
  (a) Normochromic normocytic anaemia.
  (b) Polymorphonuclear leucocytosis.
  (c) Thrombocytopaenia (occasionally).
(2) Liver function tests – raised serum alkaline phosphatase is typical.
(3) Blood cultures – at least six sets of samples should be taken for aerobic and anaerobic culture.
(4) Urinalysis – microscopic haematuria with or without proteinuria.

(5) Echocardiography – documents valvular dysfunction. Small vegetations may be missed unless transoesophageal echocardiography is used.

(6) Chest X-ray – may show signs of cardiac failure, or emboli in tricuspid or pulmonary valve disease.

(7) ECG – look for evidence of myocardial infarction secondary to emboli.

1.15

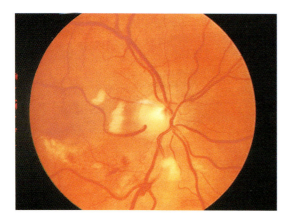

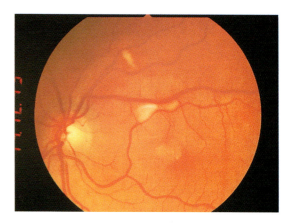

Fig. 1.15a

Q: *Describe these fundal photographs. What is the most likely cause of this fundal picture in a normotensive 35-year-old man who is visually and systemically asymptomatic? (see Fig. 1.15a)*

A: There are multiple cotton wool spots scattered throughout the posterior pole of the right eye with a few associated retinal haemorrhages. Two cotton wool spots are visible along the superior vascular arcade of the left eye. This is an example of HIV microvasculopathy; this condition is characterised by cotton wool spots accompanied by retinal haemorrhages, microaneurysms and other microvascular abnormalities. It is the most common fundal finding in patients who are HIV-positive, being seen in 50% of patients at some time during their illness. The appearance usually predates the onset of full blown AIDS and occurs when the CD4 count falls to <500 cells/μl. It is thought to be secondary to a generalised endotheliopathy caused by the HIV. This condition waxes and wanes with time and requires no treatment, although differentiation from early cytomegalovirus (CMV) retinitis may be difficult at times.

A similar fundal appearance may be seen in leukaemic patients, SLE or retinal vasculitis.

Q: *What are the other ocular manifestations of HIV infection that occur when the CD4 count is still >200 cells/μl?*

A: Figure 1.15b illustrates the common ocular conditions that are frequently seen in the HIV-positive patient and when they occur in the time course of the disease.

Although all the conditions are commonly seen in immunocompetent individuals their natural history is often significantly different in HIV-positive patients.

(1) Herpes zoster ophthalmicus often results in a prolonged keratitis with an associated severe uveitis. These often require treatment with both topical and systemic acyclovir.
(2) Herpes simplex causes a more prolonged dendritic keratitis, which tends to be peripheral rather than central and is often bilateral. Recurrences are more frequent, although lesions tend not to involve the corneal stroma. Oral acyclovir is used to minimise the frequency of recurrent episodes.

Seroconversion

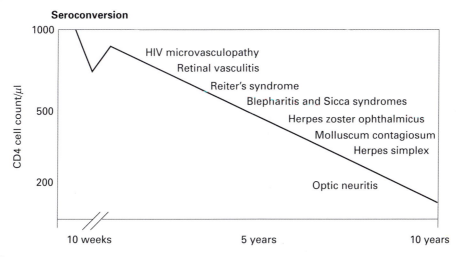

Fig. 1.15b

(3) Molluscum contagiosum produces a follicular conjunctivitis and umbilicated lesions
on the lids and face, which tend to be larger
and more numerous in HIV-positive
patients.

Recommended reading

Bloom, P., Graham, E. and Migdal, C. (1995)
Ophthalmic manifestations of HIV disease and
the acquired immune deficiency syndrome. *Recent
Adv. Ophthalmol.*, **9**, 25–58.

1.16

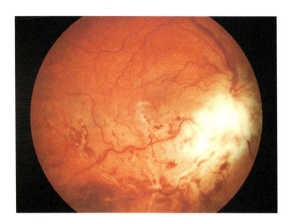

Fig. 1.16a

Q: *Describe this fundal appearance. What is the diagnosis? (see Fig. 1.16a)*

A: This photograph illustrates the classical 'pizza-pie' (tomato ketchup and mozzarella cheese) appearance of fulminant CMV retinitis. Points to note are the full thickness retinal necrosis with associated haemorrhages involving the disc and spreading along the inferior vascular arcade and the clear vitreous. CMV retinitis is not found in immunocompetent individuals, in the absence of another cause of immunosuppression it is an AIDS defining illness. It is the most common intraocular opportunistic infection in AIDS sufferers. It is not uncommon for CMV retinitis to be the presenting feature of HIV infection or more frequently the sign which heralds the development of full blown AIDS in those already known to be seropositive.

Q: *What is the other variant of CMV retinitis commonly described and how does it differ from the fulminant form?*

A: The other variant of CMV retinitis is the granular form. This has a much drier appearance, often exhibiting what is described as a 'brush fire' border. It may be difficult to distinguish this appearance from that of treated CMV retinitis.

Q: *What are the treatments of choice for CMV retinitis and what are their common side effects?*

A: The mainstays of treatment for CMV retinitis are ganciclovir and foscarnet.

(1) Ganciclovir (DHPG) is phosphorylated by the viral thymidine kinase and this phosphorylated form inhibits viral replication, i.e. it is virostatic. Induction treatment involves the insertion of an indwelling catheter (Hickman line) and a b.d. regime of 5 mg/kg is given for 2 weeks. After this time daily treatment of 5 mg/kg is given for 3–6 days/week (this varies between centres). The most common side effect is neutropaenia, which develops in one-third of patients, although this figure is higher in those patients concurrently taking zidovudine. The use of granulocyte colony stimulating factor may help maintain the neutrophil count in these patients.

(2) Foscarnet is another virostatic agent, which acts by selectively and reversibly inhibiting viral specific DNA polymerases and reverse transcriptases. The induction dose is 60 mg/kg given t.d.s. for 2 weeks. Maintenance therapy is given at a dose of 90 mg/kg in a similar regime to ganciclovir. Foscarnet is nephrotoxic especially if the patient becomes dehydrated and renal function should be closely monitored.

The morbidity and toxic effects associated with these therapies have been studied as part of a randomised trial, the results of which are summarised in Table 1.3.

Patients assigned to foscarnet were more likely to be switched to the alternative treatment (foscarnet to ganciclovir, 46%; ganciclovir to foscarnet, 11%) and most of this excess was

Table 1.3

Side effects	Ganciclovir	Foscarnet
Nephrotoxicity	34%	14%
Neutropaenia	13%	6%
Infusion related symptoms	58%	24%
Genitourinary symptoms	36%	16%
Seizures	12%	9%

attributable to toxic reactions rather than treatment failure. In 88% of cases in which treatment was switched as a result of toxic reactions, these reactions resolved after the switch.

Q: *The first photograph was taken 3 weeks after induction therapy with ganciclovir, the second illustrates the fundal changes 9 weeks post-induction. What do these pictures illustrate and how should the patient be managed? (see Fig. 1.16b)*

A: The first photograph shows that the CMV retinitis is in remission post-induction. The affected retina has a granular appearance, the haemorrhages are less numerous and the disc more clearly visible. In the second photograph there is recurrent CMV retinitis arising from the peripapillary region. The median time from induction to progression is approximately 50 days for both intravenous ganciclovir and for foscarnet, with 85% of patients developing signs of progression by 120 days. The treatment options when faced by recurrent disease are to reinduce with the same agent, reinduce with an alternative agent or to reinduce with combined therapy. In the above case the visual acuity was reduced to perception of light due to optic nerve involvement but reinduction with foscarnet was commenced because of peripheral CMV retinitis in the left eye.

Detection of recurrent CMV retinitis is not always straightforward, as demonstrated by the following photographs (Fig. 1.16c).

The first photograph demonstrates active CMV retinitis, the second photograph taken 3 months post-induction appears to show inactive retinitis. However, on closer inspection there is evidence of active granular disease along the superior border of the lesion. Despite reinduction therapy there was steady progression of the retinitis across the fovea reducing the vision to hand movements.

Q: *What other treatment modalities are available for the treatment of CMV retinitis?*

A: Ganciclovir is also available in an oral preparation with similar bioavailability as the intravenous preparation. Trials are currently underway to compare the efficacy of oral

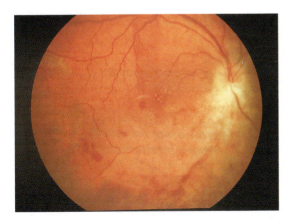
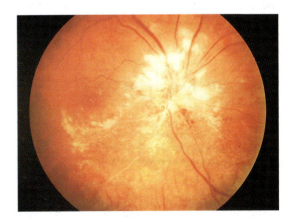

Fig. 1.16b

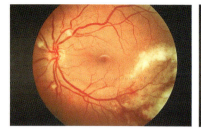 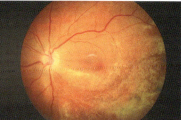 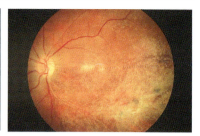

Fig. 1.16c

versus intravenous therapy and to establish the potential benefits of oral ganciclovir in a prophylactic role. Cidofovir is another virostatic agent, which has a prolonged intracellular half-life allowing it to be administered weekly for induction and biweekly for maintenance therapy. Although remission times compare favourably with ganciclovir and foscarnet, nephrotoxicity is a problem.

Local drug therapy in the form of intraocular devices that slowly release ganciclovir into the vitreous are another option. These devices are indicated in selected patients who are unable to receive systemic therapy and as a supplementary treatment in those patients whose disease is not completely controlled by maximally tolerated systemic therapy. Although these devices are relatively cheap, produce relatively long periods of remission (>200 days) and have no systemic toxicity, there is a high incidence of retinal detachment, endophthalmitis and CMV retinitis in the fellow eye. There is also a high incidence of non-ocular CMV infection.

Q: *What is the average length of survival after the diagnosis of CMV retinitis? What is the visual prognosis following treatment?*

A: The CD4 count of these patients is usually <50/µl on presentation and without treatment the average survival is <3 months, with most patients having at best counting fingers vision, at the time of death. The Studies of Ocular Complications of AIDS (SOCA) reported an increased survival time in those patients treated with foscarnet instead of ganciclovir (12.6 versus 8.5 months) – the authors concluded that these results could not be wholly explained

by the discontinuation of zidovudine in a number of patients receiving ganciclovir.

Since the introduction of Highly Active Anti-Retroviral Treatment (HAART) including protease inhibitors, survival times in patients with CMV retinitis have increased dramatically. In a study conducted in London of 147 patients with CMV retinitis the mean time from diagnosis of CMV retinitis to death was 220 days (16% 1-year survival) prior to the use of reverse transciptase inhibitors and protease inhibitors. Following the addition of a nucleoside reverse transcriptase inhibitor the mean survival rose to 353 days and in those patients also taking protease inhibitors the mean survival was 914 days.

Regarding the visual prognosis, ganciclovir and foscarnet have been shown to be equally effective in inducing a remission of CMV retinitis, preserving visual field and visual acuity. The major causes of visual loss are optic disc involvement, foveal involvement, or retinal detachment, despite the high incidence of these complications the visual acuity at the time of death in the better eye is on average 6/12.

Q: *How have anti-retroviral drugs altered the natural history of CMV retinitis?*

A: The advent of reverse transcriptase inhibitors and protease inhibitors has had a dramatic effect on the management of HIV-positive patients. Typically CD4 counts of 50/µl or less may increase to 200/µl or more with treatment. The effect this may have on CMV retinitis is 3-fold:

(1) Spontaneous improvement of CMV retinitis has been reported in patients with rising CD4 counts who are not on antiviral therapy.

(2) Sustained increases in CD4 counts achieved in the first 4 months of treatment are associated with a prolonged period of CMV retinitis quiescence. A 4-fold increase in remission times has been reported in some series. Poor initial response to treatment is associated with a high risk of CMV retinitis recurrence. However, a favourable response to protease inhibitors is dependent on which CD4 clones have been destroyed prior to therapy. If the CD4 line active against CMV has been destroyed an increase in other CD4 lines will not alter the natural history of CMV retinitis. It is therefore possible that patients with a current CD4 count of 200/μl or more may develop CMV retinitis.

(3) CMV retinitis in the pre-HAART era was characterised by the absence of significant vitreous inflammation. However, as CD4 counts recover an immune recovery vitritis (IRV) is frequently seen in patients on HAART. There appears to be a wide variation in the duration of HAART and in the rise in CD4 lymphocyte levels before the onset of IRV. The severity of visual loss in IRV is also variable, ranging from the usual mild and transient form, to a severe and persistent variant of IRV associated with cystoid macular oedema and visual loss. The latter group of patients may benefit from orbital floor steroid injections.

Q: *How should AIDS patients be screened for CMV retinitis?*

A: In most centres screening is performed by ophthalmologists, although screening may safely be undertaken by physicians familiar with the ocular manifestations of HIV-related disease using direct ophthalmoscopy. Guidelines for a physician led screening service are described below:

(1) All HIV-positive or AIDS patients with visual symptoms should undergo fundoscopy through dilated pupils (approximately 20% of patients with CMV retinitis will be asymptomatic).

(2) Patients with no visual symptoms who are deemed to have normal fundi need not be referred for an ophthalmological opinion.

(3) All HIV-positive patients with a lowest recorded CD4 count of <50/μl should be screened by physicians at two-monthly intervals.

(4) Patients with an extra-ocular focus of CMV infection need not be referred to the ophthalmologist unless there are unexplained visual symptoms or signs of a fundal abnormality.

Recommended reading

Engstrom, R. E., Jr and Holland, G. N. (1995) Local therapies for cytomegalovirus retinopathy (Review). *Am. J. Ophthalmol.*, **120**, 376–385.

Studies of ocular complications of AIDS Research Group, in collaboration with the AIDS Clinical Trials Group (1992) Mortality in patients with the acquired immunodeficiency syndrome treated with either foscarnet of ganciclovir for cytomegalovirus retinitis. *N. Engl. J. Med.*, **326**, 213–220.

Henderson, H. W. A. and Mitchell, S. M. (1999) Treatment of Immune Recovery Vitritis with local steroids. *Br. J. Ophthalmol.*, **83**, 540–545.

Walsh, J. C., Jones, C. D., Barnes, E. A., Gazzard, B. G. and Mitchell, S. M. (1998) Increasing survival in AIDS patients with cytomegalovirus retinitis treated with combination antiretroviral therapy including HIV protease inhibitors. *AIDS*, **12**, 613–618.

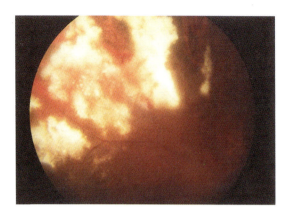

Fig. 1.17a

Q: *Describe the fundal findings seen in a 29-year-old man who gave a 2-week history of ocular discomfort, photophobia, floaters and blurred vision. He had no medical history of note. What is the most likely diagnosis? (see Fig. 1.17a)*

A: There are extensive multifocal, yellow-white, retinal infiltrates involving the peripheral retina. The remaining fundal details are unclear due to vitreous inflammation. The most likely cause of such a dramatic fundal appearance in an otherwise well patient is acute retinal necrosis (ARN).

If the diagnosis of ARN is to be considered the following features should be present:

(1) Focal areas of retinal necrosis located in the peripheral retina (outside the major temporal arcades). These may be associated with retinal haemorrhages.
(2) Rapid, circumferential progression of the necrosis over 5–10 days if untreated.
(3) Occlusive vasculopathy.
(4) Anterior granulomatous iridocyclitis and vitritis.

Patients may be immunocompetent or immu-nocompromised. ARN is more typically unilateral, but bilateral involvement is well described although the severity of the disease often differs between eyes. Typically the retinitis resolves over 4–12 weeks. However, the necrotic retina is prone to detachment.

Q: *What is the treatment of choice for ARN?*

A: ARN is thought to be secondary to Varicella-zoster virus (VZV) infection in older patients and herpes simplex in younger patients. Intravenous acyclovir is the treatment of choice, with most cases showing evidence of regression within 4 days of treatment onset. If untreated regression is noted by 3 weeks. As the retinitis regresses salt and pepper pigmentation develops in areas of retinal atrophy. If there has been no optic neuropathy or retinovascular occlusion the visual prognosis is good. Treatment of uniocular disease significantly decreases the incidence of fellow eye involvement. However, in AIDS patients there is a much higher incidence of retinal detachment (80%), bilateral involvement (90%) and recurrent disease. Fewer than 20% of AIDS patients with ARN maintain 6/6 vision.

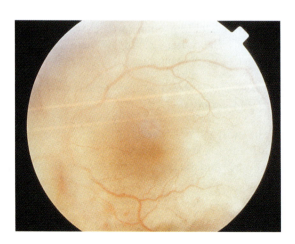

Fig. 1.17b

Q: *What is the other posterior segment manifestation of VZV infection in AIDS patients?*

A: Progressive outer retinal necrosis syndrome is a form of VZV retinitis characterised by deep retinal opacification at the posterior pole, and mid- and far-retinal periphery (Fig. 1.17b). Although there may be a mild anterior uveitis vitritis is minimal. The retinal necrosis spreads centrifugally often becoming confluent and involving the entire retina. There is a high incidence of retinal detachment, >70% of cases are bilateral and the response to antiviral treatment is limited.

1.18

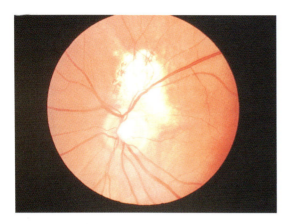
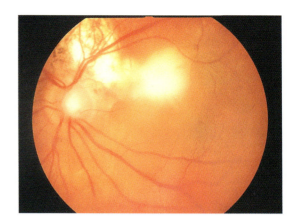

Fig. 1.18a

Q: *What is illustrated by these two fundal photographs taken 7 years apart? (see Fig. 1.18a)*

A: There is a chorioretinal scar with associated pigmentation adjacent to the superior margin of the left optic disc, the vitreous is clear. This is indicative of inactive *Toxoplasma* retinochoroiditis. The second picture, taken 7 years later, demonstrates a new focus of active retinochoroiditis arising from the temporal aspect of the old scar. The creamy, fluffy appearance and mild vitreous inflammation confirm the activity of the lesion.

Q: *Is this lesion a congenital or an acquired one?*

A: Until recently all ocular toxoplasmosis was thought to be congenital. If a pregnant mother becomes infected in the first trimester of pregnancy there is a 40% chance of passing the infection on to her offspring. If infection occurs in the third trimester the risk of vertical transmission is lower, but the resultant infection is likely to be more severe. A study looking at the incidence and aetiology of *Toxoplasma* retinochoroiditis in a population of children in the Sao Paulo region of Brazil, revealed an unexpectedly high incidence of ocular toxoplasmosis of 18%. In the same area IgM antibodies were found in <1% of cord blood samples, the ocular lesions were documented in multiple siblings, and systemic congenital toxoplasmosis was uncommon. These findings suggest that ocular toxoplasmosis is not always congenital in origin.

Q: *What are the indications for treating Toxoplasma retinochoroiditis? What therapeutic regimes are currently in use, and how do they alter the natural history of the disease?*

A: There are three main indications for treating *Toxoplasma* retinochoroiditis:

(1) Active lesions within the arcades that pose a threat to the macula or optic nerve.
(2) Any large retinal lesions >2 disc diameters, associated with an intense vitritis causing a reduction in visual acuity.
(3) Any lesion in an immunocompromised patient.

Treatment regimes usually involve two or more agents, regimes currently in favour include the following:

(1) Pyrimethamine 100 mg o.d. for 2 days then 25 mg b.d. Sulphadiazine 1 g q.d.s. with or without prednisolone 1 mg/kg to be started 3 days after commencing dual therapy, then taper off gradually.

(2) Clindamycin 150 mg q.d.s. alone or in combination with sulphadiazine therapy with or without prednisolone.

(3) Co-trimoxazole 960 mg b.d. for 2 weeks, reducing to 380 mg b.d., plus prednisolone as above.

The triple therapy regime has the highest side effect profile. Pyrimethamine treatment frequently causes anorexia and nausea, and may result in reversible bone marrow suppression (which is dose related), although this rarely develops when folinic acid supplements are taken. All patients taking clindamycin should be warned to report promptly any gastrointestinal upsets that may indicate the onset of pseudo-membranous colitis. The exact role of corticosteroids in the treatment of *Toxoplasma* retinochoroiditis remains controversial.

However, there is no evidence that any of the above regimes have any affect on the natural history of *Toxoplasma* retinochoroiditis. A prospective multicentre study in which 149 patients were treated with one of the above regimes or placebo, demonstrated that there was no difference in the duration of inflammatory activity between treated and untreated patients although a more marked reduction in the size of the retinal inflammatory lesion was seen in treated patients. The most important factor predicting the duration of inflammatory activity was the size of the lesion itself, independent of treatment. The other finding of note was that the mean recurrence rate after three years of follow-up was 49% for all groups of patients.

This patient was treated with clindamycin and prednisolone, 3 weeks later the lesion appears inactive (Fig. 1.18b) and although there is some subfoveal retinal pigment epithelial disturbance he maintains a visual acuity of 6/9.

Q: *How would your management be altered if this patient was HIV-positive with a CD4 cell count of <100/µl?*

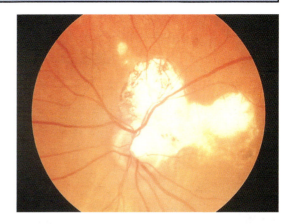

Fig. 1.18b

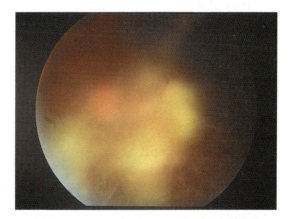

Fig. 1.18c

A: Ocular toxoplasmosis in HIV-positive patients (Fig. 1.18c) is in most cases due to reactivation of congenital disease. It is often bilateral and multifocal.

These immunocompromised patients are at risk of developing Toxoplasma encephalitis or disseminated toxoplasmosis. Therefore all active Toxoplasma lesions in such patients should be treated and systemic involvement suspected until proven otherwise. Work up should include the following:

(1) MRI of the brain to exclude cerebral toxoplasmosis. These lesions will appear hyperintense on T_2 weighted scans. A ring enhancing lesion on CT scanning is also

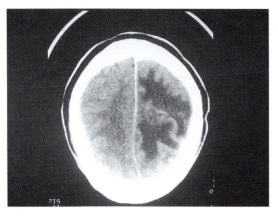
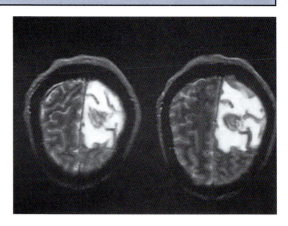

Fig. 1.18d

suggestive of cerebral toxoplasmosis (Fig. 1.18d pre- and post-contrast).
(2) Lumbar puncture.
(3) A full systemic examination looking for evidence of lymphadenopathy and/or splenomegaly that may signal disseminated toxoplasmosis.

A combination of sulphadiazine 4–6 g/day and pyrimethamine 50–100 mg/day (plus folinic acid 15 mg/day) is the treatment of choice. Clindamycin 600–1200 mg q.d.s. is an effective alternative treatment. Lifelong maintenance treatment (on half the above doses) is mandatory, although pre-existing bone marrow suppression and frequent allergies to sulphonamides often hamper this. Severe diarrhoea has been reported with low-dose clindamycin therapy in AIDS patients. Atovaquone and clarithromycin, both given with pyrimethamine may play an increasingly important role in both the treatment of established toxoplasmosis and in prophylaxis.

Recommended reading

Rothova, A. (1993) Ocular involvement in toxoplasmosis [Review]. *Br. J. Ophthalmol.*, **77**, 371–377.

Rothova, A., Meenkeen, C., Buitenhuis, H. J., Brinkman, C. J., Baarsma, G. S., Boen-Tan, T. N., *et al.* (1993) Therapy for ocular toxoplasmosis. *Am. J. Ophthalmol.*, **115**, 517–523.

1.19

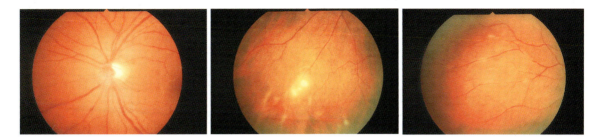

Fig. 1.19a

Q: *This 30-year-old woman presented with a gradual, painless, reduction in vision (6/18 both eyes) associated with floaters. Describe these fundal photographs. What is the differential diagnosis? (see Fig. 1.19a)*

A: The view of the disc is hazy secondary to vitreous inflammation, in the equatorial region there are numerous preretinal vitreous opacities and venous sheathing, indicative that periphlebitis is prominent. There is no evidence of choroiditis or retinitis. This is an example of retinal vasculitis associated with ocular inflammation. There are many causes of such a clinical picture but the initial differential diagnosis should include:

(1) Sarcoidosis – 28% of patients will develop a retinal vasculitis with or without choroiditis. It is probably the most common systemic condition associated with retinal vasculitis and ocular inflammation.
(2) Intermediate uveitis (pars planitis) which may be associated with multiple sclerosis.
(3) Behçet's disease associated retinal vasculitis, although there is no arterial involvement in this case.
(4) Toxoplasmosis – a retinal vasculitis without any foci of retinochoroiditis has been described in patients with high anti-toxoplasma IgM titres.

(5) Herpetic viral infection – herpes simplex and varicella zoster viruses are infectious causes of a retinal vasculitis.
(6) Lyme disease – fundal involvement is characteristically seen in stage II disease, 1–4 months after the initial infection.
(7) Idiopathic retinal vasculitis.

This patient did in fact have a previous history of granulomatous uveitis and erythema nodosum and had a proven diagnosis of sarcoidosis. There was active retinal vasculitis in both eyes with visual acuities reduced to 6/18 secondary to bilateral cystoid macular oedema.

Q: *What features of the systemic and ocular examination may help distinguish between the conditions mentioned above?*

A: Table 1.4 highlights the characteristic ocular and systemic features of conditions that commonly cause retinal vasculitis.

Q: *What other systemic conditions may cause a retinal vasculitis not associated with intraocular inflammation? (see Fig. 1.19b)*

A: There are several conditions that cause a retinal vasculopathy, which is not associated with intraocular inflammation.

(1) Wegener's granulomatosis – retinal vascular involvement is less common than scleritis.

Table 1.4

	Sarcoidosis	Intermediate uveitis	Behçet's disease	Toxoplasmosis	Lyme disease	Eales disease	Idiopathic retinal vasculitis
Anterior segment	Granulomatous uveitis, Koeppe and Busacca nodules	Low grade uveitis often asymptomatic	Hypopyon uveitis may be painless	Low grade uveitis	Keratitis; Mild-moderate uveitis	Mild uveitis	Mild-moderate uveitis
Vitreous	Vitreous cells, from a 'string of pearls' or a snowbank in severe cases	Vitreous cells with inferior snowbanks over the pars plana	Vitreous cells	Vitreous cells mild-severe	Vitreous cells; Snowbanks may be a feature	Vitreous cells; Vitreous haemorrhage	Vitreous cells
Venous sheathing	Mid-peripheral may be severe – 'candle wax drippings' (Fig. 1.19b) Venous occlusions occur rarely	Mid-peripheral usually mild; venous occlusions occur rarely	More extensive, may be associated with venous occlusions	Diffuse venous sheathing. May be seen in the absence of active foci	Mid-peripheral, usually mild	Mild-severe segmental. Sheathing. Solitary or multiple branch vein occlusions	Peripheral vascular sheathing
Arterial sheathing	None	None	Is a characteristic feature; Arterial occlusions are not uncommon	Segmental-sheathing near active foci of retinochoroiditis	None	Arteriolar sheathing	None
Retina choroid and optic nerve	Chorioretinitis or choroidal nodules often seen; Cystoid macular oedema is common; disc swelling	Cystoid macula oedema develops in 50% of cases	Focal retinal necrosis, retinal haemorrhages and macular oedema	Retinochoroiditis	No choroidal or retinal lesions; Optic neuritis	Neovascularisation of the disc and/or retina present in 80% Vitreous haemorrhage Retinal detachment	Macular oedema; diffuse capillary leakage
Systemic signs	Respiratory disease; erythema nodosum; renal disease	Demyelinating disease in 5%	Aphthous stomatitis Genital ulcers Erythema nodosum Superficial thrombo-phlebitis Arthritis-arthralgia	Nil of note	Erythema chronicum migraines Headache, malaise myalgia, arthralgia. Bells palsy Myocarditis	Hypersensitivity to tuberculin protein Sensorineural hearing loss	None

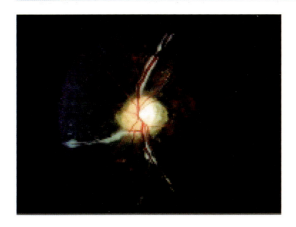

Fig. 1.19b

(2) Polyarteritis nodosa – this necrotising vasculitis involves the eye in 20% of cases. Both retinal arterioles and venules are affected.
(3) Relapsing polychondritis – retinal vasculitis is less common than scleritis, occurring in 9% of patients.
(4) SLE – in most cases the retinal vascular disease of SLE is not associated with an inflammatory infiltrate.

Q: *What initial investigations should be performed in a patient with retinal vasculitis and intraocular inflammation of undetermined aetiology?*

A: The most important step in the initial management of these patients is to take a full medical history and perform a thorough systemic examination. This is essential if systemic illnesses are not to be missed. In Caucasian patients retinal vasculitis is only confined to the eye in approximately 40% of cases.

Initial investigations will be tailored according to the history and clinical examination, appropriate tests may include:

(1) Full blood count/ESR.
(2) Urea and electrolytes, blood sugar.
(3) Liver function tests.
(4) Serum angiotensin-converting enzyme levels.

(5) Syphilis serology.
(6) Chest X-ray.
(7) Fluorescein angiography – is there evidence of cystoid macular oedema, disc swelling, diffuse or focal microvascular leakage or staining, peripheral capillary closure or neovascularisation?
(8) A Mantoux test may be useful to differentiate sarcoidosis from tuberculosis.
(9) Coagulation studies (including anticardiolipin, lupus anticoagulant, antithrombin III, protein C and S and Factor V Leiden) are indicated in cases of ischaemic retinal vasculitis.

Q: *How would you treat the sarcoid related retinal vasculitis associated with cystoid macular oedema, illustrated in Fig. 1.19a? How would you monitor visual recovery?*

A: The treatment of choice for bilateral retinal vasculitis secondary to sarcoidosis is systemic corticosteroids, provided there are no contraindications to their use. Prior to treatment the possible risks and benefits, and potential duration of steroid treatment should be discussed with the patient.

A typical treatment regime would be as follows:

(1) Prednisolone 40 mg/day for 1 week reducing by 5–10 mg/week In more severe forms of retinal vasculitis higher doses may be needed, e.g. prednisolone 80 mg for 4 days, 60 mg for 4 days and then 40 mg for 1 month. Pulsed intravenous methyl prednisolone may also be used to try and induce a remission in severe cases.
(2) Visual loss is secondary to cystoid macular oedema in the majority of these patients and the degree of oedema often provides a sensitive guide to the efficacy of treatment. Amsler grid monitoring for central distortion and micropsia will detect oedema that may not be immediately apparent on slit-lamp biomicroscopy. Treatment is tapered until there are signs of an exacerbation of the cystoid macular oedema. To minimise the side effects of corticosteroids, such as

osteoporosis, one should aim for a maintenance dose of 10 mg/day or less. If the clinical signs have been stable on the maintenance dose for 4–6 weeks this may be slowly tapered using an alternate day regime.

(3) The use of second-line immunosuppressive agents, such as cyclosporin A, is indicated if the prednisolone maintenance dose is >15 mg/day. They may also be used as an initial adjunctive treatment in severe uveitis.

(4) Cystoid macular oedema may persist even with suppression of active ocular inflammation. It may be necessary to continue with low dose (<5 mg/day) corticosteroid therapy for a year or more. Alternative treatment options that may be used in conjunction with corticosteroids are acetazolamide or non-steroidal anti-inflammatory agents, e.g. diclofenac.

(5) All patients receiving even relatively short courses of systemic corticosteroids should have their blood pressure, weight and urine monitored at each clinic visit, with periodic urea and electrolyte evaluations.

Note, a case could be made for periocular depot steroid injections in unilateral disease. Any associated anterior uveitis should be treated with topical steroids and cycloplegia as appropriate.

Q: *What is the role of conjunctival biopsy in the diagnosis of sarcoidosis and what are the characteristic histological findings?*

A: If there is a visible conjunctival mass most authorities would agree that a biopsy is a useful procedure. However, there is still debate over the role of 'blind' conjunctival biopsy in the diagnosis of sarcoidosis. The pathognomonic lesion is a non-caeseating granuloma consisting of epithelioid cells, multinucleate giant cells of the Langhans type and a thin rim of lymphocytes. Schaumann's bodies (ovoid and basophilic) and asteroid bodies (star-shaped and acidophilic) may be found in some of the giant cells.

Recommended reading

Graham, E. M., Stanford, M. R., Sanders, M. D., Kasp, E. and Dumonde, D.C. (1989) A point prevalence study of 150 patients with idiopathic retinal vasculitis: 1. Diagnostic value of ophthalmological features. *Br. J. Ophthalmol.*, **73**, 714–721.

Sanders, M. D. (1987) Retinal arteritis, retinal vasculitis and autoimmune retinal vasculitis [Duke-Elder Lecture]. *Eye*, **1**, 441–465.

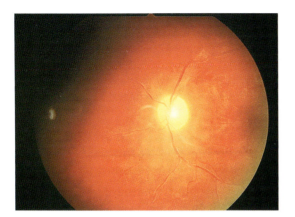

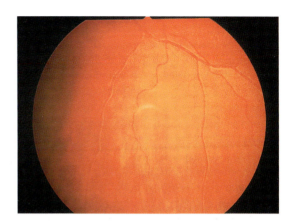

Fig. 1.20a

Q: *Describe the fundal changes seen in a 32-year-old man of Turkish descent. What is the most likely diagnosis? (see Fig. 1.20a)*

A: There is widespread sheathing of both retinal arteries and veins, with marked attenuation of the retinal arteries indicative of an extensive ischaemic retinal vasculitis. There is a degree of disc pallor, but there is no associated choroiditis, retinitis or vitritis. The most common cause of a retinal vasculitis involving both arteries and veins, in this age group is Behçet's disease. This condition has a prevalence of 80–300/100 000 in Turkey and the Middle East, and 8/100 000 in Japan. It is the leading cause of endogenous uveitis and one of the major causes of acquired blindness in these countries.

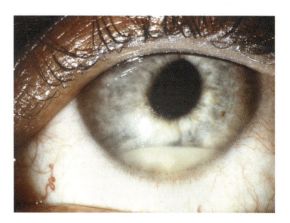

Fig. 1.20b

Q: *What are the ocular manifestations of Behçet's disease?*

A: In a large Japanese epidemiological study of over 3000 patients, 69% had ocular involvement.

(1) Bilateral acute iritis with or without hypopyon (Fig. 1.20b) – although this is the classical ocular sign of Behçet's disease a panuveitis is usually present with evidence of vitritis and macular oedema. This inflammation may run a chronic or a relapsing course in which the hypopyon waxes and wanes. A characteristic feature of the hypopyon is that it shifts with gravity as the patient's head posture changes. With recurring bouts of anterior uveitis peripheral anterior and/or posterior synechiae may form predisposing to the development of secondary angle closure glaucoma.

(2) Retinal vasculitis (Fig. 1.20a) – this is in fact more common than anterior disease and is characterised by periphlebitis, recurrent venous and arterial occlusions, retinal haemorrhages and focal regions of retinal necrosis. These vascular occlusions are the major cause of the poor visual prognosis. Retinal neovascularisation secondary to venous occlusions or inflammation may result in vitreous haemorrhage and occasionally neovascular glaucoma. In end-stage disease these florid signs are replaced by an atrophic retina and optic disc, sheathed arteries and veins and variable chorioretinal scarring.
(3) Optic disc swelling may be secondary to posterior segment inflammation (papillitis), an ischaemic optic neuropathy or raised ICP due to cerebral vein thrombosis.

The visual prognosis for individuals with posterior segment disease is poor, with <25% of patients maintaining an acuity of 6/12 or better 5 years after the onset of uveitis.

Q: *What are the systemic features of Behçet's disease?*

A: The International Study group for Behçet's Disease published their diagnostic criteria in 1990:

Recurrent oral ulceration, i.e. minor or major aphthous ulcers that have recurred at least 3 times in one 12-month period. Plus two of the following:

(1) Recurrent genital ulceration.
(2) Ocular lesions.
(3) Skin lesions – erythema nodosum, pseudo-folliculitis, paulopustular lesions or acneiform nodules.
(4) Positive pathergy test – read by a physician at 24–48 h.

The Behçet's Disease Research Committee of Japan proposed a similar list of criteria, except that the presence of aphthous mouth ulcers is not considered to be mandatory to make a positive diagnosis.

Other systemic features of Behçet's disease may include the following:

(1) Non-destructive arthritis-arthralgia affecting the ankles and wrists (52%).
(2) Obliterative thrombophlebitis and arterial occlusions (8–28%).
(3) Neurological sequelae, e.g. cranial nerve palsies and pyramidal and extrapyramidal signs (8–10%).
(4) Ulcerative haemorrhages in the gastrointestinal tract.

Q: *What systemic treatments are most commonly used in the treatment of Behçet's disease?*

A: Many immunosuppressive regimes have been tried in an attempt to alter the devastating natural history of Behçet's disease. The success or failure of these regimes appears to show a marked geographical variability; treatments that are effective in Japanese patients being less successful in Turkish patients and vice versa.

(1) Colchicine is used to inhibit neutrophil chemotaxis and migration. The aim of therapy is to prevent recurrent attacks, it is not used to treat active disease.
(2) Azathioprine does not restore compromised vision, but has been shown to maintain acuity in those with established disease and to retard the emergence of new disease. It is also an effective treatment for oral and genital ulceration.
(3) Cyclophosphamide has a similar effect to azathioprine in Japanese patients, but carries the risk of profound bone marrow suppression.
(4) Cyclosporin A at a starting dose of 5 mg/kg/day has been shown to abolish or dramatically reduce recurrent attacks of ocular disease. It has also proven to be an effective treatment in neuro-Behçet's disease. Maintenance therapy may be required for many years as treatment does not appear to induce a state of immunological tolerance.
(5) Tacrolimus (FK506), like cyclosporin A, selectively suppresses $CD4^+$ lymphocytes.

It is particularly useful in cases of refractory uveitis which have failed to respond to the other agents mentioned above. The optimum dosage is 0.10–0.15 mg/kg/day. Side effects include renal impairment, neurological symptoms, gastrointestinal upset and hyperglycaemia.

(6) Thalidomide is currently being trialled in cases of refractory uveitis including Behçet's disease.

The role of corticosteroids is a controversial one, with combination immunosuppressive regimes being favoured in the US and UK, but not in Japan.

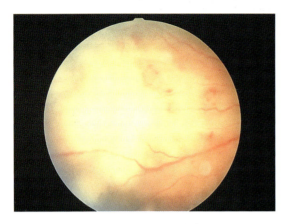

Fig. 1.21a

Q: *Describe these fundal findings seen in a 65-year-old man with a 6-week history of gradual, painless visual loss. The 'uveitis' was partially responsive to topical and systemic steroid therapy. What is the differential diagnosis? (see Fig. 1.21a)*

A: The fundal details are slightly hazy secondary to a mild vitritis. There are confluent, elevated, yellow-white chorioretinal infiltrates associated with intraretinal haemorrhages, but no evidence of retinal vasculitis. These are the appearances of an intraocular lymphoma. In this case the differential diagnosis should also include sarcoid and tuberculous choroiditis.

Intraocular lymphomas, formerly termed reticulum cell sarcomas, are high-grade B cell lymphomas of the large cell type. Ocular manifestations include:

(1) Panuveitis with a marked vitreous cellular infiltrate. The virtually pathognomonic yellow-white chorioretinal infiltrates are the most common manifestations of an intraocular lymphoma. Bilateral involvement occurs in >90% of cases.
(2) Choroidal infiltrates with or without vitreous involvement.

(3) Haemorrhagic retinal necrosis that mimics ARN and prominent perivascular infiltrates.
(4) Hypopyon uveitis – this is a rare sequela of systemic lymphoma.

Intraocular lymphoma, like leukaemia, is one of the 'masquerade' syndromes, and must be excluded in all patients >50 years of age with chronic, diffuse 'uveitis' and vitreous infiltrates.

Q: *What other investigations are indicated?*

A: Intraocular lymphoma has a strong association with CNS lymphoma, investigations should include:

(1) Vitreous biopsy – fine needle aspiration biopsy or core vitrectomy may be used to obtain a vitreous sample. The latter will have a therapeutic as well as a diagnostic role in those patients with dense vitreous infiltrates. The vitreous specimen should be sent for immediate cytologic and immunologic analysis. The diagnostic yield from vitreous biopsy is variable and repeat biopsies may be needed following negative results. However, some centres have reported this technique can establish the diagnosis in over 95% of cases.
(2) Retinal biopsy may also be helpful in selective cases. Brain MRI with gadolinium enhancement or CT scan (Fig. 1.21b).
(3) CSF cytology.
(4) Abdominal and chest CT scanning.
(5) Bone marrow aspiration and trephine (a full blood count is invariably normal).

Until recently primary intraocular-CNS lymphomas proved fatal in the vast majority of patients. However, with the advent of new intrathecal and systemic chemotherapy regimes, plus ocular and CNS radiotherapy, the prognosis has improved. A high index of suspicion in older patients with bilateral 'uveitis' remains

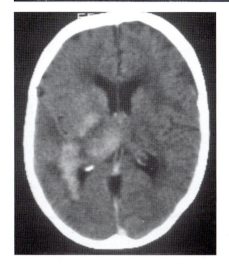
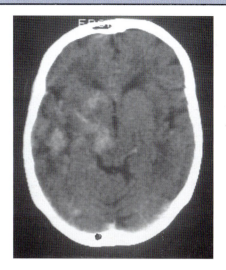

Fig. 1.21b

of paramount importance, as early diagnosis and treatment are associated with a better prognosis.

Recommended reading

Char, D. H., Ljung, B.-M., Miller, T. and Philips, T. (1988) Primary intraocular lymphoma (ocular reticulum cell sarcoma) diagnosis and management. *Ophthalmology*, **95**, 625–630.

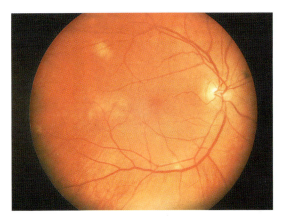

Fig. 1.22a

Q: *Describe the fundal appearance in this 35-year-old man. What is the differential diagnosis? (see Fig. 1.22a)*

A: There are several discrete, creamy-white, choroidal lesions scattered throughout the posterior pole of both eyes. There is no evidence of overlying retinitis, vasculitis or vitritis. The differential diagnosis for a patient with a multi-focal choroiditis should include the following:

(1) Infective causes:
　　(a) Tuberculous choroiditis.
　　(b) Treponemal choroiditis.
(2) Sarcoidosis – deep chorioretinal lesions of variable size may be present with minimal overlying retinitis or vasculitis (Fig. 1.22b).
(3) Presumed ocular histoplasmosis (POHS).
(4) Serpiginous choroiditis.
(5) Birdshot choroidopathy.
(6) Sympathetic ophthalmia.

This is in fact an example of choroidal tuberculosis. The appearance is variable with tubercles ranging from 1/4 to several disc diameters in size. These lesions occur most frequently at the posterior pole, are often multiple and become more pigmented with age. Associated

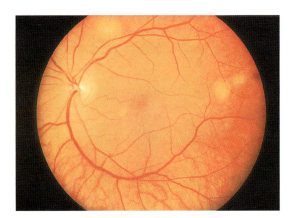

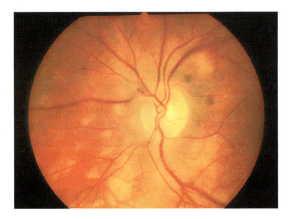

Fig. 1.22b

retinal and vitreous involvement is not uncommon.

Q: *What is the association between choroidal and systemic tuberculosis?*

A: Choroidal tubercles and tuberculomas (large solitary masses, Fig. 1.22c) are the best-documented ocular manifestations of tuberculosis. Their presence is indicative of haematogenous seeding of bacilli but is not diagnostic of miliary tuberculosis. However, choroidal

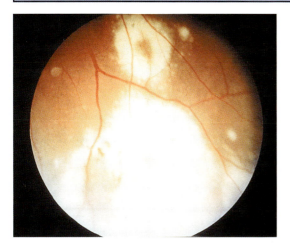

Fig. 1.22c

tubercles have been reported in 28–60% of cases of miliary tuberculosis and in 30% of cases of pulmonary tuberculosis.

Q: *What is the treatment of choice for choroidal tuberculosis? What are the ocular side effects of the agents used?*

A: The presence of tuberculous chorioditis with or without overt pulmonary involvement warrants immediate systemic treatment. The regime currently advocated by the Center of Disease Control is as follows:

An initial 2-month induction course of:

(1) Pyrizinamide 15–30 mg/kg.
(2) Rifampicin 10 mg/kg.
(3) Isoniazid 5 mg/kg.

Followed by a continuation phase of isoniazid and rifampicin for four months. As primary resistance to isoniazid is possible, ethambutol or streptomycin should be included in the initial treatment regime, until drug susceptibility studies are available. Over 95% of immunocompetent patients will be successfully treated with a full course of therapy provided compliance is optimal.

Ethambutol is known to cause an optic neuritis in 3–15% of patients treated with a continuous dose of 25 mg/kg/day. Signs of toxicity rarely appear before 6 weeks following initiation of therapy. Although the incidence of ocular toxicity is dose dependent, there is no relationship between dose and visual acuity when toxicity does occur. The pattern of visual loss is variable – in the axial type a central scotoma with reduced central and colour vision is reported in contrast to the periaxial type where pericentral or peripheral scotoma are described with preservation of central vision and colour perception. Evidence of clinical improvement is usually observed from 1–6 weeks after discontinuing ethambutol, with visual acuity returning to normal in the majority of cases by 3–12 months.

Isoniazid therapy is a rare cause of optic neuritis and optic atrophy. In reported cases the dose of isoniazid ranged from 200 to 900 mg/day with visual loss occurring 10 days to 2 months after commencing treatment. Unlike ethambutol related optic neuritis, the visual improvement on discontinuing treatment is often limited, because of the subsequent development of optic atrophy.

Q: *What screening precautions should be taken for patients receiving ethambutol or isoniazid?*

A: A complete baseline examination including refraction, colour vision assessment and visual fields is advisable prior to commencing treatment with ethambutol. Routine screening during therapy is not indicated other than monthly visual acuities and questioning regarding visual symptoms. A deterioration of two or more lines of Snellen acuity from baseline, should prompt an immediate referral to an ophthalmologist.

In the case of isoniazid therapy only those patients who are thought to be more susceptible to toxic side effects, such as alcoholics, malnourished patients and those with pre-existing cerebral damage should be monitored for visual complaints.

Q: *How would you perform a Mantoux test? What factors would you take into account when you are interpreting the results of a tuberculin skin test?*

A: A Mantoux test involves the use of a no. 26 or smaller gauge needle to inject 0.1 cm^3 (5 TU) of purified protein derivative (PPD) intracutaneously on the volar or dorsal surface of the forearm, producing a wheal of 6–10 mm. Injection should be performed within 1 h of drawing up the solution. After 48 h any induration is measured in millimetres transversely on the skin at the point of injection. The following points should be considered when interpreting a Mantoux test:

(1) What is the size of the reaction and is there a history of contact with tuberculosis?
(2) The larger the reaction the more specific the test becomes for *Mycobacterium tuberculosis*. The probability of tuberculous infection with a reaction size of 10 mm is approximately 80% for individuals with a history of exposure to tuberculosis versus 16% in those without such a history (in a Caucasian population). If reaction sizes are >22 mm all individuals will have been infected with tuberculosis irrespective of contact history.
(3) A false-negative test may arise due to an error in reporting or testing. It may also be secondary to other medical conditions such as: overwhelming tuberculosis illness (false-negatives reported in 17%), Hodgkin's disease, sarcoidosis, uraemia, corticosteroid use, elderly patients and in HIV-positive patients (in whom a reaction size of 5 mm should be considered positive).
(4) BCG vaccination induces tuberculin reactivity but the reaction tends to be smaller. It is recommended that patients with positive tuberculin reactions should be managed without regard to a history of BCG, unless it was administered within the previous year.

Helm and Holland made the following recommendations when evaluating patients for *M. tuberculosis* as a possible cause of ocular inflammation:

(1) Possible risk factors for tuberculosis, including exposure to tuberculosis and HIV status, should be investigated.
(2) The primary use of the tuberculin skin test is to provide supportive information when clinical signs and symptoms suggest tuberculosis, and its use should be limited to such patients.
(3) The size of the PPD reaction should be recorded, rather than identifying it solely as positive or negative.
(4) Isoniazid should be given concurrently when treating PPD-positive retinal vasculitis with systemic steroids.
(5) Patients should be treated only when the index of suspicion is increased by the history, examination or associated systemic findings. Treatment should be monitored jointly with a physician.
(6) There is no role for therapeutic trials of isoniazid in the management of patients with ocular inflammatory disease.

Recommended reading

Helm, C. J. and Holland, G. N. (1993) Ocular tuberculosis [Review]. *Surv. Ophthalmol.*, **38**, 229–256.

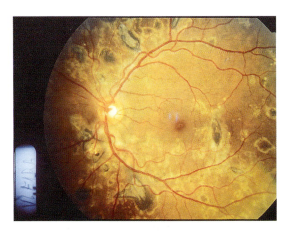

Fig. 1.23a

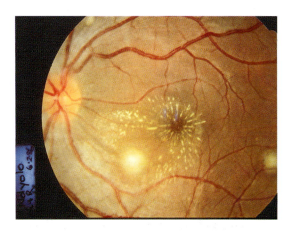

Fig. 1.23b

Q: *Describe this fundal appearance. What is the differential diagnosis? (see Fig. 1.23a)*

A: These fundal signs are typical of an inactive multifocal chorioretinitis. The differential diagnosis should include:

(1) Sarcoid related chorioretinitis.
(2) Tuberculous chorioretinitis.
(3) Treponemal chorioretinitis.

This is an example of burnt out treponemal chorioretinitis. Like systemic syphilis, ocular treponemal disease is one of the great 'imitators' and may present with a myriad of fundal appearances. As well as the more typical multifocal chorioretinitis shown above, a peri-arteritis/arteritis, neuroretinitis or papillitis (Fig. 1.23b) may also occur. Late disease may resemble retinitis pigmentosa (RP), with pigment proliferation, extensive gliosis and atrophy.

Q: *What is the role of serological investigations in the management of patients with suspected syphilis infection? What precautions should be taken when interpreting the results of these serological tests?*

A: The VDRL is a test for the anticardiolipin antibody, i.e. a non-treponemal test; it will only be positive in active treponemal infections and is a useful means by which the efficacy of treatment can be monitored (titres decrease with effective therapy). However, there is a high incidence of false-positives with conditions such as:

(1) Infections:
    (a) Bacterial endocarditis.
    (b) Infectious mononucleosis.
    (c) Leprosy.
    (d) Tuberculosis.
    (e) Mycoplasma.
    (f) Pneumonia.
    (g) Measles.
(2) Chronic liver disease.
(3) Connective tissue disease/SLE.
(4) Systemic malignancy.
(5) Advanced age.
(6) Pregnancy.

Non-treponemal tests are best suited for screening of populations as false-negatives are rare, positive results may then be confirmed by treponemal tests. Tests for treponemal antigens include the Treponemal Haemagglutination Antigen (TPHA) test and the Fluorescent

Treponemal Antibody Absorption (FTA-ABS) test, these will be positive even in inactive disease if there has been a past history of infection. False-positives are much less common with these tests, but false-negatives may be a problem. None of the above serological investigations are particularly reliable in HIV-positive patients. If syphilis is clinically suspected in such patients and serology is negative, dark-field microscopy and DFA-TP applied to lesion exudate, or direct examination of tissue with DFA-TP or silver stains can be used.

Q: *How would you investigate a patient with an active chorioretinitis and a positive VDRL and TPHA?*

A: Ocular treponemal disease especially anterior uveitis, chorioretinitis and optic neuritis have a strong association with neurosyphilis, although the exact frequency of neurosyphilis, be it asymptomatic or otherwise in patients with ocular disease is unknown. Therefore any patient with positive treponemal serology and one or more of the above ocular findings (even if neurologically asymptomatic) should be investigated for neurosyphilis, this involves:

(1) A full neurological examination looking for:
   (a) Meningism – syphilitic meningitis occurs within months to years of primary infection and may coincide with the skin rash of secondary syphilis.
   (b) Cranial nerve palsies commonly IIIrd, VIIth and VIIIth nerve palsies. Syphilitic basilar meningitis may produce multiple IIIrd, IVth and VIth nerve palsies in late neurosyphilitic disease.
   (c) Supranuclear, internuclear and gaze paretic palsies, and other pyramidal signs.
   (d) Visual field defects such as an homonymous hemianopia due to middle or posterior cerebral artery occlusion, or

bitemporal loss secondary to basilar meningitis are usually manifestations of late disease.

(2) Lumbar puncture: elevated white blood cell count and elevated protein, and CSF VDRL-positive. Unlike serum VDRLs, CSF testing rarely produces false-positive results. However, the incidence of false-negatives ranges from 19 to 50%, and a negative non-treponemal CSF test does not preclude the diagnosis of neurosyphilis. The role of CSF FTA-ABS is controversial, and there is debate over the incidence of false-negative results.

There is no consensus as to what actually constitutes a diagnosis of neurosyphilis. However, most physicians would elect to commence treatment in the presence of a CSF leucocytosis, and a raised CSF protein, in a patient with neurological symptoms at any stage of syphilis >1 year's duration, even if the CSF-VDRL was not reactive.

Q: *What is the treatment of choice for treponemal chorioretinitis or optic neuritis?*

A: The treatment of treponemal chorioretinitis and optic neuritis is controversial and the approach to treatment depends on whether one considers ocular inflammation to be a risk factor for neurosyphilis, or an actual manifestation of neurosyphilis. Many authorities would elect to treat all such patients with a regime sufficiently vigorous for neurosyphilis, irrespective of the CSF findings, i.e. a 10–14 day course of intravenous penicillin G 2–5 million IU 4 hourly.

Recommended reading

Margo, C. E. and Hamed, L. M. (1992) Ocular syphilis [Review]. *Surv. Ophthalmol.*, **37**, 203–220.

1.24

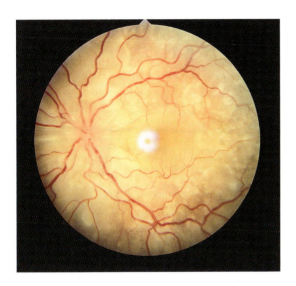

Fig. 1.24a

Q: *Describe the fundal findings of this 35-year-old, normotensive, Japanese woman who presented 4 weeks previously with headache, nausea and blurred vision. What is the most likely diagnosis? (see Fig. 1.24a)*

A: There are multifocal detachments of the sensory retina involving the entire posterior pole. These fundal signs are typical of the Vogt-Koyanagi-Harada syndrome (VKH). This rare condition is most commonly seen in Asian (particularly Japanese) and Native-American Indian patients during the fourth to sixth decades. Women are more commonly affected than men (60–70%).

Q: *What are the ocular and systemic features of VKH syndrome?*

A:

(1) Prodromal illness – this consists of headaches, nausea, fever, vertigo and meningismus (CSF examination will reveal a transient pleocytosis), lasts for several days and is followed by a uveitic phase.

(2) Uveitic phase – the most striking feature of this panuveitis is the multifocal exudative choroiditis and associated serous retinal detachments. Fluorescein angiography may reveal multiple areas of focal leakage in the early phases of the angiogram, macular oedema and disc hyperaemia. The exudative retinal detachments usually resolve spontaneously. Retinal haemorrhages and vitreous opacities are other common findings. Anterior segment involvement follows in the form of a mild to severe bilateral anterior uveitis with extensive posterior synechiae and keratic precipitates (which may be 'mutton fat').

(3) Depigmentation – perilimbal vitiligo occurs in 75% of cases and is the earliest sign of depigmentation (Fig. 1.24b). Vitiligo, alopecia and poliosis occur during the convalescent stage and correspond to fundus depigmentation. Cutaneous manifestations are rare in Hispanic patients but are present in up to 60% of Japanese patients. Depigmentation of the choroid/RPE results in the

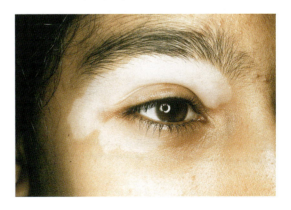

Fig. 1.24b

orange-red fundus discloration, known as 'sunset-glow' fundus.

(4) Neurological sequelae – temporary deafness and tinnitus occur early in the course of the disease in 30% of cases. Encephalopathy with seizures, hemiparesis and cranial nerve palsies are rare.

Note that cases in which exudative retinal detachments and neurological signs predominate are described as Harada's disease.

Q: *What other ocular condition may mimic the appearances described above and must be ruled out before a diagnosis of VKH syndrome can be made?*

A: Sympathetic ophthalmia produces a bilateral granulomatous panuveitis. This occurs after injury/surgery to one eye (exciting eye), followed by a latent period (between 10 days and 50 years) and the development of uveitis in the uninjured (sympathising eye). There are confluent creamy choroidal lesions (with or without overlying serous detachments) that on fluorescein angiography will exhibit hypofluorescence, due to masking, or hyperfluorescence secondary to window defects. Dysacusis, vitiligo, poliosis and aloplecia can also occur in sympathetic ophthalmia but are rare.

Histologically both conditions are characterised by a diffuse granulomatous uveal infil-

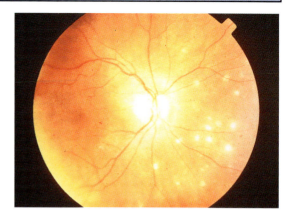

Fig. 1.24c

trate with lymphocytes and epithelioid cells predominating. However the presence of Dalen-Fuchs' nodules (Fig. 1.24c) and the absence of choriocapillaris or retinal involvement is typical of sympathetic ophthalmia. Large cell lymphoma, ocular Lyme disease and sarcoidosis should also be considered in the differential diagnosis.

Recommended reading

Moorthy, R. S., Inomata, H. and Rao, N. A. (1995) Vogt–Koyanagi–Harada syndrome. *Surv. Ophthalmol.*, **39**, 265–292.

1.25

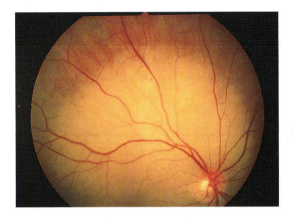

Fig. 1.25a

Table 1.5			
Male		Female	
Lung	54%*	Breast	78%
Unknown primary	25%	Lung	12%
Skin melanoma		Unknown primary	8%
Kidney		GI tract	
Testicle/prostate		Skin melanoma	
GI tract			

* Prior history of lung carcinoma was present in only 30% of these cases.

Q: *Describe the fundal lesion seen in a 56-year-old woman. What is the most likely diagnosis? (see Fig. 1.25a)*

A: There is a large raised grey-yellow subretinal lesion in the region of the superior vascular arcade. There is no overlying retinitis, vasculitis or vitreous inflammation. The most likely diagnosis is a choroidal metastatic deposit.

Q: *What is the frequency of ocular secondaries in metastatic disease? Which primary tumours are most commonly responsible for these metastases?*

A: Autopsy series report a 5–10% incidence of ocular secondaries in patients with known metastatic disease. Using data from the US, if these figures are projected to the estimated cancer deaths from carcinomas per year (approximately 300 000) there could be up to 30 000 cases of intraocular metastases per year. This is 15 times the number of primary ocular malignancies. The posterior choroid with its rich blood supply is by far the most common site for intraocular metastases. Metastases arise in the choroid 10–20 times more frequently than in the iris or ciliary body. The average age of onset of symptoms is 50–55 years of age, males and females being equally affected. The origin of the primary tumour is gender dependent. Table 1.5 outlines the data from several large series, detailing the most common primary sites for males and females.

Q: *What features of choroidal metastases will differentiate them from choroidal melanomas?*

A: The following features outlined in Table 1.6 will help distinguish choroidal metastases from primary choroidal melanomas (Fig. 1.25b).

Q: *This patient had a mastectomy 10 years previously, how would you manage both her ocular and systemic disease?*

A: The patient should be managed jointly by an oncologist/radiologist and an ophthalmologist. A full systemic examination and basic investigations such as a chest X-ray, alkaline phosphatase, liver function tests, CT scan of the brain (25% will have cerebral metastases) and an isotope bone scan should be performed to determine the extent of the metastatic disease. Any further metastatic disease should be treated on

Table 1.6

	Metastases	Primary melanoma
Fundal appearance	Relatively flat and ill defined grey-yellow or yellow-white $+/-$ clumps of overlying pigment Retinal detachments are seen earlier	Well-circumscribed elevated lesions majority are pigmented $+/-$ orange pigment overlying tumour 'Mushroom' configuration after breakthrough of Bruch's membrane
Site	Predominantly posterior pole 25% are multipe or bilateral	Most are anterior to the equator Ciliary body often involved Very rarely multiple or bilateral
Growth pattern	Fast growing	Slow growing
A-scan ultrasonography	Moderate to high internal reflectivity	Low internal reflectivity
B-scan ultrasonography	Echogenic subretinal mass sometimes lobulated with central excavation. Overlying retinal detachment	Lenticular or mushroom-shaped mass demonstrates acoustic hollowness and choriodal excavation

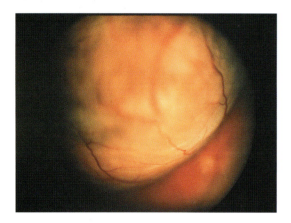

Fig. 1.25b

its merits. As this ocular lesion was causing visual disturbance the treatment of choice was 3000 rad of external beam irradiation with ^{60}Co delivered in multiple fractions over 3–4 weeks, via a lateral port. Clinical improvement should be seen in 4–6 weeks after completion of treatment. For more anterior lesions in an asymptomatic patient chemotherapy may suffice.

The proportion of patients with complete remission of visual signs and symptoms ranges from 26 to 50%, with a partial improvement or

stabilisation in a further 17–35%. The average survival time for patients with ocular metastases from breast carcinoma is 9–13 months, although survival for over 5 years has been reported. The survival times are shorter for patients with lung carcinoma, gastrointestinal or genitourinary malignancies. In these patients the ocular secondary frequently heralds the presence of the primary tumour.

Q: *This 75-year-old woman who had undergone a mastectomy 5 years earlier, presented to an ophthalmologist complaining of blurred vision. Both posterior poles exhibited the changes illustrated in Fig. 1.25c. What is the most likely diagnosis?*

A: This is an example of tamoxifen retinopathy, the characteristic features being inner retinal refractile deposits and retinal pigment epithelial disturbance. Cystoid macular oedema and optic neuropathy have also been reported. Tamoxifen is an antioestrogen drug that is the treatment of choice in metastatic breast cancer with oestrogen-positive receptors. It is also being studied for use in patients at high risk of developing breast cancer. In the 1980s a number of cases of central visual loss were

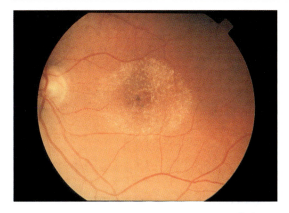

Fig. 1.25c

described in patients taking large doses of tamoxifen, e.g. 120–160 mg b.d. The current recommended dose of tamoxifen is 10–20 mg b.d., yet there have been documented cases of retinopathy and macular oedema with these lower doses. Visual recovery, with or without resolution of retinal deposits, has been reported in patients who have continued to take tamoxifen.

In a series of 135 asymptomatic patients taking tamoxifen (10 mg b.d.) only two were found to have developed retinal crystals. Both patients had 6/6 vision bilaterally with no defects on Amsler testing and normal colour vision. The cumulative dose for these two patients was 10.9 and 21.9 g, the average cumulative dose in the cohort was 17.2 g. As a result of this study the American Academy of Ophthalmologists no longer recommends screening for tamoxifen retinopathy. They suggest that in symptomatic patients with documented tamoxifen retinopathy the ophthalmologist should consult the patient's oncologist. A decision on whether to discontinue treatment can then be made, baring in mind that there is no proven additional benefit of continuing tamoxifen therapy for longer than 5 years.

Recommended reading

Albert, D. M., Rubenstein, R. A. and Scheie, H. G. (1967) Tumour metastases to the eye. I. Incidence in 213 patients with generalized malignancy. *Am. J. Ophthalmol.*, **92**, 723–726.

Ferry, A. P. and Font, R. L. (1974) Carcinoma metastatic to the eye and orbit. I. A clinicopathologic study of 227 cases. *Arch. Ophthalmol.*, **92**, 276–286.

Heier, J. S., Dragoo, R. A., Enzenauer, R. W. and Waterhouse, W. J. (1994) Screening for ocular toxicity in asymptomatic patients treated with tamoxifen. *Am. J. Ophthalmol.*, **117**, 772–775.

1.26

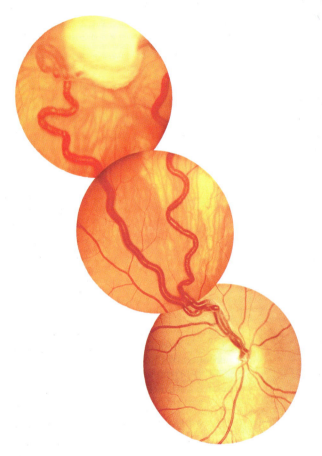

Fig. 1.26a

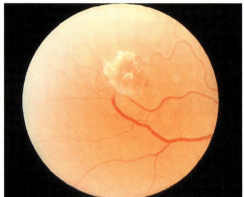

Fig. 1.26b

Q: *This asymptomatic 25-year-old man was referred by his optician. What are these retinal lesions and what is the significance of this diagnosis?(see Fig. 1.26a,b)*

A: Large feeder vessels arising from the right disc pass superotemporally into a large raised white retinal mass. A similar but smaller lesion with associated haemorrhage is found in the periphery of the left eye.

These lesions are retinal angiomas, the pres-ence of two or more such lesions is diagnostic for von Hippel-Lindau disease (VHL). This is a familial cancer syndrome caused by a germline mutation in the VHL tumour suppressor gene. VHL disease is inherited as an autosomal domi-nant trait with variable expression. Retinal angiomas are often the earliest manifestation of VHL disease and are present in approxi-mately 60% of patients. The incidence may in fact be higher, as small lesions are often only visible with the aid of fluorescein angioscopy or angiography. The mean age at time of diagnosis of retinal angiomas is 25 years, with <5% incidence in children under 10 years of age.

Q: *What are the other features of VHL disease and what baseline investigations should be performed in this patient?*

A: VHL disease is characterised by the following features:

(1) CNS haemangioblastomas. Cerebellar haemangioblastomas are the joint most frequent manifestation of VHL disease (along with retinal angiomas). Tumours are multiple or recurrent in 20% of cases (this is diagnostic for VHL disease), 30% of individuals with solitary tumours will have other manifestations of VHL disease. These lesions occur at an earlier age (mean age at diagnosis 29 years) in patients with VHL disease compared to sporadic cases. The second most common site for CNS haemangioblastomas is the spinal cord. MRI scanning is the investigation of choice for CNS haemangioblastomas. Aside from making the initial diagnosis, routine scanning is not indicated in asymptomatic patients, as surgery is only contemplated when patients develop neurological symptoms such as ataxia.

(2) Renal cell carcinoma. The majority of patients with VHL disease will develop renal cell carcinomas if they live long enough. As a result of improved neurosurgical techniques for the treatment of cerebellar lesions, renal cell carcinoma is now the main cause of death in these patients. Although the mean age at diagnosis is younger than for sporadic non-familial tumours the clinical presentation and risk of metastases are the same. In VHL disease renal cell carcinoma is often associated with renal cysts, but it is not clear what the exact nature of this relationship is. Renal ultrasonography is a suitable screening test in the majority of cases. However, if there are multiple renal cysts CT scanning is a more sensitive investigation. This patient should

have an annual renal ultrasound scan and a CT scan every 3 years (or more frequently if there are multiple renal cysts).

(3) Phaeochromocytoma. The incidence of phaeochromocytoma in VHL disease has been reported as between 7 and 19%, and in a third of these cases it may be the sole manifestation of VHL disease. Conversely the incidence of VHL disease in a group of unselected patients presenting with phaeochromocytoma has been reported as 19% (4% were also found to have multiple endocrine neoplasia type 2). Urinary VMAs and normetadrenaline levels (performed annually) can be falsely negative, so measurement of plasma catecholamines and MIBG (metaiodobenzylguanidine) scintigraphy are indicated where there is a clinical suspicion.

(4) Pancreatic cysts. These are usually asymptomatic, and as there is little evidence that they represent a premalignant condition there is no need for specific screening measures.

Q: *Which relatives of this patient would be considered 'at risk' and how should they be screened?*

A: It is essential that a full family medical history be taken with the above features of VHL disease in mind. The formulation of an accurate family tree is essential if all at risk relatives, other than first degree relatives (i.e. parents, siblings and offspring) are to be offered screening. The Cambridge screening protocol for at risk relatives is as follows:

(1) Annual physical examination and urine testing.
(2) Annual slit-lamp biomicroscopy and indirect ophthalmoscopy from age 5 until age 60 years (with or without fluorescein angioscopy or angiography from 10 years).
(3) MRI (or CT) brain scan every 3 years from age 15–40 years and then every 5 years until age 60 years.
(4) Annual abdominal ultrasound scan (kidney, adrenal, pancreas), with abdominal

CT scan every 3 years from age 15 to 65 years.

(5) Annual 24 h urine collection for VMAs and metanephrines.

Q: *How should these retinal angiomas be managed?*

A: Although some retinal angiomas may regress the majority will, if untreated, increase in size. The resultant high flow arteriovenous shunt and incompetent capillaries leads to the formation of retinal exudates and retinal detachment, with eventual visual loss. The mainstay of treatment is laser therapy with the blue-green argon laser. Treatment is applied directly over the tumour in several sessions, with attenuation of feeder vessels signalling adequate treatment. If lesions are >2 disc diameters (3 mm), are located in the extreme retinal periphery or have associated subretinal fluid, they are best managed with cryotherapy. Early detection and prompt treatment has led to a significant improvement in the visual prognosis for patients with VHL disease.

Recommended reading

Maher, E. R., Yates, J. R. W., Harries, R., Benjamin, C., Harris, R., Moore, A. T., *et al.* (1990) Clinical features and natural history of von Hippel–Lindau disease. *Q. J. Med.*, **77**, 151–163.

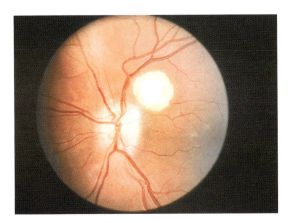

Fig. 1.27a

Q: *Describe this lesion. What is the diagnosis and what is its significance?*
(see Fig. 1.27a)

A: There is a raised, solitary white juxtapapillary lesion approximately 1 disc diameter in size superotemporal to the left optic disc. This is the classical 'mulberry' appearance of a retinal astrocytoma. These hamartomatous lesions initially have a smooth spongy appearance and are either the same colour as the background retina or a light grey-yellow. They have indistinct borders and typically evolve into the more condensed white phakoma seen in adults, the whitened appearance is caused by a combination of avascularity and calcification. They are bilateral in one-third of cases and may occur anywhere in the fundus but are usually found at the posterior pole adjacent to the disc. The significance of this diagnosis lies in the fact that retinal astrocytomas are usually considered to be pathognomonic of tuberous sclerosis. However, sporadic cases have been reported in normal individuals and in those with neurofibromatosis.

Q: *What is the role of the ophthalmologist in the investigation of a child with epilepsy?*

A: Tuberous sclerosis is the most common dominantly inherited condition causing epilepsy and mental handicap (accounting for 10% of children presenting with infantile spasms). Retinal astrocytomas are found in approximately 50% of patients with tuberous sclerosis, half of these lesions are undetected prior to ophthalmic referral. It is vital that a thorough fundal examination using indirect ophthalmoscopy be performed in all suspected cases. It is equally important to differentiate astrocytomas from other conditions that cause pale fundal lesions in infancy:

(1) Retinoblastoma – this is the most common neoplastic ocular tumour in infancy. Small tumours which are elevated pale lesions with abnormal vessels may mimic retinal astrocytomas.
(2) Optic disc drusen – these tend to be buried in younger patients, but superficial drusen may be mistaken for mulberry tumours (misleadingly described in some texts as 'giant drusen').
(3) Toxocara or toxoplasma scars are usually surrounded by pigmentary changes not seen with astrocytomas.
(4) Coats' disease – retinal vessel telangiectasis often results in the accumulation of creamy retinal exudates associated with refractive crystals.

The ophthalmologist should also be aware of other ocular findings in tuberous sclerosis:

(1) Papilloedema – secondary to intracranial tubers or occlusion of the third ventricle by giant cell astrocytomas. Figure 1.27b illustrates a disc phakoma with disc swelling secondary to raised ICP.
(2) Pseudocolobomas of the lens or iris.

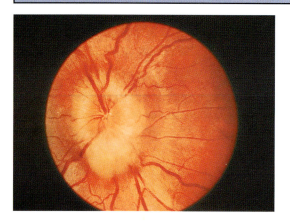

Fig. 1.27b

(3) Peripheral punched-out depigmented fundal lesions, likened to the ash-leaf patch of the skin.

Aside from retinal astrocytomas, the ophthalmologist examining a child with epilepsy should make a careful inspection for the following lesions, which may point to the aetiology of the seizures:

(1) Signs of raised ICP, e.g. papilloedema, VIth nerve palsies.
(2) Cherry red spot:
  (a) Tay–Sachs disease (GM_2 type I).
  (b) Infantile gangliosidosis (GM_1 type I and II) seen in 50% of type I cases, with or without retinal haemorrhages and corneal clouding.
  (c) Metachromatic leukodystrophy, plus optic atrophy in 30%. Seizures are not usually features of other inborn errors of metabolism associated with cherry red spots at the fovea, e.g. Niemann-Pick, Gaucher's disease (type I), sialidoses and mucolipidosis type I.
(3) Bull's eye maculopathy – all four forms of Batten's disease are characterised by visual deterioration with retinal degeneration and a severely abnormal ERG. The classical bull's eye maculopathy is seen in the early stages of the juvenile form of the disease, this is followed by more widespread RPE changes and optic atrophy. The onset of seizures between the ages of 7–16 often leads to the diagnosis.
(4) Retinal, subhyaloid or vitreous haemorrhages associated with the shaken baby syndrome. The majority of children with extensive retinal or vitreous haemorrhages will have an accompanying subdural haematoma.
(5) Ocular motility disorders – Niemann-Pick disease type C, these patients are not sphingomyelinase deficient and develop signs of neurological involvement between 2 and 10 years of age. The characteristic ocular motility disorder is a supranuclear palsy with loss of vertical voluntary saccades and fast phases of optokinetic nystagmus.
(6) Nystagmus may be a feature of Tay-Sachs disease and infantile gangliosidosis.
(7) Signs of TORCH infections.

Recommended reading

Williams, R. and Taylor, D. (1985) Tuberous sclerosis. *Surv. Ophthalmol.*, **30**, 143–154.

1.28

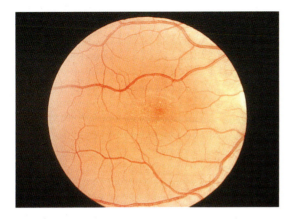

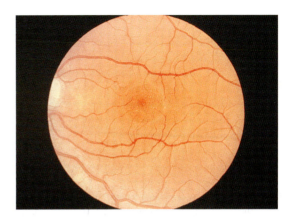

Fig. 1.29

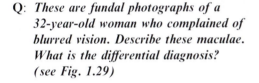

Q: *These are fundal photographs of a 32-year-old woman who complained of blurred vision. Describe these maculae. What is the differential diagnosis? (see Fig. 1.29)*

A: The most striking abnormalities are multiple, discrete subretinal lesions distributed in a symmetrical and concentric pattern in both foveas. This is an example of an early 'bull's-eye' maculopathy, the differential diagnosis should include:

(1) Stargardt's disease – this is usually inherited as an autosomal recessive condition, which typically presents in the first to second decades with decreased central vision. The macula is described as having a 'beaten-bronze' appearance but a 'bull's-eye' pattern is not uncommon. There may be flecks at the level of the RPE in the posterior pole and midperiphery.

(2) Cone-rod dystrophy – the majority of cases are inherited as autosomal dominant traits, with central visual loss occurring in the first to third decades. Temporal optic disc pallor and midperipheral pigmentation may accompany the macular changes.

(3) Familial drusen – this is an autosomal dominant disorder with variable penetrance which remains asymptomatic unless there are secondary degenerative changes.

(4) Hydroxychloroquine or chloroquine retinopathy.

Q: *What dose of hydroxychloroquine is required to produce a maculopathy? How should patients receiving hydroxychloroquine be screened/monitored?*

A: Hydroxychloroquine retinopathy is rare and toxic effects are unlikely to be seen with dosages of <6.5 mg/kg/day for over 5 years. In six case series with a total of 1500 patients treated with hydroxychloroquine only one case of retinopathy with visual loss was observed. Where doses are kept <6.5 mg/kg/day (as is current practice) no cases of toxicity were reported in a series of 973 patients followed for 7 years.

In light of this evidence the Royal College of Ophthalmologists, in conjunction with the Royal College of Physicians' Committees on Rheumatology and Dermatology, have issued new guidelines for hydroxychloroquine screening. The salient points from these guidelines are outlined below:

(1) Routine screening for hydroxychloroquine retinopathy cannot be justified. This conclusion is based on the following:

    (a) There is no evidence-based case for the cost-effectiveness of screening programmes.

    (b) There is no reliable screening test that will identify reversible toxicicty before ophthalmoscopic changes develop.

    (c) It is often difficult to distinguish hydroxychloroquine retinopathy from early age-related macular degeneration.

(2) The role of the dermatologist/rheumatologist:

    (a) Ask about visual impairment not corrected by glasses prior to treatment, and record near visual acuity of each eye. If no abnormality is detected commence treatment. If visual impairment is present refer to an optician.

    (b) Repeat the above annually.

    (c) Refer to an ophthalmologist if there is a change in acuity or blurred vision whilst on treatment and stop treatment if possible in the interim.

(3) Ophthalmological examination should include, distance and near vision, colour vision, central visual fields (preferably with a red target or red Amsler grid), corneal and retinal examination.

(4) Long-term follow-up is only likely to be needed if the patient requires long-term (>5 years) therapy.

Q: *What other medications may cause retinal pigment epithelial damage?*

A: Thioridazine (melleril) is a member of the phenothiazine family of antipsychotic medications, which if administered in doses in excess of 800 mg/day (as it may be in catatonic states) can cause retinal pigment epithelial toxicity. This may lead to blurred vision, dyschromatopsia and night blindness (nyctalopia). Initial changes are fine, deep retinal pigment epithelial stippling, which progress to widespread atrophy of the RPE and choriocapillaris.

Chlorpromazine commonly causes eyelid, conjunctival, corneal and anterior lens pigmentation; however, pigmentary retinopathy is rare unless doses exceed 1200–2400 mg/day for 12 years.

Recommended reading

The Royal College of Ophthalmologists (1998) *Ocular Toxicity and Hydroxychloroquine: Guidelines for Screening* (replacing RCOphth Guidelines, 1993). The Royal College of Ophthalmologists, London.

1.29

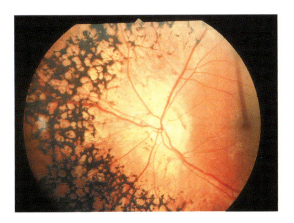
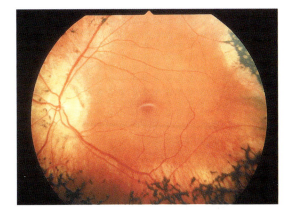

Fig. 1.29a

Q: *Describe these fundal photographs. What ocular symptoms is this patient likely to have and what is the diagnosis? (see Fig. 1.28a)*

A: There is extensive 'bone spicule' pigmentation extending from the vascular arcades to the periphery, marked arterial attenuation and waxy pallor of the optic discs. These are the classical features of retinitis pigmentosa (RP). The patient has marked nyctalopia (night blindness) and grossly constricted visual fields.

Q: *Why may patients with pigmentary retinopathies present to a neurologist?*

A: Pigmentary retinopathies can broadly speaking be divided into two groups, those with purely ocular disease and those with associated single or multisystem disease. A number of patients in the latter group will have neurological symptoms, the most common of which is ataxia. The following are syndromes in which pigmentary retinopathy and neurological disease coexist:

(1) Autosomal dominant syndromes:

(a) Olivopontocerebellar atrophy ataxia, external ophthalmoplegia may also occur.

(b) Charcot-Marie-Tooth disease – degeneration of lateral horn of spinal cord, optic atrophy.

(2) Autosomal recessive syndromes:

(a) Refsum's disease – cerebellar ataxia, partial deafness and ichthyosis. This is the only pigmentary retinopathy that is amenable to treatment.

(b) Batten's disease – all three forms are associated with CNS deterioration.

(c) Cerebrohepatorenal (Zellweger's) syndrome – muscular hypotonia, nystagmus and cerebral demyelination are the neurological features.

(d) Friedreich's ataxia – spinocerebellar degeneration, limb incoordination, neuronal deafness and optic atrophy.

(e) Chronic progressive external ophthalmoplegia – ptosis (may be mistaken for myasthenia gravis) and heart block (Kearns-Sayre-Daroff).

(f) Pallidal degeneration and RP – extrapyramidal rigidity, dysarthria.

(g) Usher's syndrome type I – congenital total deafness, absent vestibular function.

Q: *What conditions may mimic RP?*

A: The following conditions may have a similar ophthalmoscopic appearance to RP:

(1) Congenital infections:
    (a) Rubella, there may be associated congenital cataracts, glaucoma, cardiac defects, deafness and mental retardation.
    (b) Varicella zoster.
    (c) Herpes simplex.
    (d) Syphilis, the typical 'salt-and-pepper' fundus may be associated with normal vision.
(2) Acquired infections:
    (a) Measles.
    (b) Onchocerciasis.

(3) Atypical RP:
    (a) Unilateral RP.
    (b) Sectorial RP (usually non-hereditary but may be autosomal dominant).
    (c) Pericentral RP.
    (d) Paravenous retinal dystrophy.
(4) Toxic retinopathy:
    (a) 4-Amino-quinolones.
    (b) Phenothiazines.
    (c) Desferrioxamine.
(5) Miscellaneous:
    (a) Post-exudative retinal detachment, e.g. Harada's disease or hypertensive crises.
    (b) Trauma.
    (c) Central retinal artery occlusion.

Most cases of pseudo-RP can with the aid of a careful history, and psychophysical or electrophysiological testing, be distinguished from true RP.

Section 2

Optic discs

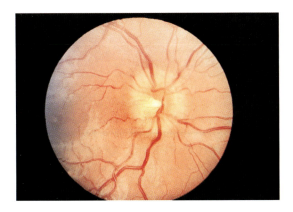 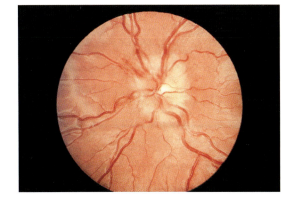

Fig. 2.1a

Q: *Describe the optic discs of this 25-year-old woman who presented with a 2-month history of headaches, her visual acuities were 6/6 in both eyes. She was normotensive. What is the differential diagnosis? (see Fig 2.1a)*

A: There is bilateral disc swelling with obscuration of the disc margins and vessels. The retinal veins have a choked appearance and the optic nerve head capillaries are distended. The disc cups are still visible and there is a small nerve fibre layer haemorrhage on the supero-nasal aspect of the left disc. A feature not evident from these photographs is the absence of spontaneous venous pulsation. The appearance of bilateral disc swelling with no symptomatic visual loss is typical of papilloedema, i.e. bilateral disc swelling secondary to raised intracranial pressure (ICP). The differential diagnoses for conditions producing papilloedema include:

(1) Intracranial space-occupying lesion.
(2) Pseudotumour cerebri.
(3) Idiopathic intracranial hypertension (IIH):
    (a) Steroid withdrawal.
    (b) Steroid therapy.
    (c) Tetracycline therapy.
    (d) Endocrine dysfunction.
(4) Sagittal sinus thrombosis.
(5) Aqueductal stenosis or other causes of hydrocephalus.
(6) Sudden onset severe hypertension.

Note, a transient unilateral or bilateral disc swelling with minimal if any visual symptoms may occur in young insulin-dependent diabetics. This tends to resolve spontaneously over several weeks with no residual field loss.

Q: *How might one differentiate bilateral disc swelling secondary to raised ICP from that caused by demyelination, by examination alone?*

A: Patients with bilateral disc swelling secondary to papilloedema often have surprisingly few visual symptoms whereas demyelination will usually produce rapid and marked visual loss. On examination the following parameters will differ (Table 2.1):

Table 2.1.

	Papilloedema	Demyelination
Visual acuity	Usually normal or minimally decreased unless chronically increased ICP; transient visual obscurations	Rarely normal; 6/9 – no light perception
Colour vision	Usually normal colour vision	Markedly reduced colour vision, often only able to see Ishihara control plate

Note that bilateral optic neuritis, especially causing disc swelling, is a relatively uncommon finding.

Q: *How would you investigate this patient?*

A: The first step is to rule out an intracranial space-occupying lesion by performing a CT scan or MRI of the brain.

In this case a CT scan showed no such mass and the ventricles were considered to be of normal size. An MRI scan was also normal with no evidence of sagittal sinus thrombosis or a posterior fossa mass, both of which may be missed with CT scanning. A lumbar puncture was then performed; CSF analysis was normal and the CSF opening pressure was 35 cmH$_2$O. Goldmann visual field testing showed early constriction of both visual fields with enlarged blind spots. Urea, electrolytes and calcium were within the normal range (hypoparathyroidism and Addison's disease have been associated with pseudotumour cerebri), and a full blood count and clotting screen did not reveal any blood dyscrasias. There was no drug history of note such as oral contraceptives, corticosteroids, tetracycline, psychotherapeutic drugs, vitamin A or anti-inflammatory drugs. The diagnosis, which is one of exclusion, is IIH, formerly known as benign intracranial hypertension or pseudotumour cerebri.

Q: *What are the medical treatment options for IIH?*

A: Therapy is indicated if the patient has persistent headaches or if there is evidence of visual field loss. Various therapeutic regimes have been used including diuretics (e.g. frusemide or acetazolamide) and corticosteroids. The latter is not recommended as a first-line treatment as the ICP often rises again after steroid withdrawal. Several small series have shown that pulsed intravenous methylprednisolone (250 mg q.d.s.) for 5 days followed by an oral taper, in combination with acetazolamide, can be effective in cases where there is severe visual loss. Weight loss should be an integral part of all regimes. The role of the oral contraceptive pill in IIH is still a subject of debate, but is probably a chance association. Repeat lumbar punctures are of dubious benefit and are not only painful but also technically demanding in view of the size of many of these patients. All patients should have baseline visual fields with repeat perimetry at regular intervals. β-Blockers or amitriptyline have proved effective in treating persistent headaches in patients with and without visual field loss.

Q: *Why might this patient complain of diplopia?*

A: Unilateral or bilateral VIth nerve palsies are not uncommon in cases of IIH. These are false localising signs and as a general rule are the only neurological signs that are compatible with a diagnosis of IIH.

Q: *How would you manage a patient with progressive visual field loss despite medical treatment?*

A: A significant minority of patients despite medical treatment will continue to have progressive visual field loss. In these cases decisive action must be taken before extensive and permanent field loss occurs. The surgical treatment of choice for visual loss in IIH is optic nerve sheath decompression or fenestration. This technique has now superseded lumbar-peritoneal shunts which have a high failure and complication rate. In addition, lumbar-peritoneal shunting has failed to halt progressive visual field loss in several well-documented cases.

Following optic nerve sheath fenestration an improvement in visual fields can be expected in approximately one-third of eyes, a stabilisation in one-third and one-third will exhibit continuing visual field deterioration. The probability of failure from 3 to 5 years is approximately 35%. However, failure with visual field deterioration can occur at any time after surgery and patients should therefore be followed up routinely with automated perimetry.

Q: *How does optic nerve sheath fenestration work?*

A: The exact mechanism by which optic nerve sheath fenestration relieves papilloedema secondary to IIH remains unclear. Possible mechanisms include:

(1) Creation of a filtering bleb through which CSF may exit the nerve sheath.
(2) Scarring in the subarachnoid space with shifting of the pressure gradient from the nerve head to the retrobulbar portion of the nerve.

The fact that papilloedema frequently resolves after unilateral fenestration favours the former hypothesis. Cyst-like structures adjacent to the site of fenestration have also been imaged postoperatively. A model simulating fluid spaces corresponding to the intracranial vault, chiasm and optic nerves has been used to demonstrate initiation of fluid flow along the nerve sheath with a subsequent drop in pressure in both nerve sheaths following unilateral fenestration. An additional puzzling feature of this procedure was that resolution of the papilloedema often occurred despite recurrence of raised ICP in the postoperative period. This phenomenon can be explained by Bernoulli's equation of fluid dynamics, which states that as the velocity of a fluid increases, the pressure it exerts decreases. When the ICP in the above model was increased to pathological levels after fenestration the reduced intrasheath pressure persisted as long as active fluid flow continued along the nerve sheath.

Recommended reading

Corbett, J. J. and Thompson, H. S. (1989) The rational management of idiopathic intracranial hypertension [Review]. *Arch. Neurol.*, **46**, 1049–1051.

Radhakrishnan, K., Ahlskog, J. E., Garrity, J. A. and Kurland, L. T. (1994) Idiopathic intracranial hypertension (Review). *Mayo Clin. Proc.*, **69**, 169–180.

Spoor, T. C. and McHenry, J. G. (1993) Long-term effectiveness of optic nerve sheath decompression for pseudotumour cerebri. *Arch. Ophthalmol.*, **11**, 623–625.

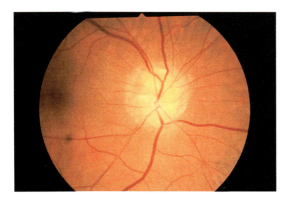 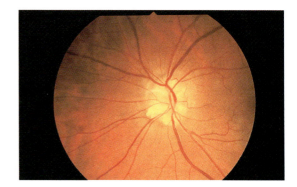

Fig. 2.2a

Q: *Describe the optic discs of this visually asymptomatic, 18-year-old girl who presented with a 2-month history of intermittent frontal headache. What is the cause of this disc swelling? What simple investigations would confirm the diagnosis? (see Fig. 2.2a)*

A: The optic discs appear swollen; however, their appearance is not typical of papilloedema. Specific features to note include:

(1) Irregular but relatively distinct disc margins and loss of the central cup.
(2) Areas of creamy-yellow discoloration within the discs.
(3) Anomalous vascular pattern of retinal vessels at the optic nerve head.
(4) Absence of disc hyperaemia, capillary dilatation or retinal venous dilatation.
(5) Another feature of these discs not apparent from these photographs was the presence of spontaneous venous pulsation.

It should be noted that the presence of spontaneous venous pulsation does not rule out intracranial pathology as ICP may fluctuate.

The appearances described above are typical of the pseudopapilloedema produced by optic disc drusen. The diagnosis may be confirmed by either:

(1) Fundus photography with fluorescein filters *in situ* but without injection of fluorescein – optic disc drusen exhibit autofluorescence (Fig. 2.2b). Over 50% of buried drusen will not be detected by preinjection fundal photography.

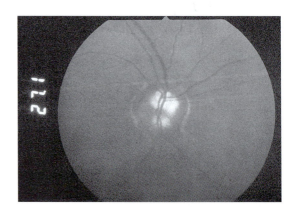

Fig. 2.2b

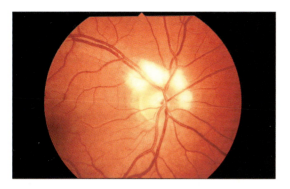 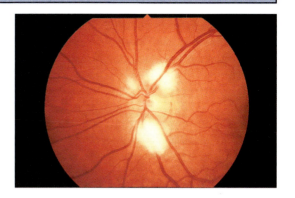

Fig. 2.2c

(2) CT scan of the orbits – the calcific drusen are visible as white lesions at the optic nerve head (calcareous deposits may also develop in cases of chronic papilloedema).
(3) B-scan ultrasonography – this is the most reliable and straightforward method of detecting optic nerve head drusen.
(4) Optical coherence tomography (OCT) is also effective in detecting buried drusen. Prompt recognition of this condition will prevent the patient being subjected to unnecessary and invasive investigations for 'papilloedema'.

Q: *What are the ocular complications and associations of optic nerve drusen?*

A: Optic nerve drusen are equally common in males and females, are bilateral in two-thirds of patients, and have an incidence of between 5 and 20/1000. They may be familial, being inherited as an autosomal dominant trait with variable penetrance. Disc drusen are thought to arise as a result of axonal degeneration caused by disruption of axonal transport and tend to move more superficially with age. As a rule visual acuity is unaffected by drusen of the disc; however, associated visual field defects (which may be progressive) occur in 70% of cases where the drusen are visible. Lower nasal field defects are most common followed by sectorial defects, arcuate scotomas and marked concentric narrowing of the visual field. Optic disc drusen may be associated with haemorrhagic sequelae, these are usually sub-

retinal or subpigment epithelial and frequently arise from areas of subretinal neovascularisation. Superficial disc and vitreous haemorrhages have also been reported.

There have been a number of conditions associated with optic disc drusen reported in the literature (e.g. compressive lesions of the anterior visual pathways). However, the only true associations are with retinitis pigmentosa (in such cases the drusen often lie just off the disc margin in the superficial retina) and with anterior ischaemic optic neuropathy (AION). Both optic disc drusen and AION are associated with small discs. AION may occur in younger patients in the presence of disc drusen.

Q: *What other conditions may cause the appearance of pseudopapilloedema?*

A: Although optic nerve drusen are the most common cause of pseudopapilloedema, a number of other conditions may simulate disc swelling:

(1) Myelinated nerve fibres (Fig. 2.2c). These appear as distinctive bright white feathery areas in the nerve fibre layer. They frequently are adjacent to the optic nerve head and may obscure the disc margins at this point. The remainder of the disc architecture and vasculature is normal. They are an innocent finding and aside from occasional localised field defects are not a cause of significant visual morbidity. They may

occasionally be associated with unilateral high myopia; in these cases the visual prognosis is poor despite correction of the refractive error and amblyopia therapy.

(2) Hypermetropia. Hypermetropic eyes are usually small eyes, which typically have small and 'crowded' optic discs that may appear swollen. The absence of capillary dilatation, venous tortuosity and the presence of a distinct disc margin and spontaneous venous pulsation are reassuring signs in these eyes.

Recommended reading

Kurz-Levin, M. M. and Landau, K. A. (1999) Comparison of imaging techniques for diagnosing drusen of the optic nerve head. *Arch. Ophthalmol.*, **117**, 1045–1049.

Tso, M. O. M. (1981) Pathology and pathogenesis of drusen of the optic nervehead. *Ophthalmology*, **88**, 1066–1079.

2.3

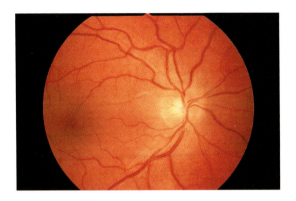
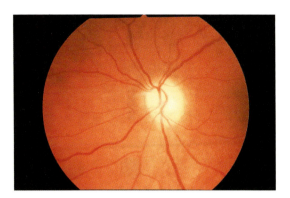
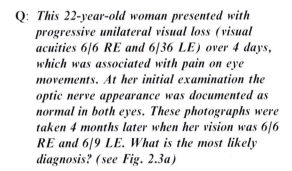

Fig. 2.3a

Q: *This 22-year-old woman presented with progressive unilateral visual loss (visual acuities 6/6 RE and 6/36 LE) over 4 days, which was associated with pain on eye movements. At her initial examination the optic nerve appearance was documented as normal in both eyes. These photographs were taken 4 months later when her vision was 6/6 RE and 6/9 LE. What is the most likely diagnosis? (see Fig. 2.3a)*

A: The right optic disc is normal and there is marked pallor of the left optic disc. The most common cause of this clinical picture and fundal appearance in a 22-year-old female is demyelinating optic neuritis. This may present in one of two forms:

(1) Retrobulbar optic neuritis – as in the case above, the optic disc appears normal at presentation. In the absence of disc changes the diagnosis is made on the pattern of the visual loss. Although the history of rapid visual loss is typical of demyelinating disease, craniopharyngiomas and pituitary tumours may occasionally cause fairly rapid visual loss, usually without any subsequent visual recovery. A potential pitfall that may occur if these patients are not reviewed by an ophthalmologist is that other causes of visual loss such as central serous retinopathy (CSR) may be missed and an erroneous diagnosis of retrobulbar neuritis made.

(2) Bulbar optic neuritis – disc swelling is seen at the time of presentation, although the natural history of visual loss is the same as that seen with retrobulbar optic neuritis. Again these patients should be reviewed by an ophthalmologist as unilateral disc swelling may also be a feature of intermediate uveitis and a careful inspection of the fundus looking for periphlebitis, vitreous inflammation and snowbank opacities is mandatory in these patients.

Note, periphlebitis may be a feature of bulbar optic neuritis and there is an increased incidence of future demyelinating disease in patients with intermediate uveitis.

Q: *What is the most useful clinical sign when assessing patients with suspected unilateral optic nerve dysfunction?*

A: Most patients with optic neuritis will have some degree of impaired visual acuity with or without a colour vision or a visual field defect. Many patients will also describe a subjective

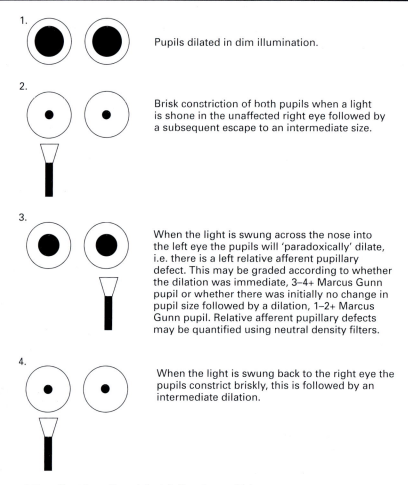

1. Pupils dilated in dim illumination.

2. Brisk constriction of both pupils when a light is shone in the unaffected right eye followed by a subsequent escape to an intermediate size.

3. When the light is swung across the nose into the left eye the pupils will 'paradoxically' dilate, i.e. there is a left relative afferent pupillary defect. This may be graded according to whether the dilation was immediate, 3–4+ Marcus Gunn pupil or whether there was initially no change in pupil size followed by a dilation, 1–2+ Marcus Gunn pupil. Relative afferent pupillary defects may be quantified using neutral density filters.

4. When the light is swung back to the right eye the pupils constrict briskly, this is followed by an intermediate dilation.

Fig. 2.3b Testing for a relative afferent pupillary defect (left optic neuritis).

difference in the brightness of a stimulus between the affected and unaffected eye. As mentioned above, there may or may not be optic nerve head swelling, depending on whether the demyelination is retrobulbar or not.

However, the sine qua non is a relative afferent pupillary defect (RAPD; first described by Marcus Gunn in 1904) which may be detected with the swinging flash light test (Fig. 2.3b).

Some neurology textbooks describe a trace Marcus Gunn pupil in which there is an initial constriction followed by an escape to a larger intermediate size than when the light is swung back to the normal eye. However, this is a particular subtle observation that is subject to considerable inter-observer variability and its clinical significance is also a matter of some debate.

The test is a relative assessment of the anterior afferent visual pathways and is simply a comparison of the direct and consensual light reflexes. Lesions posterior to the anterior optic tract will not produce a RAPD nor will opacities of the ocular media. (Certain cataracts may produce scattering of incident light causing stimulation of a larger retinal area than in the contralateral eye. This may occasionally result in a contralateral 'paradoxical RAPD'.) This test is equally effective if there is only one functioning pupil (e.g. if one pupil has been pharmacologically dilated).

Q: *In cases of suspected retrobulbar optic neuritis what features of the patient's history may point to demyelination being the underlying pathology?*

A: As well as a characteristic pattern of visual loss, the presence of any of the following is suggestive of demyelinating disease:

(1) A history suggestive of a Uhtoff's phenomenon (neurological symptoms exacerbated by temperature rises, e.g. when having a hot bath).
(2) A previous history of self-resolving visual loss.
(3) Other neurological symptoms past or present:
    (a) Limb parasthesia and/or weakness.
    (b) Cerebellar symptoms such as ataxia.
    (c) Urinary frequency and/or incontinence.
    (d) Electric-shock-like sensation radiating down the trunk and limbs produced by neck flexion (Lhermitte's phenomenon).
(4) A family history of similar visual loss.

Q: *What is the role of corticosteroid therapy in the management of optic neuritis?*

A: The Optic Neuritis Treatment Trial (ONTT) commenced in 1988 and recruited over 450 patients with a first episode of optic neuritis who were then randomised into three groups:

(1) Intravenous methylprednisolone 500 mg q.d.s. for 3 days followed by prednisolone 1 mg/kg for 11 days.
(2) Oral prednisolone 1 mg/kg for 14 days.
(3) Placebo.

Initial reports showed a more rapid visual recovery in the first two groups; however, after 12 months there was no significant difference in visual outcome between all three groups. More importantly the patients who received oral prednisolone alone appeared to have a higher incidence of recurrent optic neuritis. The relative risk for oral prednisolone versus placebo was 1.79. The investigators concluded that oral corticosteroids alone (in the dose range used in the trial) should not be used in the treatment of optic neuritis. The most recent data from the ONTT has thrown up another surprising result; of those patients who received intravenous and oral therapy only 7% went on to develop further episodes of demyelination over a 2-year period, as opposed to 14 and 16% in the oral and placebo groups, respectively. Combination therapy was thought to be especially beneficial in those patients who had three or more plaques of demyelination evident on MRI of the brain and were thus deemed as being at high risk for developing future demyelinating episodes.

Despite these results there is ongoing debate as to which patients with optic neuritis should be treated with intravenous methylprednisolone. However, most clinicians would agree that patients incapacitated by severe visual loss (<6/60) or those with poor vision in the fellow eye would benefit from an expedited visual recovery.

Q: *What is the role of CSF analysis and MRI in cases of clinically isolated optic neuritis?*

A: Isolated optic neuritis may represent a 'forme fruste' of multiple sclerosis (MS). CSF changes in optic neuritis are similar to those in MS, with elevations in IgG and oligoclonal banding being reported in between 24 and 55% of optic neuritis patients. Similarly, MRI scans of the brain show evidence of more widespread demyelination in 60% of optic neuritis cases. However, CSF and MRI abnormalities do not necessarily predict whether the patient will develop subsequent demyelinating episodes.

If the clinical course is typical for optic neuritis there is no need for further investigation. If there is a suggestion of collagen vascular disorders the following investigations may be considered:

(1) Antinuclear antibody titres.
(2) Erythrocyte sedimentation rate (ESR) and/or C-reactive protein (CRP). CSF analysis and MRI scanning are only indicated if the course becomes atypical (progressive visual loss >10 days or persistent pain) or if the

patient requests that all investigations that might further define a diagnosis of MS be performed.

Q: *What is the visual prognosis? What percentage of these patients will go on to develop MS?*

A: The visual prognosis following an episode of optic neuritis is good. The visual acuity in the affected eye at 5 years, reported in the ONTT was as follows:

>20/25 or better	87%
20/25–20/40	7%
20/50–20/190	3%
<20/200	3%

These results did not significantly differ by treatment group.

Despite good Snellen visual acuities, defects in colour perception, brightness and contrast sensitivity and stereopsis often persist, as does the RAPD. A recurrence of optic neuritis in either eye occurred in 28% of patients, but was more common in patients with MS.

The ONTT reported that the 5-year cumulative probability of clinically definite MS after an episode of optic neuritis was 30% and this probability did not differ by treatment group. In those patients with a normal MRI at presentation 16% developed MS at 5 years. In those patients with three or more lesions on MRI the risk rose to 51%. Lack of pain, the presence of disc swelling and mild visual loss were features of the optic neuritis that were associated with a low risk of MS, in patients with a normal MRI. Previous clinical trials, with longer follow-up, have shown that as many as 60% of patients with optic neuritis will at some point have a second demyelinating episode, i.e. will develop MS. Demyelinating optic neuritis occurs in 100% of patients with long-standing MS, although only 55% will present with symptomatic visual impairment.

Recommended reading

Beck, R. W., Cleary, P. A., Anderson, M. M., Jr, Keltner, J. L., Shults, W. T., Kaufman, D. I, *et al.* (1992) A randomised, controlled trial of corticosteroids in the treatment of acute optic neuritis. The Optic Neuritis Study Group. *N. Engl. J. Med.*, **326**, 581–588.

Beck, R. W., Cleary, P. A., Trope, J. D., Kaufman, D. I., Kuppersmith, M. J., Paty, D. W., *et al.* (1993) The effect of corticosteroids for acute optic neuritis on the subsequent development of multiple sclerosis. The Optic Neuritis Study Group. *N. Engl. J. Med.*, **329**, 1764–1769.

Rizzo, J. F. and Lessel, S. (1988) Risk of developing multiple sclerosis after uncomplicated optic neuritis: a long-term prospective study. *Neurology*, **38**, 185–190.

The Optic Neuritis Study Group (1997) Visual function 5 years after optic neuritis: experience of the Optic Neuritis Treatment Trial. *Arch. Ophthalmol.*, **115**, 1545–1552.

The Optic Neuritis Study Group (1997) The 5-year risk of MS after optic neuritis: experience of the Optic Neuritis Treatment Trial. *Neurology*, **49**, 1404–1413.

2.4

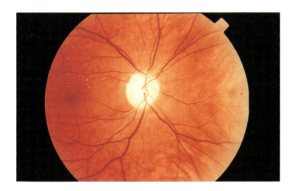

Fig. 2.4a

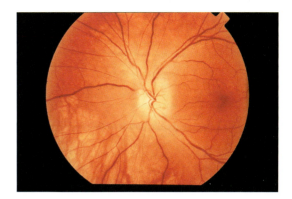

Q: *Describe the discs of this 53-year-old man. What is the differential diagnosis? (see Fig. 2.4a)*

A: There is optic atrophy of the right disc with no evidence of glaucomatous cupping. The left disc is swollen superiorly with obscuration of the disc vessels. The discs are also rather small. The differential diagnosis should include the following:

(1) Acute AION in the left eye and optic atrophy in the right secondary to a previous AION. In this age group this is likely to be a non-arteritic optic neuropathy.
(2) Acute demyelinating optic neuritis in the left eye and disc pallor in the right eye secondary to previous retrobulbar or bulbar optic neuritis. This usually occurs in younger patients.
(3) Frontal lobe mass causing optic atrophy secondary to compression of one optic nerve and disc swelling in the other secondary to raised ICP, i.e. the Foster-Kennedy syndrome. Although this syndrome is much beloved of examiners it is extremely uncommon in clinical practice.

(4) Compressive lesions – sphenoidal ridge meningiomas are more common in women, and will only cause disc swelling if there is intraorbital spread. The disc swelling may then be associated with opto-ciliary shunt vessels. Thyroid eye disease could in theory produce these disc appearances with asymmetrical orbital involvement.
(5) Infiltrative lesions – haematological malignancies, metastatic carcinoma, sarcoidosis and tuberculosis may all cause disc swelling which may result in optic atrophy.

This case of pseudo-Foster–Kennedy syndrome was secondary to bilateral non-arteritic AION.

Q: *How does the pattern of visual loss differ between non-arteritic AION, demyelinating optic neuritis and compressive optic neuropathy?*

A: Figure 2.4b illustrates the natural history of visual loss in these optic neuritides.

(1) Non-arteritic AION:
 (a) Sudden painless visual loss which may vary from mild to severe, one-third of

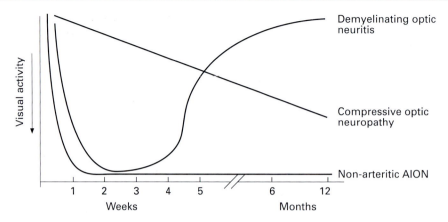

Fig. 2.4b

cases will have no significant drop in acuity (VA 6/6).

  (b) Field defects are often altitudinal or arcuate and correspond to the disc swelling which is usually sectorial (the superonasal sector is most commonly involved). Both the visual acuity loss and the visual field deterioration tend to be permanent and non-progressive.

  (c) Some visual improvement will occur in approximately 10% of cases.

(2) Demyelinating optic neuritis:

  (a) Visual loss is variable (visual acuities may range from 6/6 to no light perception), occurs over 1–5 days and may be associated with pain on eye movements.

  (b) Central scotomas are common but any form of field loss is possible. The ONTT reported that two-thirds of fellow eyes had asymptomatic field defects and that 13% of patients had chiasmal or retrochiasmal field defects at some point during the first year of follow-up.

  (c) Visual acuity typically begins to improve after 2–3 weeks with visual acuity and fields returning to normal in the majority of patients by 1 year.

(3) Compressive optic neuropathy:

  (a) Slowly progressive and initially asymptomatic visual loss is the rule. Sudden visual loss may follow haemorrhage within the compressive lesion.

  (b) Central scotomas are typical with contralateral superotemporal field loss heralding anterior chiasmal involvement.

Q: *What medical conditions are associated with non-arteritic AION? How should AION be treated?*

A: The aetiology of non-arteritic AION remains unclear. With the exception of diabetes no systemic disorders are firmly associated with non-arteritic AION. In fact the prevalence of systemic disorders known to predispose patients to vaso-occlusion appears to be lower among patients with non-arteritic AION than in patients with cerebrovascular and ischaemic heart disease. The few histopathological studies of non-arteritic AION have also failed to show significant atherosclerotic changes in the optic nerve head vessels. Likewise, non-arteritic AION is not particularly associated with disorders that predispose to embolisation of the cranial circulation. Many studies have tried to find an association between non-arteritic AION and abnormalities of the coagulation cascades or other haematological disorders; to date, none has been proven. The best documented anatomical correlation is with small cup:disc ratios and small disc cross-sectional areas. Events such as an episode of systemic hypotension (e.g. gastrointestinal haemorrhage), cardiac

surgery and cataract surgery have all been identified with AION. In the latter case the development of AION is not thought to be linked
with local anaesthesia, intraoperative complications or a postoperative rise in intraocular
pressure.

No treatment has proven to be efficacious in
established non-arteritic AION. Some series
have shown a marginal short-term protective
effect of aspirin in reducing the risk of non-
arteritic AION in the fellow eye, but by 5
years this effect is negligible. Patients should
be warned that there is a 15–25% risk of
fellow eye involvement. The recent vogue for
optic nerve sheath fenestration has been short
lived following the curtailment of a large randomised trial because of unfavourable visual outcomes in those patients who had undergone
surgery.

Recommended reading

Boghen, D. R. and Glaser, J. S. (1975) Ischaemic
optic neuropathy. The clinical profile and natural
history. *Brain*, **98**, 689–708.

Beck, R. W., Hayreh, S. S., Podhajsky, P. A., Tan, E.
S. and Moke, P. S. (1997) Aspirin therapy in non-
arteritic anterior ischaemic optic neuropathy. *Am.
J. Ophthalmol.*, **123**, 212–217.

Lessell, S. (1999) Non-arteritic anterior ischaemic
optic neuropathy: enigma variations [Editorial].
Arch. Ophthalmol., **117**, 386–388.

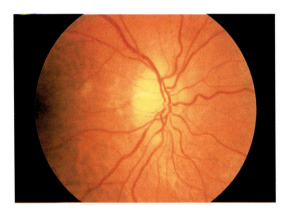 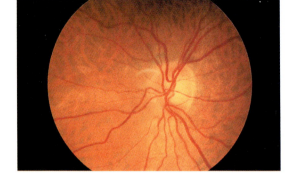

Fig. 2.5a

Q: *This 75-year-old man presented with a sudden unilateral loss of vision in his right eye associated with an occipital headache, general malaise and weight loss. What is the most likely diagnosis? What would be your initial management? (see Fig. 2.5a)*

A: The finding of pallid swelling of the optic disc associated with sudden and profound visual loss in an elderly patient is secondary to arteritic AION until proven otherwise. Giant cell arteritis (GCA) may present with sudden visual loss and no other prodromal visual or systemic symptoms; however, characteristic prodromal symptoms include:

(1) Headache, which is typically temporal and is associated with scalp tenderness, is present in 80% of cases and is the initial symptom in 25% of cases. Occipital headaches are also common. Particular attention should be paid to any new headaches or a change in the pattern of an old headache. Jaw claudication is another characteristic and relatively specific feature of GCA.
(2) Polymyalgia rheumatica, which almost exclusively affects patients >55 years is a prodromal finding in up to 40% of cases.

(3) Weight loss, depression and fatigue may predate the onset of focal symptoms by several months, and are the presenting complaints in 40–50% of cases.

If untreated, bilateral ocular involvement will occur in 35–65% of cases.

The history described above is highly suggestive of GCA and therefore immediate steroid therapy is indicated irrespective of the ESR result. The patient should be admitted and an intravenous 1 g intravenous infusion of methylprednisolone given followed by a 5–7 day course of high-dose oral prednisolone (1 mg/kg). A confirmatory temporal artery biopsy should ideally be performed within 48 h of commencing steroid therapy.

Q: *What is the significance of the ESR in cases of suspected GCA? What factors other than GCA will influence the ESR?*

A: The ESR in healthy individuals is known to increase with age and is slightly higher in females than in males of a similar age. There have been several attempts to define what is the upper limit for a normal ESR. Miller in a study of 27 000 healthy individuals devised a formula for calculating this according to the age and sex of the patient:

- Males = age in years/2
- Females = (age in years +10)/2

The ESR will be influenced by a number of systemic and haematological factors.

An elevated ESR may be caused by the following:

(1) Rouleaux formation by red blood cells.
(2) Elevated plasma fibrinogen, immunoglobulins, plasma proteins or lipids.
(3) Inflammatory disease, malignancy, infection and connective tissue disease.
(4) Pregnancy.

An artificially low ESR may be caused by:

(1) Microcytic hypochromic anaemia.
(2) Polycythaemia.
(3) Low serum fibrinogen.
(4) Congestive cardiac failure.

Physicians should be aware that 15–20% of patients with GCA will not have an elevated ESR. The diagnosis of GCA should be a clinical one that may be supported by an elevated ESR, but should not be refuted solely because of a 'normal' ESR. Conversely, an alternative diagnosis such as a urinary tract or chest infection, or metastatic, primary or haematological malignancy should be considered in the elderly patient with no symptoms suggestive of GCA, who happens to have an elevated ESR.

Q: *What is the role of the CRP in the management of patients with suspected and proven GCA?*

A: The ESR and the CRP are both measures of the acute phase response, and like the ESR, the CRP will be elevated in the presence of tissue necrosis, inflammation, infection, malignancy and rheumatic disease. Unlike the ESR, the CRP is not influenced by the age or sex of the individual, and will rise and fall rapidly (within 4–6 h) in response to fluctuations in inflammatory stimuli. Recent studies have shown that a CRP of >5 mg/l is a more sensitive and specific test for GCA than an elevated ESR alone. The

specificity of diagnosis was improved further when an elevated ESR and CRP were the criteria used. As changes in the CRP level mirror fluctuations in the inflammatory state more closely than does the ESR, it is the more useful investigation for monitoring the activity of GCA and its response to treatment.

Q: *What is the role of temporal artery biopsy in the management of GCA? What would be the significance of a negative biopsy in the above case?*

A: The role of temporal artery biopsy in the management of suspected GCA is a controversial topic.

The following case scenarios illustrate some of the potential dilemmas:

(1) Is a biopsy needed if there is a clear-cut history of GCA with an elevated ESR?
(2) A positive biopsy will confirm the clinical diagnosis but will a negative biopsy mean that steroid therapy can be withdrawn? In the latter case the biopsy should be repeated on the contralateral side as 'skip areas' of entirely normal artery may have been biopsied.
(3) In patients with a history strongly suggestive of GCA and an equivocal ESR a positive biopsy may help maintain the physician's enthusiasm for long-term treatment with a debilitating drug. However, the dilemma whether to treat remains if the biopsy is negative.
(4) In the elderly patient who presents with vague symptoms and an elevated ESR in whom a diagnosis of GCA is deemed possible but unlikely, a negative biopsy may enable the physician to withhold steroid therapy with confidence.
(5) What exactly constitutes a positive biopsy is also a subject of debate; the American College of Rheumatology defined a positive biopsy as one that showed necrotising arteritis characterised by a predominance of mononuclear cell infiltrates or a granulomatous process with multinucleate giant cells. Traditional teaching states that a

temporal artery biopsy should be performed within 48 h of commencing corticosteroid therapy. A study of over 500 consecutive temporal artery biopsies (performed at the Mayo clinic) concluded that the biopsy positivity rate was unrelated to previous corticosteroid therapy. They also found evidence of arteritis in biopsy specimens after more than 14 days of corticosteroid therapy.

Finally, when requesting a temporal artery biopsy, physicians should be aware that this is not a risk-free procedure as complications such as scalp necrosis although rare, are well described.

Q: *How would you manage a case of biopsy proven GCA if there was no ocular involvement?*

A: There has recently been a trend in the rheumatological literature to recommend treatment of such cases with low dose prednisolone, i.e. 20–40 mg/day, and to reserve higher dosages for those who develop visual symptoms. The rationale behind such an approach is flawed on two counts. Firstly, this regime is based on two small series (<35 patients) in which two patients developed an AION on the low-dose treatment. Secondly, it is impossible to predict which patients with GCA will go on to develop ocular symptoms and, although prodromal ocular symptoms may occur, the most common presenting symptom is profound irreversible visual loss.

Ophthalmologists are aware of the potentially debilitating effects of high-dose corticosteroids in elderly patients, but most would recommend that visually asymptomatic patients with GCA be treated initially with at least 1 mg/kg prednisolone. This can then be rapidly tapered to lower maintenance levels. Treatment is usually required for 18 months or more and

should be titrated against the patient's symptoms and the ESR/CRP.

Q: *What are the other ocular presentations of GCA?*

A: Ocular presentations of GCA include the following:

(1) Sudden visual loss:
   (a) AION in 90% of cases.
   (b) Central or branch retinal artery occlusions 10% of cases. The finding of a central retinal arterial occlusion and a contralateral AION is thought to be pathognomonic of GCA.
   (c) Anterior or global ocular ischaemic syndromes are rarer causes of visual loss.
   (d) Hemianopic or other patterns of visual field loss.
   (e) Focal neurological deficits will develop in 25–30% of untreated cases.
(2) Diplopia. Between 10 and 15% of patients will develop diplopia, this may be secondary to a microvascular cranial neuropathy or to muscular ischaemia. Cranial nerve palsies secondary to GCA characteristically resolve within 2–3 weeks, whereas other microvascular palsies usually take 2–3 months to resolve.

Recommended reading

Hayreh, S. S. (1990) Anterior ischaemic optic neuropathy: differentiation of arteritic from non-arteritic type and management. *Eye*, **4**, 25–41.

Hayreh, S. S., Podhajsky, P. A., Raman, R. and Zimmerman, B. (1997) Giant Cell Arteritis: validity and reliability of various diagnostic criteria. *Am. J. Ophthalmol.*, **123**, 285–296.

Hayreh, S. S, Podhajsky, P. A. and Zimmerman, B. (1998) Ocular manifestations of giant cell arteritis. *Am. J. Ophthalmol.*, **126**, 742–744.

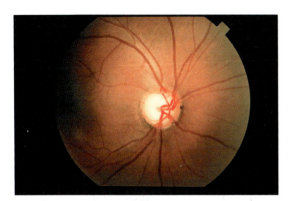

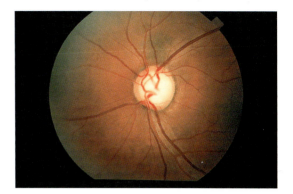

Fig. 2.6a

Q: *This 75-year-old man presented to his physician with a 3-month history of exertional dyspnoea. He had no past medical history of note and was a non-smoker. Describe his optic discs. What is the relevance of these disc changes in this clinical setting? (see Fig. 2.6a)*

A: There is bilateral disc cupping with a cup: disc ratio of 0.8 in both eyes. The neuroretinal rim which is pink is thinned temporally in both eyes and is notched inferiorly in the right disc. There is nasal displacement of the vessels. These appearances are consistent with the diagnosis of glaucomatous optic neuropathy.

The incidence of primary open-angle glaucoma increases with age; 0.5 – 1.0% of the population aged >40 in the US have this form of glaucoma and this increases to between 3.5 and 7.5% in the >80 age group. In fact the single most important risk factor for the development of primary open-angle glaucoma is increasing age. The first-line medical treatment for open-angle glaucoma is a topical non-selective β-blocker, usually in the form of timolol or levobunolol.

A large epidemiological study of a predominantly white, inner-city population in the north of England found a 37% prevalence of airways obstruction in the >65 year olds; of these 86%

had lability of respiratory function suggesting that a deterioration could be expected with β-blocker therapy.

Spirometric investigations have been performed on elderly patients with glaucoma but no history of airways disease.

More than a quarter of the patients in this study were found to have undiagnosed obstructive airways disease. Patients may have been using topical β-blockers for many years before developing serious respiratory side effects, which are often precipitated by a respiratory tract infection. Ophthalmologists and physicians involved with the care of the elderly should therefore be mindful of the use of topical β-blockers by elderly patients even if there is no apparent history of obstructive airways disease. They should also be aware of studies which have shown that <10% of such patients admit to adverse drug effects in response to a general question, athough this increases to 30% when they are asked specific questions about common side effects.

Q: *What measures can be taken by ophthalmologists to minimise the respiratory side effects of topical β-blockers?*

A: The following steps will minimise the risk of respiratory complications in elderly patients:

(1) Take a careful respiratory history before commencing treatment with a topical β-blocker. A positive history of airways disease is an absolute contraindication to the use of non-selective β-blockers. Ophthalmologists should also be aware that the term 'selective' β-blocker is not entirely accurate. Preparations such as betaxolol are in fact 'relatively selective' β-blockers and significant dose-related β₂-blocking activity has been associated with respiratory compromise.

(2) If there is any suggestion of respiratory compromise prior to treatment, or after direct questioning on subsequent visits, spirometric evaluation including peak flow and FEV_1/FVC ratios should be performed. If obstructive airway disease is confirmed β-blocker therapy should not be commenced or it should be discontinued. Changing to a relatively selective agent is not recommended as <25% of patients will show a significant improvement in respiratory function.

(3) All patients should be instructed in the technique of digital lacrimal sac occlusion in order to minimise the passage of topical medications into the nasal cavity, so reducing systemic absorption via the nasal mucosa.

Q: *What are the other systemic side effects of topical β-blockers?*

A: Topical β-blockers which are systemically absorbed via the nasal mucosa are not subject to first pass liver clearance and may be responsible for the following side effects:

(1) Cardiovascular:

(a) Bradycardias other arryhthmias and syncope. Topical β-blockers have been implicated as the greatest single risk factor for falls in the elderly glaucoma patient.
(b) Congestive cardiac failure.
(c) Some ocular β-blockers may have a negative effect on serum lipid profiles.

(2) Depression is more common in glaucoma than other chronic ocular conditions and this may in part be related to β-blocker therapy.

(3) Impotence.

(4) Polypharmacy – serious drug interactions may be overlooked, such as augmentation of cardiac depressant drugs.

Q: *Aside from glaucoma what other conditions may cause optic disc cupping?*

A: Arteritic AION (GCA) may eventually cause disc cupping; other optic neuritides characteristically produce optic atrophy without cupping. In glaucoma the neuroretinal rim remains pink until very late in the disease although the cup may be pale. In optic atrophy both the cup and the neuroretinal rim are pale.

Recommended reading

Diggory, P., Cassels-Brown, A., Vail, A., Abbey, L. M. and Hillman, J. S. (1995) Avoiding unsuspected side-effects of topical timolol with cardio-selective or sympathomimetic agents. *Lancet*, **345**, 1604–1606.

O'Donoghue, E. (1995) β-blockers and the elderly with glaucoma: are we adding insult to injury? [Commentary]. *Br. J. Ophthalmol.*, **79**, 794–796.

Ocular motility and lid disorders

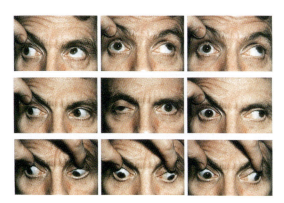

Fig. 3.1a

Q: *Describe the ocular motility signs. What is the diagnosis? (see Fig. 3.1a)*

A: In the primary position the right eyelid is ptotic and there is a manifest divergent squint. The right eye does not adduct past the midline, there is marked reduction of elevation and depression, but abduction appears full. Both pupils are of equal size, i.e. there is no aniso-coria. This is the appearance of a pupil sparing right IIIrd nerve palsy.

Q: *What associated findings would be of interest when examining a patient with a IIIrd nerve palsy?*

A: A IIIrd nerve palsy may be caused by a lesion anywhere between the brainstem and the orbit. However, the most common aetiology is a microvascular one that results in an isolated palsy with no other associated signs. Despite this, an examination should include the following:

(1) The most crucial associated finding will be whether there is pupillary involvement. An efferent pupillary defect, which manifests as a fixed dilated pupil, is highly suggestive of a compressive aetiology, e.g. a posterior communicating artery aneurysm or an intracranial space-occupying lesion. Clinicians should be aware that pupillary involvement is not pathognomonic of compressive lesions (present in 95%) as up to 20% of microvascular palsies will have an associated efferent pupillary defect.

(2) Is there evidence of papilloedema that may point to an intracranial event?

(3) Is there involvement of other cranial nerves? If the IVth and VIth cranial nerves are involved (with or without internal ophthalmoplegia), this may indicate a cavernous sinus or an orbital apex syndrome. In both of these scenarios there may be associated proptosis and venous congestion.

(4) Are there any pyramidal or cerebellar signs? Brainstem pathology such as ischaemic or demyelinating episodes may produce a IIIrd nerve palsy in conjunction with a contralateral hemiparesis (Weber's syndrome), with ipsilateral cerebellar signs (Nothnagel's syndrome) or with contralateral hemitremor (Benedikt's syndrome).

(5) The blood pressure should always be measured and the urine checked for glucose.

(6) Temporal tenderness or other signs suggestive of giant cell arteritis.

The most common causes of an acquired IIIrd nerve palsy are ischaemia (20%), aneurysm (14–30%), trauma (8–16%) and neoplasia (4–15%). Up to one-quarter of all cases will be of undetermined aetiology.

Q: *If this patient was a 70-year-old hypertensive who appeared to have an isolated IIIrd nerve palsy what investigations would be appropriate? What follow-up arrangements should be made?*

A: Work-up for a presumed microvascular IIIrd (IVth or VIth) nerve palsy should include:

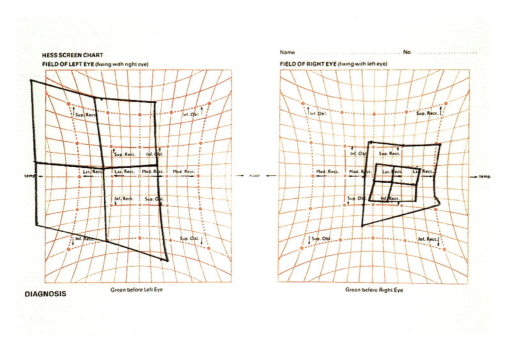

Fig. 3.1b

(1) Full blood count.
(2) Erythrocyte sedimentation rate.
(3) Blood glucose.
(4) VDRL (Venereal Disease Research Laboratories) test and Fluorescent Treponemal Antibody Absorption (FTA-ABS) tests.
(5) Antinuclear antibodies to exclude a systemic vasculitis should be considered in younger patients with no microvascular risk factors.
(6) Hess chart (with or without field of binocular single vision) and full orthoptic assessment to document extent of ocular motility deficit. Figure 3.1b illustrates this patient's Hess chart.

The majority of patients with microvascular cranial nerve palsies show signs of improvement within 1 month and may have a complete recovery by 3 months.

During this recovery period troublesome diplopia (in cases without a pupil covering ptosis) may be improved by fitting fresnel prisms to spectacles (although this rarely elim-

inates the diplopia) or fogging of one spectacle lens. Recovery should be monitored with serial orthoptic and Hess chart examinations.

If there are no signs of recovery after 3 months, if there is progression of the palsy or if additional signs develop, neuroimaging including cranial CT or MRI and MRA or cerebral angiography are recommended.

If the nature of the motility disorder appears to fluctuate, myasthenia gravis should be considered and a tensilon test performed.

Q: *This 10-year-old girl has evidence of a left IIIrd nerve palsy. Describe the physical signs demonstrated by these photographs. What is their relevance regarding the aetiology of this IIIrd nerve palsy? (see Fig. 3.1c)*

A: The left eye appears hypotropic and the lid ptotic in the primary position. Elevation of the left eye is reduced in all positions. Adduction of the left eye is also slightly reduced. The ptosis decreases markedly on right gaze (i.e. on adduction of the left eye). This is an example of a lid-gaze dyskinesis where nerve fibres from the

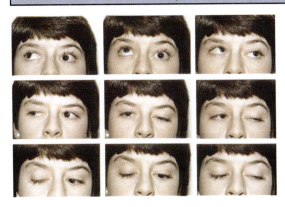

Fig. 3.1c

medial rectus supply some of the innervation to the levator muscle resulting in an inverse Duane's syndrome. Such aberrant regeneration is never seen after a microvascular cranial neuropathy and is indicative of a compressive or traumatic aetiology.

Q: *What other signs of aberrant regeneration may occur following a IIIrd nerve palsy?*

A: Other examples of aberrant regeneration following IIIrd nerve palsies include:

(1) Pseudo-von Graefe's sign – retraction of the lid on attempted downgaze. This is another example of lid-gaze dyskinesis.
(2) Pupil-gaze dyskinesis:
    (a) Pupillary constriction on depression of the eye caused by inferior rectus fibres innervating the pupillary sphincter.
    (b) Pupillary constriction on adduction (or convergence) of the eye secondary to misdirection of fibres from the medial rectus to the pupillary sphincter.

If signs of aberrant regeneration develop in a presumed microvascular palsy neuroimaging is mandatory to rule out a compressive aetiology.

Q: *What is the likely underlying pathology if these signs of aberrant regeneration develop de novo?*

A: Aberrant regeneration is most commonly seen as a secondary phenomenon following an established IIIrd nerve palsy. However, this is not the only clinical presentation. Primary aberrant regeneration may occur without any preceding palsy, in such cases signs of misdirection develop alongside signs of insidious IIIrd nerve paresis. The underlying lesion is invariably an intracavernous meningioma or aneurysm.

3.2

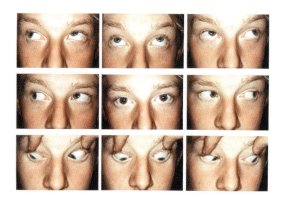

Fig. 3.2a

Q: *Describe these ocular movements. What is the most likely diagnosis? How would you confirm this on examination? (see Fig. 3.2a)*

A: There is a degree of left hypertropia in the primary position, this increases in right gaze and is absent in left gaze. The underacting muscle can be identified by performing the Parks–Bielschowsky three-step test. This test is often the cause of much confusion, some of which may be alleviated by the summary diagram below and Figure 3.6.

Step 1: *Which is the higher eye?* In this case it is the left eye, the underacting muscle may therefore be a depressor of the left eye (inferior rectus or superior oblique), or an elevator of the right eye (superior rectus or inferior oblique). Having narrowed the search to four muscles Step 2 is performed.

Step 2: *Is the vertical deviation greater on left or right gaze?* In this case the hypertropia is greater on right gaze (*contralateral side*), the underacting muscle will therefore be a depressor of the left eye whose action is maximal on adduction (left *superior* oblique) or an elevator of the right eye whose action is greatest on

abduction (right superior rectus). *Remember contralateral side = superior.* In reality superior oblique palsies are much more common than isolated superior rectus palsies; however, the diagnosis should be confirmed by performing Step 3 of the Parks–Bielschowsky test.

Step 3: *The head tilt test. Is the vertical deviation greater on left or right head tilt?* The superior obliques and the superior recti produce incyclotorsion of the globe. In the normal eye there is no vertical deviation of the globe as their opposing vertical actions cancel each other out. The inferior obliques and inferior recti produce excyclotorsion, and again their opposing vertical actions cancel each other out. In the case of a left superior oblique palsy the left hypertropia will be increased by tilting the head to the left. This is because the left superior rectus will be the sole intorter of the eye and its elevating action will not be counteracted by the paretic left superior oblique. *Remember ipsilateral = oblique.* Conversely if the right superior rectus was the paretic muscle the left hypertropia would be increased on right head tilt, as the depression caused by the intorting right superior oblique would not be opposed by the paretic right superior rectus. *Remember contralateral = rectus.*

Q: *What will be the characteristics of the compensatory head posture adopted by this patient? (see Fig. 3.2b)*

A: Patients with incomitant squints frequently adopt a compensatory head posture to place the eyes in position of least deviation and to minimise cyclotropia. The head posture may have

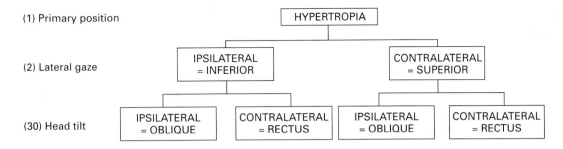

(1) Primary position — HYPERTROPIA

(2) Lateral gaze — IPSILATERAL = INFERIOR / CONTRALATERAL = SUPERIOR

(30) Head tilt — IPSILATERAL = OBLIQUE / CONTRALATERAL = RECTUS / IPSILATERAL = OBLIQUE / CONTRALATERAL = RECTUS

Fig. 3.2b

up to three components: a head tilt, a face turn and chin elevation or depression. The simple way to determine the head posture for a given palsy is that the head is placed into the field of action of the paretic muscle, e.g.:

(1) Left VIth nerve palsy – primary action is abduction of the globe therefore there is a face turn to the left.
(2) Left IVth nerve palsy – the superior oblique has the following actions:
    (a) Depressor of the globe in adduction → chin down with face turn to the right.
    (b) Incyclotorter of the globe → head tilt to the right.

The detection of a compensatory head posture can therefore yield valuable information about the nature of an ocular motility disorder before commencing the ocular motility examination proper.

Q: *What are the common causes of IVth nerve palsies in adults?*

A: Approximately one-third of IVth nerve palsies in adults are decompensated congenital palsies. The common causes of acquired isolated IVth nerve palsies are:

(1) Trauma (40%) – damage to the nerve normally occurs as it exits the dorsal aspect of the brainstem. Bilateral involvement is common. The prognosis is reasonably good with >50% recovering spontaneously within 3–6 months.
(2) Undetermined (30%).

(3) Microvascular (20%).
(4) Neoplasm–aneurysm (10%).

Q: *How would you distinguish between a unilateral and a bilateral IVth nerve palsy?*

A: All IVth nerve palsies should be considered bilateral until proven otherwise. Features that will help differentiate between the two include:

(1) The compensatory head posture of a unilateral palsy is chin depression, with a head tilt and face turn to the contralateral side. In bilateral palsies a chin down head posture is adopted.
(2) There is often a marked 'V' pattern esotropia in bilateral IVth nerve palsies with little deviation in the primary position.
(3) There will be a positive head tilt test to both sides in bilateral palsies.
(4) Greater than 10° of excyclotortion is suggestive of a bilateral IVth nerve palsy. Torsion may be measured on the synoptophore or with double Maddox rods.

The absence of a manifest vertical deviation in the primary position may explain why many cases of bilateral fourth nerve palsies are missed by neurologists, despite the patient's complaints of persistent torsional diplopia.

Q: *How may an acute IVth nerve palsy be differentiated from a decompensated congenital IVth nerve palsy?*

A: Table 3.1 outlines how a decompensated congenital IVth nerve palsy may be distinguished from an acquired palsy.

Table 3.1

	Congenital	Acquired
History	Duration of diplopia is uncertain; diplopia is intermittent and not particularly troublesome	Definite time of onset; diplopia is constant and is troublesome
Head posture	Often a long-standing head posture seen in old photographs which patient is unaware of	Patient is aware of compensatory head posture which is frequently uncomfortable
Comitance	Is usually well established* Primary = Secondary deviation Hess charts – equal-sized fields	Only overaction of the contralateral synergist (inferior rectus) Secondary > primary deviation Hess charts – field of affected eye will be obviously smaller
Fusion amplitude	Vertical fusion range $10^\triangle$; relatively large field of binocular single vision	Normal vertical fusion range of $2–3^\triangle$
Torsion	Extremely rare	Rarely absent

*Comitance develops as a result of the muscle sequelae following paralytic strabismus. These muscle sequelae are governed by Hering's and Sherrington's laws.

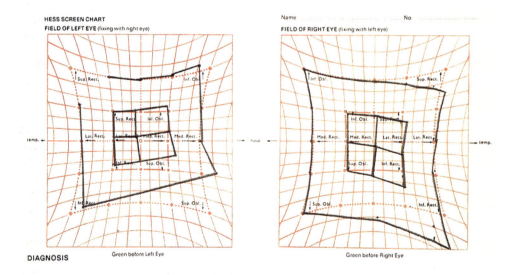

Fig. 3.2c

In the case of a left IVth nerve palsy the muscle sequelae will be as follows:

(1) Overaction of the contralateral synergist – right inferior rectus.
(2) Contracture of the ipsilateral antagonist – left inferior oblique.
(3) Secondary inhibition of the contralateral antagonist – right superior rectus. These muscle sequelae are demonstrated in the Hess chart of the above patient (Fig. 3.2c).

3.3

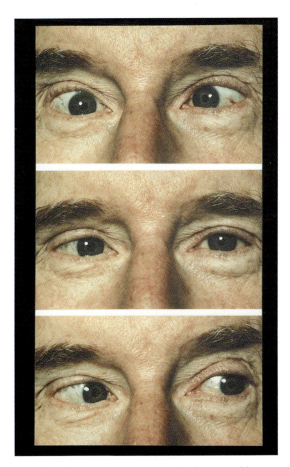

Fig. 3.3a (top) right gaze; (centre) primary position; (bottom) left gaze

Q: *This 60-year-old man presented with a 3-day history of horizontal diplopia. What is the diagnosis? (see Fig. 3.3a)*

A: In the primary position there appears to be a right esotropia, the angle of which increases on attempted right gaze as the right eye fails to abduct. There is no manifest squint visible in left gaze with full adduction of the right eye and full abduction of the left eye. This is an example of a right VIth nerve palsy. The esotropia will be larger when the patient fixates with the paretic eye, i.e. the secondary deviation

is greater than the primary deviation. Another point to note is that the deviation will also be larger when the patient views a distant object, mild VIth nerve palsies may be missed if the examiner only uses a near target when performing a cover test.

Q: *What features help differentiate between a neurological and a restrictive abduction deficit? What conditions may mimic a VIth nerve palsy?*

A: The following features will help differentiate between a neurological and a restrictive abduction deficit:

(1) Saccadic velocities: in neurogenic palsies the saccadic velocity is depressed throughout the field of action of the palsied muscle. A restrictive aetiology is characterised by normal saccadic velocities with a sudden deceleration as the restrictive field is entered.

(2) In neurogenic palsies the range of movement is generally greater on duction testing compared to versions. There is no such difference between ductions and versions in restrictive disease.

(3) If there is marked restriction of the extraocular muscles retraction of the globe may be noted on attempted abduction.

(4) If the intraocular pressure is >8 mmHg higher in abduction than in the primary position this would point to a restrictive aetiology.

(5) Forced duction and force generation testing may help determine the degree of restriction and residual muscular function, respectively.

(6) EMG recordings will also help differentiate between these two aetiologies.

An abduction deficit may also be secondary to:

(1) Thyroid eye disease.

(2) Medial orbital wall fractures.
(3) Duane's syndrome (typical form). In this congenital motility disorder there is reduced abduction, with cocontraction of the medial and lateral recti on attempted adduction causing retraction of the globe (and subsequent narrowing of the palpebral fissure). It is usually a unilateral disorder, which predominantly affects the left eye.
(4) Myasthenia gravis can masquerade as a VIth nerve palsy and should always be suspected if the character of the abduction deficit is variable.
(5) Spasm of the near reflex causing tonic convergence may simulate bilateral VIth nerve palsies, in this condition an apparent inability to abduct the eyes is accompanied by prompt constriction of the pupils with attempted lateral gaze. Saccadic movements elicited with an optokinetic nystagmus (OKN) drum are invariably normal.

Q: *Having determined that this abduction deficit is a neurological one what other features of the ocular and systemic examination may point to the site of the underlying pathology?*

A: The VIth cranial nerve passes from the brainstem through the subarachnoid space, over the apex of the petrous temporal bone before entering the cavernous sinus. It then enters the orbit via the superior orbital fissure before innervating the lateral rectus. Lesions anywhere along this route may result in an abduction deficit, associated physical signs to look for include the following:

(1) Ipsilateral – horizontal conjugate gaze palsy.
    (a) Internuclear ophthalmoplegia.
    (b) Horner's syndrome.
    (c) Vth, VIIth and VIIIth nerve palsies.
(2) Contralateral – hemiparesis.

Any combination of the above points to a brainstem (lower pontine) lesion as the cause of the VIth nerve palsy.

(3) Auricular signs:

(a) Severe otitis media may lead to an extradural abscess of the petrous apex with associated ipsilateral facial pain and facial paralysis (Gradenigo's syndrome).
(b) Haemotympanum and CSF otorrhoea are suggestive of a basal skull fracture.
(c) Decreased hearing in combination with ataxia and Vth nerve paresis is typical of acoustic neuromas.
(4) Papilloedema – a VIth nerve palsy may be a false localising sign of raised intracranial pressure (ICP) or it may arise as a direct result of the lesion that has caused the increased intracranial pressure (ICP), e.g. an acoustic neuroma.
(5) Ipsilateral
    (a) IIIrd nerve palsy.
    (b) IVth nerve palsy.
    (c) Ophthalmic division of Vth nerve palsy.
    (d) Horner's syndrome.
    (e) Optic nerve involvement.
    (f) Proptosis and chemosis.

All of the above are common features of both cavernous sinus and orbital syndromes.

In these conditions there is invariably a constellation of signs, which may make it difficult to distinguish neurological from restrictive palsies.

Q: *What is the role of botulinum toxin in the management of VIth nerve palsies?*

A: Botulinum toxin may be used both in a diagnostic and a therapeutic role in the management of VIth nerve palsies. However, before its use is contemplated in any capacity it is essential that the patient has been fully investigated and that the aetiology of the palsy is known. This is because botulinum toxin can mask the progression of a palsy that has been misdiagnosed as being of microvascular origin.

(1) Diagnostic uses. By paralysing the medial rectus the degree of residual function in the lateral rectus can be assessed. This is important when considering the nature of surgery for unresolved palsies. It is

particularly helpful if forced duction and force generation tests are equivocal.

(2) Therapeutic uses. Peroperative botulinum toxin to the ipsilateral medial rectus allows surgery to be confined to a vertical recti transposition procedure, thus significantly reducing the risk of anterior segment ischaemia. Postoperatively, if successful realignment is achieved, this may be maintained by either repeating this injection or by medial rectus recession, performed 4–6 months after the initial surgery.

In children a large esotropia may persist even after full recovery of lateral rectus function. In some cases botulinum toxin to the medial rectus may obviate the need for esotropia surgery.

There is no evidence that medial rectus botulinum toxin significantly influences the speed or degree of recovery following VIth nerve palsy.

Recommended reading

Fitzsimons, R., Lee, J. and Elston, J. (1989) The role of botulinum toxin in the management of sixth nerve palsy. *Eye*, **3**, 391–400.

3.4

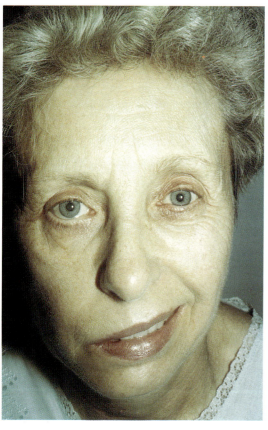
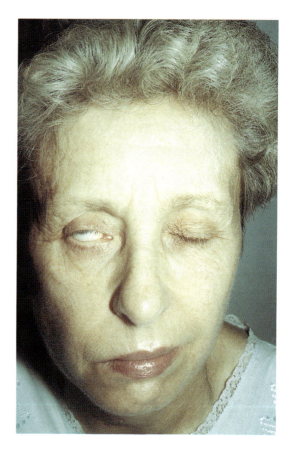

Fig. 3.4a

Q: *What is the diagnosis? What features of the examination may point to the aetiology and sequelae of this condition?*

A: This is a right lower motor neurone VIIth nerve palsy, the brow ptosis is evidence of uni-lateral frontalis involvement. The examination should be tailored to ascertain both the aetiology and the sequelae of the palsy, it should include the following:

(1) Assess the extent of the VIIth nerve weak-ness, especially inadequacy of lid closure

(lagophthalmos). The presence and extent of a Bell's phenomenon (upward deviation of the globe on attempting lid closure) should be noted. The above photographs demonstrate incomplete lid closure and a good Bell's phenomenon, therefore despite incomplete lid closure this eye is not at high risk of developing exposure keratitis. Bilat-eral VIIth nerve involvement is a more ominous sign as approximately 25% of such patients will have a pontine or menin-geal neoplasm. Lyme disease, sarcoidosis and treponemal, mycobacterial or crypto-coccal meningitis are other causes of bilateral facial nerve palsies.

(2) Corneal examination:

  (a) Reduced corneal sensation indicating involvement of the Vth cranial nerve. Corneal sensation is lost early in patients with acoustic neuromas.

  (b) Is there evidence of fluorescein staining over the inferior cornea indicating epithelial loss?

  (c) The tear film should also be assessed as nervus intermedius involvement can reduce the lacrimal secretions.

  (d) Corneal anaesthesia, an abnormal tearfilm, lagophthalmos and a reduced Bell's phenomenon will all contribute to the development of ocular surface disease. Orbicularis weakness will reduce the efficacy of the lacrimal pump and may cause a functional block of nasolacrimal outflow resulting in epiphora. This may be demonstrated by a positive fluorescein dye disappearance test in the presence of a patent nasolacrimal outflow system.

(3) If there is diminished taste over the anterior two-thirds of the tongue this would suggest involvement of the nervus intermedius or the chorda tympani.

(4) Auricular examination. Check for evidence of Herpes zoster involving the post auricular skin, the auditory canal or the palate. If present the VIIth nerve palsy could be due to the Ramsay–Hunt syndrome. An auroscopic examination should also be performed to rule out any middle ear pathology. The VIIIth nerve should be formally examined and any reduced sensitivity or hyperacusis noted. Any scars from previous mastoid or intracranial surgery may also give clues to the aetiology of the palsy.

(5) Ocular motility examination. VIth nerve involvement would suggest pathology in the floor of the fourth ventricle. Demyelination in this region may cause gaze palsies associated with VIIth nerve weakness.

(6) A full neurological examination is indicated especially in younger patients as unilateral facial weakness may be the presenting sign of the Guillain–Barré syndrome (especially the Miller–Fisher variant).

(7) General examination – look for evidence of the ocular and systemic features of Lyme disease or a generalised lymphadenopathy which may indicate HIV infection.

The patient in Fig. 3.3a had a Bell's palsy of recent onset.

Q: *What is the role of corticosteroid therapy in the treatment of Bell's palsy?*

A: In 80% of cases a reversible conduction block interrupts the function of the nerve and a full recovery within 1–2 months is the rule. However, in 20% of cases axonal degeneration occurs which results in some degree of permanent weakness. Bad prognostic signs include a complete palsy, loss of taste, hyperacusis and advanced age. In these cases corticosteroid treatment should be considered. Corticosteroid therapy has been variously reported to be effective or ineffective in reducing the severity and duration of the denervation. If there are no contraindications a short rapidly tapering course of prednisolone (80 mg/day initially decreased over 10 days) should be instigated as soon as possible, ideally within 4 days of the onset of symptoms. The use of acyclovir in combination with corticosteroids has recently been reported as producing a more rapid and complete recovery of facial nerve function compared with corticosteroids alone in patients with Bell's palsy. This raises the possibility that Bell's palsy may be secondary to Herpes simplex infection.

Q: *This 14-year-old boy developed a left facial palsy following surgery for an acoustic neuroma. What other neurological sequelae have arisen as a result of this lesion and its treatment? (see Fig. 3.4b)*

A: The most obvious abnormality is the injected conjunctiva of the left eye, this in combination with a temporal tarsorrhaphy suggests

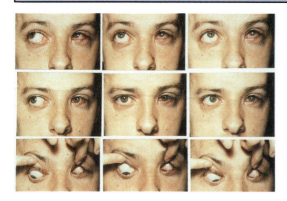

Fig. 3.4b

that there is significant ocular surface disease, caused by an iatrogenic VIIth nerve palsy.

The second feature of note is the presence of a left esotropia (manifest convergent squint) in the primary position. The most likely cause for this is a left lateral rectus palsy – this is confirmed by the inability to abduct the left eye past the midline.

The third point of note is the markedly reduced adduction of the right eye with otherwise normal ocular motility. This finding in combination with a left-sided abduction deficit is indicative of a left horizontal gaze palsy, caused by damage to the ipsilateral pontine paramedian reticular formation.

Isolated pontine gaze palsies do not cause manifest squints and are best demonstrated by examining ipsilateral saccades, which are of reduced amplitude and speed, and do not carry the eyes past the midline.

Q: *What are the manifestations of aberrant regeneration following a facial nerve palsy?*

A:

(1) Facial grimacing with up turning of the mouth on attempted lid closure is a par-
ticularly distressing consequence of aberrant regeneration following facial nerve palsies. Botulinum toxin injections into the affected muscles often provide symptomatic relief. Facial myokymia may be confused with the above condition, it is characterised by intermittent involuntary movements of the facial muscles but is not caused by aberrant regeneration. It is usually a benign and self-limiting condition; however, if symptoms persist for months brainstem glioma, stroke or demyelination should be considered.

(2) 'Crocodile tears' describes the excessive lacrimation stimulated by eating or even the smell of food. There are two explanations for this phenomenon:

(a) Fibres from the nervus intermedius destined for the chorda tympani (and then on to the submandibular and sublingual glands) are redirected into the greater petrosal nerve as it leaves the middle ear. These fibres will eventually supply the lacrimal gland via the pterygopalatine ganglion.

(b) Fibres from Jacobsen's nerve (a branch of the IXth cranial nerve travelling in the middle ear) contribute to both the greater and lesser petrosal nerves. The lesser petrosal nerve carries parasympathetic fibres destined for the parotid gland via the otic ganglion.

The finding of an apparent XIIth nerve palsy ipsilateral to the facial weakness points to previous surgery (usually for an acoustic neuroma). Hypoglossal nerve transposition may be attempted to reinnervate the facial musculature in cases of long-standing facial weakness. Sural nerve grafts have also been used at the time of the primary surgery or as secondary procedures.

3.5

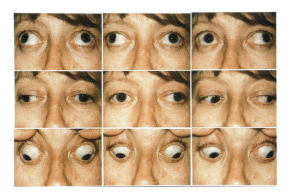

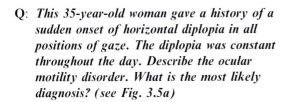

Fig. 3.5a

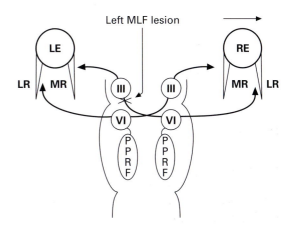

Fig. 3.5b

Q: *This 35-year-old woman gave a history of a sudden onset of horizontal diplopia in all positions of gaze. The diplopia was constant throughout the day. Describe the ocular motility disorder. What is the most likely diagnosis? (see Fig. 3.5a)*

A: There is an exotropia in the primary position. The left eye does not adduct past the midline and adduction of the right eye is significantly reduced. There is full abduction, elevation and depression of both eyes. The most likely diagnosis given the history and these photographs is a bilateral internuclear ophthalmoplegia secondary to demyelination. Although from the above evidence myasthenia gravis cannot be ruled out.

Q: *What other features of the ocular motility examination would confirm this diagnosis?*

A: An internuclear ophthalmoplegia is characterised by an adduction deficit on the ipsilateral side and nystagmus of the contralateral abducting eye. Vertical nystagmus is also a common feature of both unilateral and bilateral internuclear ophthalmoplegias (INOs). Other features to look for are a reduction in the saccadic velocity of the adducting eye causing it to lag behind the abducting fellow eye – this is best demonstrated with an OKN drum. This may enable the examiner to detect a subclinical INO before there is an obvious adduction deficit. All INOs should be considered bilateral until proven otherwise. Convergence should also be assessed as this may be intact in a so-called Cogan's posterior INO. The presence of a pale disc or discs, signifying previous optic neuritis, may also point to a demyelinating aetiology.

Adduction deficits in myasthenia are typically variable and may be associated with other ocular signs such as ptosis. The saccades will initially be of normal velocity and abducting nystagmus may be present.

Q: *What is the anatomical explanation for the motility disturbance seen in this condition?*

A: An INO is caused by a lesion in the medial longitudinal fasciculus (MLF). This structure is responsible for the integration of information between the IIIrd, IVth and VIth cranial nerve nuclei (see Fig. 3.5b). The VIth nerve nucleus is connected to the contralateral medial rectus subnucleus via the MLF and therefore lesions in this region will produce an adduction deficit. The lesion is ipsilateral to the eye with impaired adduction. A number of theories exist to explain the abducting nystagmus, the most popular of which is an altered inhibitory input to the lateral rectus muscle.

Q: *What would be the result if the above lesion extended to involve the ipsilateral paramedian pontine reticular formation (PPRF)?*

A: The result of such a lesion will be a left gaze palsy in addition to reduced adduction of the left eye. In the horizontal plane only the right lateral rectus will be fully functional and it will exhibit abducting nystagmus. This combination of an internuclear ophthalmoplegia and an ipsilateral gaze palsy, caused by a lesion of the MLF that extends caudally to include the PPRF, is known as the one-and-a-half syndrome. In the initial period after such a lesion the contralateral PPRF is unopposed and the eyes will be conjugately deviated away from the lesion (to the right), the INO will, however, prevent the left eye adducting and the right eye is tonically abducted. This transient phenomenon is known as a paralytic pontine exotropia.

Q: *What is the natural history of INOs secondary to demyelination?*

A: INOs secondary to demyelination are usually transient phenomena that resolve over a period of 6–12 weeks. In patients >50 years of age INOs are invariably secondary to a brainstem vascular event; in these patients the ocular motility abnormalities tend to persist.

3.6

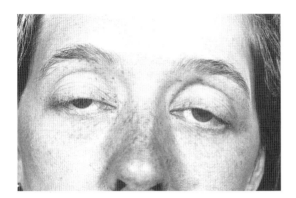

Fig. 3.6a

Q: *Describe the appearance of this 30-year-old woman. What aspects of the history may point to the underlying pathology? (see Fig. 3.6a)*

A: This photograph illustrates bilateral asymmetrical ptoses in a young woman. This finding especially if of recent onset should suggest the possibility of myasthenia gravis. Appropriate questions would include:

(1) Full history of the ptosis, i.e. duration, variability (is it present first thing in the morning, is it worse in the evenings or when tired?), is the asymmetry constant?
(2) Other neurological symptoms suggestive of myasthenia:
   (a) Variable diplopia.
   (b) Dysphagia and/or dysphasia
   (c) Generalised weakness, i.e. difficulty rising from a chair.
   (d) Drug history, e.g. penicillamine use in rheumatoid arthritis.
   (e) General medical history – is there evidence of other autoimmune disease, e.g. thyrotoxicosis or hypothyroidism (dysthyroid ophthalmopathy may mimic ocular myasthenia), rheumatoid arthritis, systemic lupus erythematosus, pernicous anaemia or Sjögren's syndrome.

Q: *If this is a myasthenic ptosis what other characteristic lid signs may be present other than fatiguability?*

A: The classical sign of a myasthenic ptosis is fatiguability. This is best demonstrated on prolonged upward or lateral gaze. Other signs which if present would suggest a myasthenic aetiology include:

(1) Cogan's lid twitch. This refers to the excessive elevation of the ptotic lid when after a period of downgaze the patient is asked to return their gaze quickly to the primary position. Fluttering of the lids may occasionally be observed with lateral gaze.
(2) If the more ptotic eyelid is elevated to the normal position by the examiner the contralateral eye may become more ptotic. This is because the frontalis muscle (whose overaction is trying to compensate for the more ptotic eye) relaxes with this manoeuvre and the contralateral lid, which had been held in a seemingly normal position by this overaction, now becomes ptotic. This phenomenon is often a feature of involutional ptoses.
(3) Always remember to check for orbicularis weakness/fatiguability in all ptotic patients as this may confirm your suspicions of myasthenia. The 'peep' sign is elicited by asking the patient to gently close their eyes, in the myasthenia patient fatiguability of the orbicularis often results in a subtle opening of the lids.

Q: *How would you perform a tensilon test? What are the limitations of this test in the investigation of myasthenia gravis?*

A: There are a number of steps that should be followed to ensure that the tensilon test is a safe and instructive one.

(1) The test must be performed with full resuscitation facilities at hand and with 400 µg of atropine already drawn up in a 1 ml syringe. Asthma and cardiac arrhythmias, e.g. Wolff–Parkinson–White syndrome, are considered relative contra-indications.

(2) The patient should be warned about the short-term gastrointestinal, lacrimal and salivatory side effects of the test.

(3) The physician should also have a definite end point in mind which will signify a positive result:

    (a) An improvement in the degree of ptosis as documented by photographs or videotape.

    (b) An improvement in ocular motility as documented by pre and post test Hess charts. This requires two experienced and speedy orthoptists as the effects of the edrophonium only last for 5 min. Alternatively the ocular motility examination may be videoed.

(4) Having established a secure intravenous access a 2 mg test dose of edrophonium is given followed by a saline flush. A positive effect should occur within 30–45 s. If there is no response after one minute and if there are no adverse side effects, the remaining 8 mg may be given. It should be noted that larger doses are unlikely to produce a significant response if there has been no improvement with the initial 2 mg dose. Injection of a saline placebo as a pretest measure can be used to rule out functional disorders.

The tensilon test is not a fool-proof one, ptosis tends to respond better than ophthalmoplegia and false-negative results may be seen in long-standing myasthenia which is refractory to anticholinesterases. False positive results have been reported in a diverse range of conditions including brainstem tumours, orbital apex syndromes, multiple sclerosis, the Eaton–Lambert syndrome and Guillain–Barré syndrome.

Q: *What percentage of patients will have purely ocular symptoms? Why are the extraocular muscles (EOM) particularly susceptible to myasthenic involvement?*

A: Approximately 90% of all patients with myasthenia will have ocular involvement at some stage during their life. Patients with purely ocular myasthenia account for approximately 15% of myasthenic patients. Unlike general myasthenia, men are more frequently affected, especially after the age of 40. If generalised disease is going to develop it will have done so in 80% of patients within 1 year of presentation and in 94% within 3 years of presentation. Many patients with clinical ocular myasthenia have reduced numbers of acetylcholine receptors and abnormal electromyographic responses in clinically unaffected muscles. The limb muscle end-plates in these patients also show similar ultrastuctural changes to those in patients with generalised myasthenia. Such subclinical generalised disease does not appear to predict which patients will later develop clinically generalised disease.

There are a number of reasons why EOM are more susceptible to myasthenia than other skeletal muscles:

(1) Extremely rapid contraction kinetics and high firing frequencies of twitch EOM may increase susceptibility to fatigue.

(2) There are less prominent secondary synaptic folds in twitch EOM fibres than extremity twitch fibres. This may mean there are fewer acetylcholine receptors on the postsynaptic membrane.

(3) The mean quantal content of twitch EOM is less than half that of extremity muscle.

(4) EOM fibres receive multiple synapses per fibre, a configuration that is more susceptible to fatigue than the single-terminal fibres of other muscles.

Aside from these physiological reasons, one of the most important factors influencing the predominance of ocular involvement is that even minimal dysfunction of an EOM will result in ocular misalignment with resultant diplopia.

Q: *What is the role of anticholinergics and other agents in the treatment of ocular myasthenia?*

A: Pyridostigmine, 60–120 mg orally every 3 h except at night, is the initial treatment of choice. However, the response in ocular myasthenia is often unsatisfactory and complementary treatment with corticosteroids may be beneficial. The initial dose should be small (e.g. 10 mg) and this is increased by increments of 5–10 mg/week until there is a symptomatic improvement or an alternate day regime of up to 1–1.5 mg/kg is reached. This dose can then be tapered to 20–30 mg on alternate days; if this taper is too rapid a relapse may be precipitated. Although most physicians prefer to commence treatment with a low dose of prednisolone, acute exacerbation of myasthenic weakness is rarely seen with doses of <60 mg/day and this may be prevented by pretreatment with intravenous γ-globulin.

Ocular myasthenia may be controlled on long-term, low-dose steroid therapy, i.e. 5–10 mg prednisolone on alternate days. If higher doses are required a second-line immunosuppressive agent such as azathioprine (2–3 mg/kg/day maintenance dose) may be added to enable the steroid dose to be reduced and/or eventually discontinued. The immunosuppressive effects of azathioprine will not be evident for 3–6 months and joint therapy should therefore be continued for this period of time. Thymectomy is rarely beneficial in ocular myasthenia.

Recommended reading

Drachman, D. B. (1994) Myasthenia gravis [Review]. *N. Engl. J. Med.*, **330**, 1797–1810.

Weinberg, D. A., Lesser, R. L. and Vollmer, T. L. (1994) Ocular myasthenia: a protean disorder [Review]. *Surv. Ophthalmol.*, **39**, 169–210.

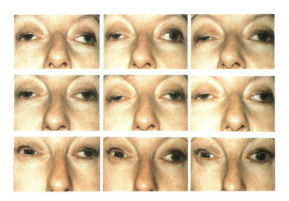

Fig. 3.7a

Q: *This 42-year-old woman gave a 10-year history of slowly progressive bilateral ptoses. What is the differential diagnosis? (see Fig. 3.7a)*

A: The photograph depicts bilateral and slightly asymmetrical ptosis, associated with a divergent squint and complete external ophthalmoplegia. The differential diagnosis of a ptosis, which is long-standing and slowly progressive, should include the following:

(1) Myotonic dystrophy.
(2) Myasthenia gravis; however, the symmetry of the ptosis and the history of slow progression over 10 years deems this unlikely.
(3) Chronic progressive external ophthalmoplegia (CPEO). The associated ocular motility abnormalities point to this diagnosis in the above case.

Q: *What are the other ocular and systemic features of this condition?*

A: The usual presenting sign of CPEO is a symmetrical ptosis. This is then followed by a slowly progressive restriction of extraocular movements with vertical muscle involvement being followed by that of the horizontal muscles. Diplopia is surprisingly rare considering the often gross restriction of extraocular movement. A pigmentary retinopathy may also be present and if associated with heart block this is known as the Kearns–Sayre syndrome. Diabetes and hypogonadism are also associated with CPEO. Neurological sequelae such as cerebellar disorders causing ataxia are not uncommon.

Q: *What is the inheritance of this condition and what are its characteristics?*

A: CPEO exhibits mitochondrial inheritance, i.e. the gene responsible for its transmission is found in the mitochondrial (mt) DNA. All our mtDNA is maternally inherited because the mitochondria of the sperm are lost after fusion with the egg. An affected mother passes the defect to all her children, but only her daughters will transmit the trait to subsequent generations.

Q: *How can the often considerable variation in phenotype between affected siblings be explained?*

A: Each mitochondrion contains between two and 10 DNA molecules, and there are multiple mitochondria in each cell allowing both normal and mutant DNA to coexist within the same cell. This condition is known as heteroplasmy. The proportion of normal to mutant DNA will fluctuate through the process of replicative segregation. The proportion of mutant mtDNA required to produce a disease phenotype is known as the threshold effect, and varies from organ to organ and person to person. In pedigrees of families with mitochondrial diseases there is often a variable mixture of mutant/normal mtDNA in the offspring, the severity of the disease being related to the proportion of mutant to healthy DNA. This explains why not all children of carrier females are affected.

Q: *What factors cause mutations to arise in the mitochondrial genome? Why is mtDNA more susceptible to these factors than nuclear DNA?*

A: Endogenous factors causing mutations in mtDNA:

(1) DNA polymerase misincorporation – the β and γ DNA polymerases are highly inaccurate, accounting for a substitution of 1/3000–8000 base pairs causing random misincorporations.
(2) Oxidative stress is the term used to describe DNA damage caused by superoxide radicals, hydrogen peroxide and hydroxyl radicals. Not only do mitochondria use 90% of cellular oxygen, but mtDNA is not bound to histones and is therefore more susceptible to damage by these oxidised species.
(3) Deamination causing DNA point mutations.
(4) Depurination which increases the misincorporation of non-complementary nucleotides when the damaged DNA template is copied by DNA polymerases.

Exogenous factors causing mutations in mtDNA:

(1) Alkylating agents – some of these agents have been shown to modify the mtDNA five times more efficiently than nuclear DNA *in vitro*.
(2) Ultraviolet radiation.
(3) Irradiation (X-rays).

The 'DNA repair repertoire' is underdeveloped in comparison with that of nuclear DNA. Although a rudimentary excision repair mechanism capable of preventing mutations does exist the mitochondrial polymerase is unable to proof-read and remove certain modified bases. The mtDNA is devoid of introns and therefore a random mutation is more likely to strike a coding DNA sequence.

All of the above factors contribute to a mtDNA mutation rate 10–17 times higher than that of the nuclear genome.

Q: *What other ophthalmological and neurological conditions exhibit mitochondrial inheritance?*

A:

(1) Leber's hereditory optic neuropathy (LHON) – this condition is characterised by sudden painless visual loss, which may progress over days to weeks. Simultaneous involvement is rare, but the fellow eye is normally affected within 2–3 months.
(2) The visual loss is usually severe with acuities of 6/60 to finger counting, central scotomas and reduced colour vision. The discs are initially swollen, the hyperaemic appearance often preceding the visual loss. The condition typically affects individuals between the ages of 15 and 25 and has a 4:1 male:female ratio. The disease is linked to heritable point mutations in the mtDNA. Four mutations at nucleotide positions 11 778, 3460, 15 257 and 14 484 have primary pathogenetic importance. The probability of visual recovery (seen in <10% of cases) is dependent on the type of primary mtDNA mutation.
(3) The MELAS syndrome – this syndrome consists of **m**itochondrial **e**ncephalomyopathy, **l**actic **a**cidosis and **s**troke-like episodes. In 80% of cases there is a point mutation at nucleotide position 3243 in the $tRNA^{Leu(URR)}$ gene.
(4) Myoclonic epilepsy with ragged-red fibres – myoclonus, seizures, cerebellar ataxia and mitochondrial myopathy are typical features. Myoclonic epilepsy with ragged red fibres has been linked to mutations at nucleotide positions 8344 and 8356 in the $tRNA^{Lys}$ gene.
(5) Neuropathy, ataxia, retinitis pigmentosa and maternally inherited Leigh disease – proximal-muscle weakness, developmental delay and dementia are other features of

this condition that is associated with mutations at position 8993 in the ATPase 6 gene.

Recommended reading

Johns, D. R. (1995) Mitochondrial DNA and disease [Review]. *N. Engl. J. Med.*, **333**, 638–644.

3.8

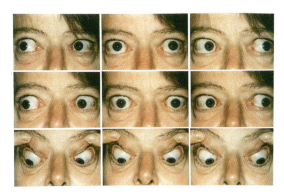

Fig. 3.8a

Q: *Describe the extraocular movements illustrated in these photographs. What is the most likely diagnosis? (see Fig. 3.8a)*

A: There is no manifest deviation in the primay position. There is gross restriction of elevation in both eyes and abduction is also restricted bilaterally. Note also the symmetric upper and lower lid retraction. These findings are characteristic of the restrictive myopathy associated with Graves' disease. The most commonly involved muscles are the inferior recti followed by the medial recti (the superior and lateral recti are rarely significantly involved).

Q: *What is the pathophysiology of extraocular muscle involvement in thyroid eye disease?*

A: The following scheme has been proposed for the chain of events leading to Graves' ophthalmopathy:

(1) Initiation – circulating T cells in patients with Graves' disease directed against an antigen on thyroid follicular cells recognise and cross-react with this antigen on orbital (and pretibial fibroblasts).

(2) Release of inflammatory mediators – as a result of interaction between these CD4 T cells and orbital fibroblasts, cytokines such

as interferon-γ, interleukin (IL)-1α, transforming growth factor (TGF)-β and tumour necrosis factor (TNF) are released into the surrounding tissue.

(3) Propagation – the autoimmune response in orbital connective tissue is perpetuated by these cytokines which induce the expression of immunomodulatory proteins (the 72-kDa heat-shock protein, intercellular adhesion molecules and HLA-DR4) in orbital fibroblasts.

(4) Glycosaminoglycan (GAG) deposition – the cytokines mentioned above and insulin-like growth factor I stimulate GAG production (mainly hyaluronic acid) by fibroblasts and fibroblast proliferation. GAG deposition leads to the passive accumulation of interstitial fluid in the extraocular muscles and orbital fat with a resulting increase in volume and motility dysfunction.

(5) Chronic oedema and inflammation of the orbital tissues may progress to fibrosis of the endomysial connective tissues investing the muscle fibres. Fibrosis begins when a tissue fibroblast is transformed into a myofibroblast. These then secrete a proteoglycan matrix and subsequently infiltrate it with collagen. The transformation of fibroblasts into myofibroblasts is directed by TNF-α and TGF-β secreted by macrophages. The deposition of matrix and collagen is known to be promoted IL-1, TNF-α, TGF-β and platelet-derived growth factor. The muscle cells themselves remain intact but may become atrophic and fibrotic in longstanding disease as a result of chronic compression.

(6) The humoral immune responses associated with thyroid eye disease, e.g. antimuscle and antifibroblast antibodies, are now thought to be a secondary phenomena arising as a result of T cell-mediated

inflammatory responses in the orbit and are not themselves primarily pathogenic.

Q: *What is the role of surgery in the treatment of Graves' restrictive myopathy.*

A: There are a number of guiding principles when dealing with the surgical management of this condition:

(1) No surgical intervention for strabismus should be considered while there is active orbital inflammation.

(2) The signs of ocular motility dysfunction should ideally be stable for at least 6 months (as documented by serial Hess charts, uniocular fields of fixation, fields of binocular single vision and/or cover testing in the nine positions of gaze) before contemplating surgery.

(3) If orbital decompressive surgery is indicated for either compressive optic neuropathy, corneal exposure or for disfiguring proptosis this should be carried out first as the nature of the motility disorder may alter following orbital decompressive surgery (e.g. A-pattern esotropias).

(4) The ophthalmologist should have a sound understanding of what are the indications for and the aims of surgery. These should be discussed fully with the patient pre-operatively. The most common indication for surgery is persistent diplopia in the primary position with a reduced and de-centred field of binocular single vision. The aim of surgery is to improve the size and position of the field of binocular single vision rendering the patient free of diplopia in the primary position. Surgery rarely produces a dramatic improvement in the range of extraocular movement and persistent diplopia in extremes of gaze is the rule rather than the exception.

(5) It is advisable to avoid resecting muscles in patients with thyroid eye disease. Recessions are the procedure of choice, ideally with an adjustable suture technique. In cases of vertical misalignment the surgeon should be careful not to overcorrect with excessive recession of the inferior rectus as this may result in reversal of the vertical diplopia, which is not well tolerated. To avoid this complication the operated eye should ideally be hypotropic after adjustment, although even then late slippage may still occur.

Recommended reading

Bahn, R. S. and Heufelder, A. E. (1993) Pathogenesis of Graves' ophthalmopathy. [Review]. *N. Engl. J. Med.*, **329**, 1468–1475.

3.9

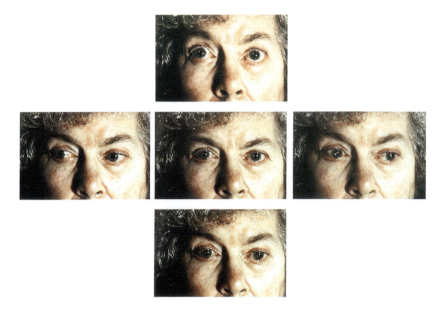

Fig. 3.9

Q: *Describe the ocular motility deficit in this 75-year-old woman. What is the differential diagnosis? (see Fig. 3.9)*

A: There is gross reduction of movement in all positions of gaze with vertical versions being affected more than horizontal versions. There is no evidence of a deviation in the primary position nor of ptosis. The differential diagnosis should include the following:

(1) Thyroid eye disease.
(2) Progressive supranuclear palsy (PSNP).
(3) Myasthenia gravis.
(4) Chronic progressive external ophthalmoplegia.
(5) Ocular fibrosis syndromes.

On examination there was no evidence of fatiguability, restriction of ocular movements, or proptosis. The mask like Parkinsonian facies and these motility signs point to the diagnosis of progressive supranuclear palsy.

Q: *How would you confirm that this is a supranuclear disorder?*

A: In cases of true supranuclear palsy fast eye movements (voluntary saccades) and slow eye movements (pursuits) will be reduced. Vestibular induced slow eye movements which bypass these supranuclear pathways will be unaffected. In the case of PSNP the initial and most severe deficit is one of voluntary downgaze. Doll's head testing is the most practical way of assessing suspected supranuclear vertical gaze palsies. The patient's head is clasped in the examiner's hands and the neck is then extended fully (although this may be limited by underlying rigidity), this will produce a reflex downgaze in patients with PSNP by stimulation of the vestibular system.

Horizontal movements may also be assessed using the doll's head technique or by caloric testing. To test the horizontal eye movements the patient's head should be inclined at 60° to the horizontal, so placing the horizontal semi-circular canal in an upright position. By injecting warm water into the external auditory meatus the endolymph in the canal rises stimulating the end organ (this is equivalent to an ipsilateral headturn). This causes the eyes to deviate slowly to the opposite side followed by a rapid corrective movement to the same side (this corrective movement is not under the influence of the vestibular system). The reverse is true if cold water is used. **C**old **O**pposite **W**arm the **S**ame (**COWS**) is a useful mnemonic which refers to the direction of the corrective fast eye movements.

Q: *What is the most common cause of a PSNP and what are the other clinical features of this condition?*

A: Over 75% of cases of PSNP are due to Steele–Richardson–Olszewski disease (typical PSNP). This condition usually affects patients in their 60s and 70s; initial symptoms include instability and falls, and a gruff dysarthria, which is followed by dysphagia. Frontal lobe deficits are common although the degree of dementia is variable, perseveration with repetition of words and phrases is typical. Axial rigidity and gait problems are features shared with true Parkinsonian patients. However, distal limb akinesia and rigidity are uncommon and classical rest tremor is almost never seen. The median survival for this condition is six to seven years.

Q: *What is the underlying pathology in cases of Steele–Richardson–Olszewski disease?*

A: The characteristic lesions of typical PSNP are cell loss and a high density of neurofibrillary tangles and neuropil threads in the brainstem and basal ganglia (principally the globus pallidus, the subthalamic and dentate nuclei). Atypical PSNP describes variants in which the severity or distribution of the abnormalities differs from the typical pattern. The diagnosis of typical or atypical PSNP is not valid if any of the following pathological features are present:

(1) Large or numerous infarcts.
(2) Marked diffuse or focal atrophy.
(3) Lewy bodies.
(4) Changes indicative of Alzheimer's disease.
(5) Diffuse spongiosis or prion protein-positive amyloid plaques.

In such cases a diagnosis of combined PSNP has been proposed.

Recommended reading

Hauw, J. J., Daniel, S. E., Dickson, D., Horoupain, D. S., Jellinger, K., Lantos, P. L., *et al.* (1995) Preliminary NINDS neuropathological criteria for Steele–Richardson–Olszewski syndrome (progressive supranuclear palsy) [Review]. *Neurology*, **44**, 2015–2019.

Quinn, N. (1995) Parkinsonism-recognition and differential diagnosis [Review]. *Br. Med. J.*, **310**, 447–452.

3.10

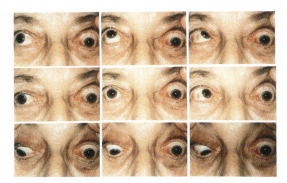

Fig. 3.10a

Q: *This 75-year-old lady presented with a sudden onset of diplopia, pulsating proptosis, ocular discomfort and 'noises in her head'. She was otherwise well with no past medical or ophthalmic history of note. What signs are demonstrated by these photographs? What is the differential diagnosis? (see Fig. 3.10a)*

A: In the primary position the left eye is hypotropic and slightly exotropic. There is a complete external ophthalmoplegia of the left eye; the extraocular movements of the right eye appear full. There is no significant anisocoria. The other features of note are the chemosis and dilated conjunctival and episcleral vessels of the left eye. Slit-lamp examination of the episcleral and conjunctival circulation demonstrated reversal of flow in these vessels.

The differential diagnosis should include the following:

(1) Carotid-cavernous sinus fistula.
(2) Orbital apex syndrome.
(3) Cavernous sinus thrombosis – this usually complicates cases of orbital cellulitis, and the patient is invariably pyrexial and unwell.

Q: *What other features of the ocular examination may confirm the diagnosis of a carotid-cavernous sinus fistula?*

A: The symptoms and signs associated with arteriovenous fistulae involving the cavernous sinus will vary according to the nature of the fistula. In general carotid-cavernous sinus fistulae may be divided into two groups:

(1) High-flow shunts. These are usually post-traumatic (i.e. major head trauma, often associated with a basal skull fracture) and result from a tear within the cavernous portion of the internal carotid artery. High-flow shunts may also be found in older patients following rupture of an intra-cavernous carotid artery aneurysm.
(2) Low-flow shunts. The exact aetiology of dural arteriovenous fistulae of the cavernous sinus is not known. They probably develop following an insidious thrombosis of the sinus. Recanalisation then occurs with pre-existing arteries in the walls of the dural sinus becoming sufficiently enlarged to form a haemodynamic shunt. These lesions are most commonly seen in post-menopausal women.

Other ophthalmic signs of a high-flow fistula include:

(1) Pulsatile proptosis, this may be subtle and may be missed on manual palpation of the globe. If in doubt the presence of pulsatile exophthalmos may be confirmed using the handheld Perkins tonometer, which will allow the examiner to detect the subtle increase in amplitude of the ocular pulse.
(2) A bruit which is best heard over the lateral orbital wall (often heard by the patient).
(3) Elevated intraocular pressure due to a raised episcleral venous pressure or secondary angle closure glaucoma.
(4) Retinal vascular dilatation.

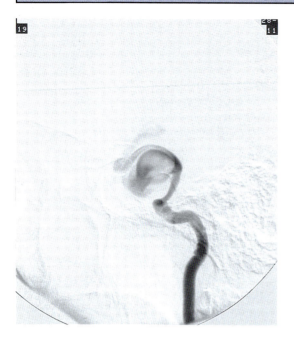 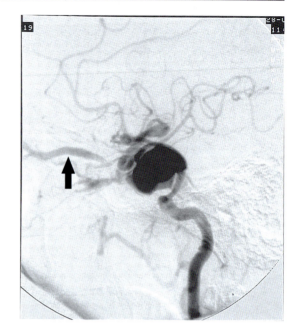

Fig. 3.10b

All of these signs were present in the above patient.

Signs may be bilateral but are invariably less marked in the contralateral eye. Low-flow fistulae will exhibit similar signs but to a lesser degree. Unlike high-flow lesions, they are prone to a chronic-relapsing course with occasional exacerbations.

Q: *What would be the investigation of choice in the above patient?*

A: A CT scan will demonstrate proptosis and enlargement of the EOM in proportion to the degree of shunting; the superior ophthalmic vein will also be enlarged. However, the definitive investigation in cases of suspected arteriovenous shunts is angiography. Selective catheterisation of both left internal and left vertebral arteries was performed in the above patient. Figure 3.10b illustrates two frames from the angiogram.

The early frame outlines a large intracavernous carotid artery aneurysm which has ruptured into the cavernous sinus. The dilated superior ophthalmic vein is clearly visible in the later frame. These findings explain why this elderly women presented with a history and physical signs typical of a high-flow fistula.

Q: *What are the treatment options in patients with carotid-cavernous sinus fistulae?*

A: The decision to treat is dependent on the nature of the fistula. In high-flow fistulae the incidence of visual loss without treatment is approximately 50%, therefore treatment is almost always indicated. Detachable balloon embolisation has now superseded invasive neurosurgical procedures as the treatment of choice. It allows safe occlusion of the fistula while preserving flow in the internal carotid artery in the majority of cases.

Intervention in low-flow dural fistulae is only indicated in the presence of impending visual loss, persistently raised intraocular pressure refractory to medical treatment, marked chemosis and lid swelling (with or without exposure) or an intrusive bruit. An initial ploy that can be tried is intermittent compression of the ipsilateral carotid artery with the opposite hand. This simple manoeuvre may be enough to close some low-flow shunts. If this proves unsuccessful intravascular embolisation is the treatment of choice using either particles or liquid tissue adhesives.

Section 4

Visual fields

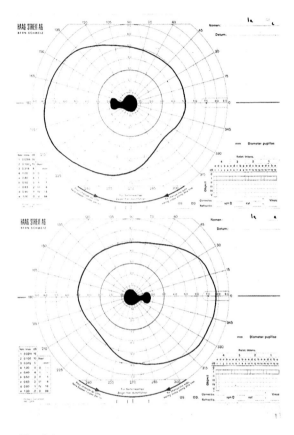

Fig. 4.1a

Q: *These are the visual fields of a 30-year-old man (of no fixed abode) who gave a 2-month history of bilateral visual loss. His visual acuities were 6/18 in both eyes. Describe the visual field defects. What is the most likely diagnosis? What will be the appearance of his optic discs? (see Fig. 4.1a)*

A: This is an example of bilateral centrocecal scotomas, note the field loss extends from the blind spot to involve fixation. Centrocecal scotomas are secondary to defects in the nerve fibre bundle (NFB). Other field defects associated with NFB lesions are central scotomas that do not involve the blind spot and paracentral sco-

tomas, which lie next to but do not involve fixation.

The most likely cause for this clinical scenario is nutritional optic neuropathy, also known as tobacco–alcohol amblyopia. This is a less satisfactory term, because although a significant number of patients with this condition are heavy smokers and have a history of alcohol abuse, there is no direct evidence proving a causative link between these habits and the development of this optic neuropathy.

The optic discs in this condition initially appear normal before developing subtle temporal pallor.

If nutritional optic neuropathy is not suspected from the history, other causes of progressive bilateral visual loss, with NFB field defects in this age group should be considered:

(1) Drug toxicity:
   (a) Ethambutol/isoniazid.
   (b) Heavy metals.
   (c) Methanol.
(2) Leber's hereditary optic neuropathy.
(3) Infiltrative optic neuropathy:
   (a) Carcinomatous.
   (b) Lymphoreticular.
   (c) Granulomatous (sarcoidosis, tuberculosis, syphilis).
(4) Compressive lesions such as meningiomas are uncommon in this age group.
(5) Cone dystrophy.

Q: *How should this patient be investigated?*

A: The following routine investigations should be performed:

(1) Full blood count – is there evidence of macrocytosis?
(2) Vitamin B12 and folate levels.
(3) Venereal Disease Research Laboratories (VDRL) test.
(4) Chest X-ray to look for evidence of neoplasia, sarcoidosis or tuberculosis.

(5) If a nutritional cause was not suspected a heavy metal screen, a lumbar puncture and a CT scan should be performed. Screening for Leber's mitochondrial mutations should also be considered.

Q: *What is the mechanism of optic nerve damage?*

A: The exact mechanism of optic nerve damage is not fully understood. Following the cessation of Soviet aid to Cuba in 1991 an epidemic of optic neuropathy and peripheral neuropathy affected over 50 000 people across the island. This tragic episode was an ideal opportunity to study risk factors for the development of nutritional optic neuropathy. Investigators found that the risk was reduced among subjects with higher dietary intakes of methionine, vitamin B12, riboflavin and niacin, and in those people with higher serum concentrations of antioxidant carotenoids. Tobacco use (particularly cigars) was associated with an increased risk of optic neuropathy, although many non-smokers were affected. The number of new cases fell steadily after Castro initiated vitamin supplementation for the entire population.

Q: *How should this patient be managed and what is the visual prognosis?*

A: These patients should be actively encouraged to give up smoking and drinking with the help of rehabilitation programmes and to eat a well-balanced diet. This should be supplemented by a daily regime of B complex vitamins with monthly intramuscular injections of hydroxycobalamin (1000 mg). Nutritional optic neuropathy is in part reversible, with a degree of visual recovery occurring in most cases over several months, provided patients comply with the above regime.

Recomended reading

The Cuba Neuropathy Field Investigation Team (1995) Epidemic optic neuropathy in Cuba – clinical characterization and risk factors. *N. Engl. J. Med.*, **333**, 1176–1182.

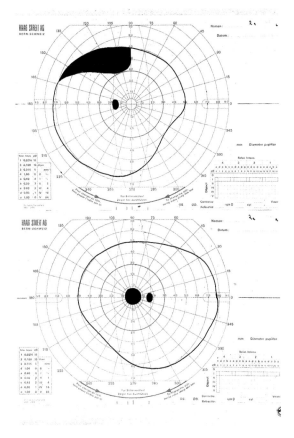

Fig. 4.2a

Q: *This 45-year-old patient presented with slowly progressive unilateral visual loss (6/60 RE 6/6 LE) and the following field defect. Describe this visual field defect. Where is the visual pathway lesion likely to be?*
(see Fig. 4.2a)

A: The finding of a dense unilateral central scotoma on confrontational testing should always alert the examiner to the possibility of field loss in the other eye. On testing the visual field of the left eye, finger counting was accurate in all four quadrants, but there was evidence of red desaturation in the superotemporal quadrant. This field defect is known as a junctional scotoma, and is the result of pathology in the distal optic nerve and anterior chiasm. The superotemporal loss in the left eye is caused by destruction of the decussating inferonasal fibres from the left eye which lie in the anterior chiasm. Historically, these decussating fibres were thought to pass forward into the distal portion of the contralateral optic nerve in a configuration known as von Wilbrand's knee. However, anatomical studies have shown that this is not the case and that von Wilbrand's knee is in fact an artefactual phenomenon, which is seen in the distal optic nerve of enucleated eyes.

If the crossed macular fibres are involved there may be an upper temporal paracentral scotoma instead of the more peripheral upper temporal loss illustrated above.

The lesion in this case was in fact a right optic nerve/chiasmal granuloma secondary to sarcoidosis.

Q: *What would be the most likely diagnosis if this pattern of field loss was found in*
(1) a 7-year-old child or
(2) a 50-year-old woman?

A: If this pattern of field loss is seen in a child anterior visual pathway imaging is mandatory to exclude intrinsic optic nerve. Chiasmal lesions such as a chiasmal glioma or suprasellar lesions including craniopharyngiomas and dysgerminomas.

Similar field loss in a 50-year-old woman may be secondary to the following conditions:

(1) Meningiomas are the most common cause of anterior chiasmal/optic nerve compression in women of this age.
(2) Pituitary tumour.
(3) Vascular occlusion.
(4) Anterior communicating artery aneurysm.
(5) Demyelinating disease.
(6) Granulomatous disease, e.g. sarcoidosis, syphilis and histiocytosis X.

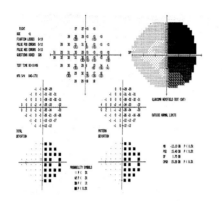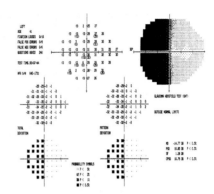

Fig. 4.3a

Q: *A 35-year-old woman presented with this pattern of visual field loss and headaches. What features of this patient's history might point to the aetiology of the underlying lesion? (see Fig. 4.3a)*

A: This bitemporal hemianopia that respects the vertical midline is highly suggestive of a pituitary tumour. The most likely diagnosis in view of the field defects and the history of headache is a macroadenoma. As the pituitary fossa is situated 1 cm below the chiasm the tumour must be at least this size to cause chiasmal compression. Pituitary adenomas may be secreting or non-secreting, prolactinomas are the most common pituitary secreting adenoma. The following questions may help confirm this diagnosis:

(1) Is there a history of menstrual irregularity or amenorrhoea?
(2) Has there been a loss of libido?
(3) Is there a history of galactorrhoea?

Loss of libido and menstrual irregularity are features of hyperprolactinaemia and hypopituitarism.

Q: *How should patients with suspected prolactinomas be managed?*

A: All such patients should have a serum prolactin performed at the first clinic visit to exclude a prolactinoma. The normal prolactin level is approximately 100 mU/l; a level of 5000 mU/l suggests a macroadenoma. Levels of 2500 mU/l in the presence of a macroadenoma are likely to be secondary to a non-secreting tumour compressing the pituitary stalk. Neuroimaging in the form of a CT scan or MR should be performed. (see Fig. 9.4c).

Bromocriptine is the first-line treatment for macroprolactinomas; initial therapy begins with doses of 1.25 mg/day. In most patients this is usually sufficient to reduce galactorrhoea, restore menstruation and return serum prolactin levels to normal. In large adenomas there is often a rapid and dramatic improvement in the visual fields over a period of days to weeks. Side effects such as nausea/vomiting, mood changes and fatigue can be minimised by taking a low dose at bedtime or by administering the tablets intravaginally. Most patients require bromocriptine indefinitely as discontinuation of therapy frequently leads to a sudden expansion of the tumour.

Alternative agents that may be used in cases of bromocriptine intolerance include, pergolide (50 μg to 1 mg t.d.s.), cabergoline (50 μg to 1 mg orally twice weekly) or quinagolide (75–600 mg in divided doses daily).

Neurosurgery is only indicated in those patients who fail to respond to medical therapy or for those patients with rapidly progressive visual loss who cannot tolerate medical therapy. There is no evidence that the results of surgery are improved by pretreating with bromocriptine; in fact, chronic bromocriptine therapy may cause pituitary fibrosis that will make surgery technically more difficult.

Q: *How would your management change if this patient became pregnant?*

A: Although bromocriptine reduces the chances of conception the physician and ophthalmologist should be aware that pituitary adenomas, especially prolactinomas (16%) may increase in size rapidly during pregnancy. No teratogenic side effects have been reported with bromocriptine; nevertheless, most physicians elect to discontinue treatment during pregnancy and monitor for visual field deterioration at regular intervals. Bromocriptine therapy can be recommended if necessary.

Q: *Aside from microprolactinomas, what are the other causes of a moderately elevated serum prolactin?*

A: If the serum prolactin level is only marginally elevated the following conditions should be considered:

(1) Pregnancy and lactation.
(2) Stress or anxiety.
(3) Any hypothalamic or pituitary tumour which compresses the pituitary stalk.
(4) Drugs:
    (a) Oestrogens.
    (b) Dopamine antagonists, e.g. phenothiazines and metaclopromide.
    (c) Methyldopa.
    (d) Cimetidine.
(5) Severe primary hypothyroidism.
(6) Polycystic ovarian syndrome.
(7) Hepatic or renal failure.

The finding of hyperprolactinaemia should be interpreted with caution as levels may be misleadingly elevated during sleep (therefore samples should be taken 2–3 h after waking). Even the minor stress of venepuncture may stimulate prolactin secretion.

Q: *What other field defects may be produced by chiasmal lesions.*

A: Approximately 85% of chiasms are situated directly above the pituitary fossa, 5% are prefixed (i.e. they lie anterior to the fossa) and 10% are postfixed (i.e. they lie posterior to the fossa). It therefore follows that a junctional scotoma is more likely to occur if the chiasm is postfixed because the expanding tumour mass will impinge on the anterior chiasmal fibres. The optic tracts may be compromised by a pituitary tumour if the chiasm is prefixed resulting in an incongruous homonymous hemianopia. Macular crossing fibres are distributed throughout the chiasm and if they are primarily affected by a chiasmal lesion the result is a central bitemporal hemianopia.

Q: *What other visual symptoms may trouble a patient with a bitemporal hemianopia?*

A: As well as bitemporal field loss such patients may complain of:

(1) Postfixational blindness, i.e. when fixating on a near target, objects distal to this target lie in the affected overlapping temporal visual fields.
(2) The 'hemifield slide phenomena' (Fig 4.3b).

If patients have a pre-existing exophoria or intermittent exotropia there will be overlapping of the intact nasal fields causing diplopia.

In cases of a pre-existing esophoria or intermittent esotropia separation of the nasal hemifields will result in a central blind area.

If there is a vertical deviation patients will complain of vertical separation of images crossing the vertical meridian.

Q: *What are the optic disc appearances associated with long-standing compressive chiasmal lesions?*

A: Long-standing compressive chiasmal lesions will either result in a 'bow-tie' or 'band' optic

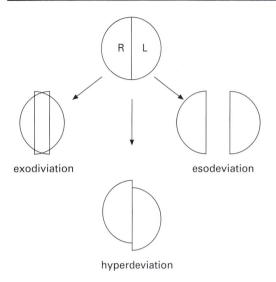

exodiviation   esodeviation

hyperdeviation

R = right temporal projection
L = left temporal projection

Fig. 4.3b

atrophy. There is loss of nerve fibres from the ganglion cells nasal to the fovea supplying the central temporal field, which pass to the temporal disc margin, resulting in atrophy of this temporal portion of the disc. Ganglion cells from the nasal retina supplying the peripheral temporal field are also affected, producing nasal disc pallor with relative sparing of the superior and inferior arcuate bundles. Bow-tie atrophy is also seen in pregeniculate optic tract lesions. Although patients with 'band' atrophy may recover both acuity and visual field following successful decompression those with normal optic discs should have virtually complete return of visual function within 14 days of surgery.

Q: *What other neuro-ophthalmological signs may be associated with chiasmal syndromes? (see Fig. 4.3c)*

A: Aside from the variable patterns of visual field loss and optic atrophy described above, what other neuro-ophthalmic signs may be associated with chiasmal lesions.

(1) Papilloedema is frequently associated with suprachiasmal tumours (due to involve-

ment of the third ventricle) but rarely intrasellar lesions.

(2) Extraocular muscle palsies may occur with prechiasmal tumours.

(3) See-saw nystagmus characterised by alternate intorsion and elevation of one eye and extorsion and depression of the fellow eye is a well-described feature of diencephalon and chiasmal tumours.

Q: *Describe this visual field defect. What are the possible causes of this pattern of visual field loss? (see Fig. 4.3c)*

A: At first glance this appears to be an example of a bitemporal hemianopia. However, the important point to note is that the field loss does not respect the vertical midline and therefore cannot be due to a chiasmal lesion.

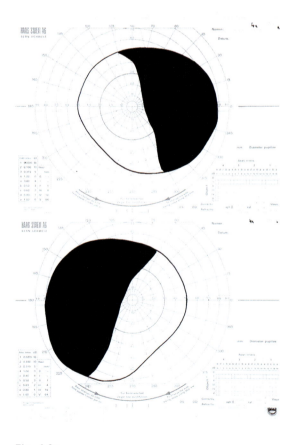

Fig. 4.3c

This pseudo-bitemporal hemianopia may be caused by:

(1) Tilted optic discs.
(2) Optic disc drusen.
(3) Sectorial retinitis pigmentosa or another sectorial pigmentary retinopathy.
(4) Retinal detachments.

By correctly diagnosing this pattern of field loss the patient may be spared unnecessary neurological investigations.

Recomended reading

Klibanski, A. and Zervas, N. T. (1991) Diagnosis and management of hormone-secreting pituitary adenomas [Review]. *N. Engl. J. Med.*, **324**, 822–831.

Levy, A. and Lightman, S. L. (1994) Diagnosis and management of pituitary tumours [Review]. *Br. Med. J.*, **308**, 1087–1091.

4.4

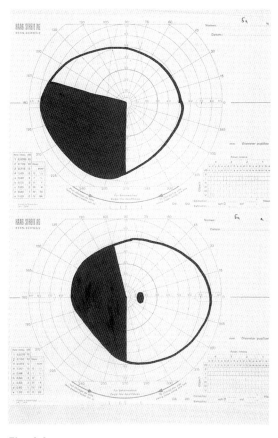

Fig. 4.4

Q: *Describe this pattern of visual field loss, which was associated with bilateral optic atrophy. What is the likely anatomical site of the lesion? (see Fig. 4.4)*

A: These fields show a left-sided incongruous homonymous hemianopia. The hemianopic field loss means that the lesion must be retro-chiasmal. The very incongruous nature of the field loss and the associated bilateral optic atrophy point to a right optic tract lesion.

Q: *What other ocular signs may be caused by an optic tract lesion?*

A: The classical signs of an optic tract lesion include:

(1) Incongruous homonymous hemianopia, although complete homonymous hemianopias have been reported. If the causative lesion involves the posterior chiasm, fibres from the ipsilateral superior retina (which cross in this region) may be involved resulting in an additional ipsilateral inferotemporal field defect.
(2) Bilateral retinal nerve fibre layer atrophy or optic atrophy, which may be of the 'bow-tie' variety.
(3) Relative afferent pupillary defect in the eye with temporal field loss (i.e. contralateral to the side of the lesion), despite normal visual acuity and colour vision in that eye.
(4) Light stimulation of the 'blind' retina produces no pupillary reaction, but normal constriction is present when functioning retina is stimulated (Wernicke's pupil).

4.5

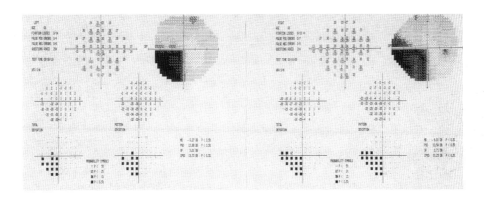

Fig. 4.5a

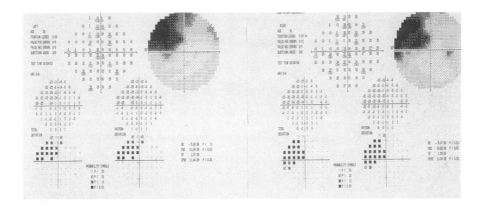

Fig. 4.5b

Q: *Describe this pattern of field loss. Where is the site of the lesion? (see Fig. 4.5a)*

A: This is a left inferior homonymous quadrantanopia, note that the field loss involves fixation and not the blind spot, this points to a retrochiasmal rather than an optic nerve lesion. The involvement of the inferior visual field is characteristic of a parietal lobe lesion. A relatively congruous homonymous hemianopia with denser field loss inferiorly may also be seen with parietal lesions.

The term congruous describes *incomplete* homonymous hemianopias in which field loss extends to the same angular meridian in both eyes. By definition complete homonymous hemianopias cannot therefore be described as congruous. The nearer a lesion is to the occipital cortex the closer nerve fibres from corresponding retinal points run together and the more congruous the resultant field defect.

Temporal lobe lesions do not usually involve fixation and have a characteristic 'pie in the sky' pattern of superior field loss (Fig. 4.5b).

Q: *What ocular motility and neurological sequelae may be associated with parietal lobe lesions?*

A: A number of supranuclear ocular motility disturbances may be caused by parietal lobe lesions:

(1) Patients with parietal or temporal lobe lesions may exhibit conjugate deviation of the eyes superiorly and away from the side of the lesion during forced lid closure (Cogan's sign). This spasticity of conjugate gaze is solely a lateralising, and not a localising sign.

(2) Another feature of parietal lobe lesions is that there is often defective pursuit eye movements to the side of the lesion. This results in asymmetric optokinetic nystagmus (OKN), with a slower OKN response being elicited when the drum is rotated to the side of the lesion. OKN is normal in occipital lobe lesions.

Neurological textbooks often expound in great depth the various signs of parietal lobe dysfunction. The list of apraxias, dysgraphia, dyscalculia, astereognosis, sensory inattention, etc., is often quite bewildering! However, although there is no general consensus on this subject, most physicians would agree that loss of two-point discrimination and the presence of dressing apraxia are reliable tests of dominant and non-dominant parietal lesions, respectively.

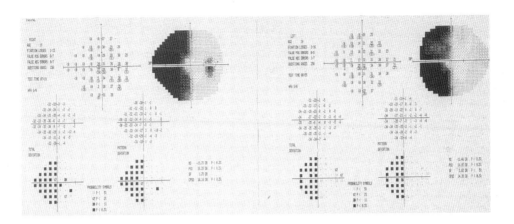

Fig. 4.6a

Q: *Describe this pattern of visual field loss. Where is the site of the lesion? (see Fig. 4.6a)*

A: This is an example of a complete homonymous hemianopia with macular sparing, the causative lesion is therefore in the occipital lobe. If there was no macular sparing it would be impossible to localise the underlying lesion from this visual field alone. For true macular sparing to be present at least 5° of the macular field must be spared in both eyes, artefactual macular sparing may be produced by wandering fixation during perimetry! It should also be noted that the majority of patients with occipital lobe lesions exhibit splitting of the macula.

Q: *How can the phenomenon of macular sparing be explained?*

A: The macular region of the visual cortex is located at the tip of the occipital lobe, and represents a watershed zone between the circulations of the posterior and middle cerebral arteries. The midperipheral and peripheral field is supplied solely by the posterior cerebral artery, whereas the visual cortex subserving the central field is supplied by terminal branches of both posterior and middle cerebral arteries. These terminal branches of the middle cerebral artery are thought to continue perfusing the macular cortex after posterior cerebral occlusion.

Q: *What other field defects are characteristic of occipital lobe lesions?*

A:

(1) The macular cortex which is supplied by these terminal branches is often the first area to be affected in hypoperfusion states, this results in a central homonymous hemianopia.
(2) Fibres from the nasal periphery of the contralateral retina relay to the anterior calcarine fissure. A lesion in this area will result in a monocular, contralateral visual field defect known as a temporal crescent. This is the only pattern of monocular field loss seen with a retrochiasmal lesion. It should be noted that these defects begin approximately 60° from fixation, in which case central field testing will not identify them.

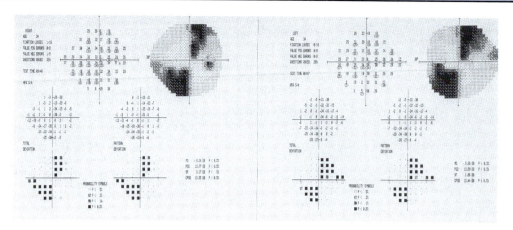

Fig. 4.6b

(3) 'Tubular' fields secondary to bilateral occipital lobe infarction with macular sparing.

(4) Crossed quadrant hemianopias or 'checkerboard' fields (Fig. 4.6b). This pattern of visual field loss is caused by either simultaneous or consecutive lesions, one above the calcarine fissure the other below the contralateral calcarine fissure.

Faces

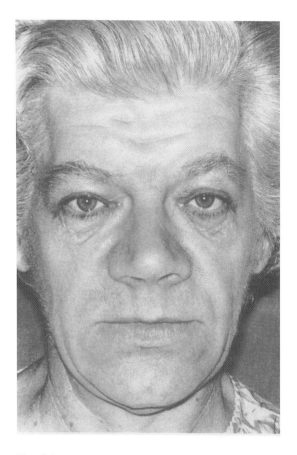

Fig. 5.1

Q: *Describe the facial features of this 56-year-old woman. What is the most likely diagnosis? (see Fig. 5.1)*

A: This is an example of an acromegalic facies. Note the prominent supraorbital ridges, the square jaw line and the broad nose. Sebhorroeic changes over the cheeks and rhinophyma are other facial features commonly seen in cases of acromegaly.

Q: *What investigations would help confirm the diagnosis?*

A: In cases of suspected acromegaly the following investigations may be helpful:

(1) Basal plasma growth hormone (GH) >5 ng/ml (GH secretion is pulsatile, and acromegaly should not be ruled out or diagnosed on the basis of a single random GH measurement).
(2) Failure of suppression of serum GH to <2 ng/ml after 100 g of glucose is considered to be diagnostic for acromegaly.
(3) An elevated insulin-like growth factor (ILGF)-I level is an excellent screening tool as it reflects the average GH secretion over a 6–12 h period.

If these investigations point to the diagnosis of acromegaly the following investigations are indicated:

(4) Dynamic pituitary function tests to determine the extent of pituitary gland destruction. Partial or complete anterior hypopituitarism is seen in approximately 20% of cases.
(5) Hyperprolactinaemia has been reported in a similar proportion of cases. CT or MRI of the pituitary fossa and optic chiasm. There is no longer any role for plain skull radiography in the investigation of suspected pituitary fossa lesions.
(6) Glucose tolerance test – this will be abnormal in 25% of patients with acromegaly.
(7) ECG with or without echocardiography, the left ventricular mass is generally increased and there is a subsequent reduction in diastolic function even in the absence of hypertension or coronary artery disease.

Q: *What explanation would account for elevated growth hormone titres in the absence of a pituitary mass on CT or MRI?*

A: Growth hormone hypersecretion in acromegalic patients is secondary to a pituitary adenoma in over 99% of cases. However, there are well-documented cases of secondary pituitary hyperplasia induced by excess growth hormone releasing hormone secreted from the hypothalamus or from an ectopic source. Although many tumours are known to secrete GH (lung, breast and ovary) there has only been a single reported case of frank acromegaly secondary to ectopic GH secretion, the source being a pancreatic islet cell tumour.

Q: *What features of the ocular examination are of particular relevance in acromegalic patients?*

A: If the underlying pituitary adenoma is >1 cm in diameter there is a risk of anterior visual pathway compression. The exact nature of this visual loss is dependent on the size of the adenoma and the position of the optic chiasm. Relevant features of the ocular examination include:

(1) Signs of optic nerve compression:
    (a) Reduced visual acuity.
    (b) Diminished colour vision (Ishihara plates).
    (c) A relative afferent pupillary defect.
    (d) Optic atrophy.
(2) Signs of visual pathway compression (see Section 4):
    (a) Junctional scotoma (anterior chiasmal).
    (b) Bitemporal hemianopia (chiasmal).
    (c) Incongruous hemianopia (optic tract).

Although confrontational visual fields may provide some information on visual field loss automated or Goldmann perimetry should be performed for all acromegalic patients.

Recommended reading

Krishna, A. Y. and Philips, L. S. (1994) Management of acromegaly: a review. *Am. J. Med. Sci.*, **308**, 370–375.

Wass, J. A. (1993) Acromegaly: treatment after 100 years [Editorial]. *Br. Med. J.*, **307**, 1505–1506.

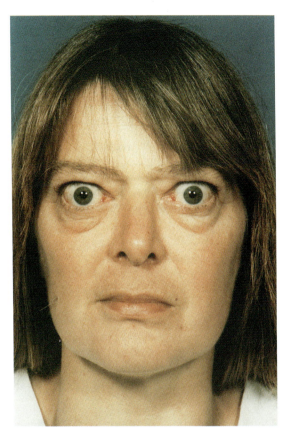

Fig. 5.2

Q: *Describe the ocular signs visible in this photograph. What is the most likely diagnosis? (see Fig. 5.2)*

A: There is bilateral upper and lower lid retraction, periorbital oedema, and mild injection of the conjunctiva over the insertions of the lateral rectus muscles. There is no manifest ocular deviation in the primary position. Although there is a degree of proptosis bilaterally (as measured by a Hertel exophthalmometer) it is not possible to comment on this without a lateral facial photograph.

These are the typical features of Graves' disease.

Q: *What classification systems may be used to describe the severity of thyroid eye disease?*

A: The modified Werner (NOSPECS) classification of thyroid eye disease:

Grade	Suggestions for grading
Class 0	**N**o physical signs or symptoms
Class 1	**O**nly signs (limited to upper lid retraction, stare, and lid lag)
Class 2	**S**oft tissue involvement with symptoms and signs
0	absent
a	minimal
b	moderate
c	marked
	Signs include, resistance to retropulsion of the globe, oedema and/or injection of the conjunctiva and caruncle, oedema and fullness of the lids and lacrimal gland enlargement.
Class 3	**P**roptosis 3 mm or more in excess of upper normal limits
0	absent
a	3–4 mm increase above upper normal
b	5–7 mm increase
c	8 mm or more increase
Class 4	**E**xtraocular muscle involvement, usually with diplopia
0	absent
a	limitation of motion of extreme gaze
b	evident restriction of motion
c	fixation of globe or globes
Class 5	**C**orneal involvement (primarily due to lagophthalmos)
0	absent
a	stippling of the cornea
b	ulceration
c	clouding, necrosis, perforation

Class 6	**S**ight loss due to optic nerve involvement
0	absent
a	disc pallor or choking, or visual field defect; vision 6/6–6/18
b	same, but vision 6/24–6/60
c	blindness, i.e. vision <6/60

Approximately 90% of cases are described as non-infiltrative and fall into classes 0 or 1. Classes 2–6 describe infiltrative disease which accounts for the remaining 10% of patients. There are two major limitations of this classification:

(1) It does not take into account whether the disease is active or inactive.
(2) Patients with thyroid eye disease do not develop clinical signs in a stepwise linear fashion, i.e. patients may have compressive optic neuropathy (class 6) but have no significant proptosis (class 4) or corneal exposure (class 5).

Attempts have been made to grade disease activity in order to predict which patients may benefit from medical treatment. The system proposed by Mourits *et al.*, outlined below, has been shown to be modestly predictive of active disease when scores are greater than 4. For each item present one point is given.

Pain	1 Painful, oppressive feeling on or behind the globe, during last 4 weeks
	2 Pain on attempted up, side or down gaze, during the last 4 weeks
Redness	3 Redness of the eyelid(s)
	4 Diffuse redness of the conjunctiva covering at least one quadrant
Swelling	5 Swelling of the eyelid(s)
	6 Chemosis
	7 Swollen caruncle
	8 Increase of proptosis of ≥2 mm during a period of 1–3 months
Impaired function	9 Decrease of eye movements in any direction of ≥5 during a period of 1–3 months

10 Decrease of visual acuity of ≥1 line(s) on the Snellen chart (using a pinhole) during a period of 3 months.

Q: *What are the drug therapies used in the treatment of Graves' disease?*

A: The majority of patients with Graves' disease will initially be treated using antithyroid drugs often in combination with a β-blocker. The most commonly used regimes are as follows:

(1) Block and replace regime. Carbimazole 40–60 mg/day is given to completely suppress the hyperactive thyroid gland and thyroxine 100 µg/day is taken to replace the thyroid hormones. This is usually continued for 12–18 months.
(2) Gradual dose titration. Initially carbimazole 10–20 mg t.d.s. is given and after 4–6 weeks this is reduced according to the clinical status of the patient and the thyroid function tests. After 2–3 months this may be reduced to a once-daily dose. Further step wise reductions are continued until the patient has been successfully rendered euthyroid on a maintenance dose of 5 mg/day. Treatment is normally continued for 18 months.

Thyroid stimulating hormone (TSH) levels may remain low for weeks or months after serum thyroxine and tri-iodothyronine concentrations have returned to normal. Therefore TSH levels alone should not be used to monitor therapy in the initial treatment period.

β-Blockers are used in conjunction with antithyroid drugs in the initial phase of treatment for two reasons. Thyroxine has a half-life of 7 days and therefore treatment with carbimazole alone will not provide any symptomatic relief for 7–10 days. However, blockade of the sympathetic nervous system will rapidly reduce many of the manifestations of Graves' disease such as anxiety, palpitations, and tremor. β-blockers will also prevent the peripheral conversion of T4 to T3. Propranolol is the β-blocker most commonly used as it is non-selective and has no intrinsic sympathomimetic activity. Nadolol is intrinsically long acting and may be more useful than propranolol.

Q: *What are the methods of action and side effects of carbimazole?*

A: Methimazole is the active metabolite of carbimazole, it disrupts the synthesis of T3 and T4 at a number of points:

(1) Reduction of iodine uptake into the follicular cells of the thyroid.
(2) Reduction of thyroglobulin synthesis.
(3) Blocks formation of di-iodotyrosine in the colloid.
(4) Carbimazole is thought to reduce serum concentrations of thyrotropin-receptor antibodies and increase suppressor T cell activity. This mild immunosuppressive action may be beneficial in Graves' disease.
(5) Unlike propylthiouracil it does not block the conversion of T4 to T3.

Mild side effects such as rashes, arthralgia, nausea and vomiting are common and respond to reducing the dose of carbimazole. Serious side effects occur in approximately 3/1000 patients.

(1) Agranulocytosis (granulocyte count $<500/mm^3$) is an idiosyncratic reaction that occurs rapidly, irrespective of dose or duration of treatment. It may develop in patients of any age, but is seen more frequently in patients >40 years of age and occurs within 3 months of initiating treatment. All patients should be warned that if they develop a sore throat or unexplained temperature they should stop the tablets and seek immediate medical advice. The majority of patients recover within 2–3 weeks of discontinuing the drug although fatalities still occur despite appropriate isolation and prophylactic antibiotic therapy.
(2) Cholestatic jaundice (very rare).
(3) Lupus-like syndromes (very rare).

Q: *How will pregnancy alter the management of the thyrotoxic patient?*

A: Although Graves' disease is uncommon during pregnancy if present it poses a number of management problems:

(1) Carbimazole crosses the blood–placental barrier and the smallest dose necessary should be used. Alternatively propylthiouracil may be used, as little crosses the blood–placental barrier and it only appears in breast milk in small amounts. A block and replace regime should not be used as little of the thyroxine will cross the blood–placental barrier.
(2) Foetal hyperthyroidism may be a problem in mothers with pre-existing Graves' disease even if they are now euthyroid. This is because thyroid stimulating immunoglobulins may still be circulating and will stimulate the foetal thyroid. A foetal tachycardia of 160 b.p.m. is strongly suggestive of foetal hyperthyroidism. Maternal treatment with carbimazole should be commenced in such cases and supplementary thyroxine may be given to prevent the mother becoming hypothyroid.

Q: *What proportion of patients will relapse on discontinuing antithyroid medications and how should they be managed?*

A: There are no reliable tests for predicting which patients are going to relapse on discontinuing treatment. Relapse is more likely within 6 months after withdrawal, but it may occur many years later. There is some evidence to suggest that the rate of relapse is lower if initial treatment is continued for 2 years, and it tends to be lower with block and replace regimes. A recent Japanese study reported a relapse rate of 1.7% in patients treated with methimazole for 6 months, followed by a combination of methimazole and thyroxine for 1 year, and a further 3 years of thyroxine therapy alone. The relapse rate in those patients not receiving thyroxine was 35%.

Recurrent Graves' disease can be treated in a number of ways:

(1) Radioiodine is the treatment of choice (when there are no contraindications) for recurrent hyperthyroidism after medical therapy. The aim of treatment is to destroy sufficient thyroid tissue to render the patient euthyroid or hypothyroid, but there is little consensus regarding the most appropriate dose schedule. Pre-treatment with antithyroid drugs or β-blockers is advisable in most cases as a euthyroid state is usually not achieved for several months after treatment. Radioiodine should be used with caution in those with established thyroid eye disease or those patients with risk factors for ophthalmopathy (e.g. smokers and/or age >40 years), in view of the results of the randomised trial published by Bartalena *et al*. In this study 443 patients with Graves' disease and mild or no ophthalmopathy were treated with methimazole until euthyroid. They were then randomised into three groups: (a) continued methimazole therapy, (b) radioiodine and (c) radioiodine with adjuvant prednisolone cover. After radioiodine treatment 15% of patients developed new ophthalmopathy or worsening of pre-existing ophthalmopathy. This occurred in only 3% of the methimazole group and in no patients who received radioiodine and adjuvant corticosteroids. This study has proven what many ophthalmologists have long suspected, that is, radioiodine predisposes to the development of ophthalmopathy and may exacerbate pre-existing disease. A course of prednisolone 0.4–0.5 mg/kg daily for 1 month, tapered over 2 months, was the regime used in this study.

(2) Reinstigation of antithyroid drugs. Very long-term therapy is safe provided regular review is maintained.

(3) Subtotal thyroidectomy should be reserved for those patients in whom radioiodine therapy is contraindicated or for cases where there is a large goitre.

Recommended reading

Bartelena, L., Marcocci, C., Bogazzi, F., Manetti, L., Tanda, M. L., Dell'Unto, E., *et al*. (1998) Relation between treatment for hyperthyroidism and the course of Graves' ophthalmopathy. *N. Engl. J. Med.*, **338**, 73–78.

Franklyn, J. A. (1994) The management of hyperthyroidism [Review]. *N. Engl. J. Med.*, **330**, 1731–1738.

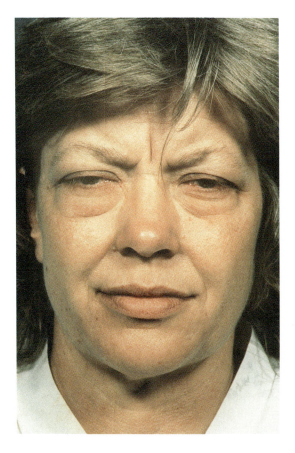

Fig. 5.3

Q: *Describe these facial features. What is the most likely diagnosis? (see Fig. 5.3)*

A: This is a characteristic example of a myxoedematous facies. Note the coarse dry skin, the 'peaches and cream' complexion, the thinning of the lateral two-thirds of the eyebrows.

Q: *What questions would you ask this patient to confirm the diagnosis?*

A: A systematic history may elicit the following symptoms typical of hypothyroidism:

(1) Cold intolerance.
(2) Weight gain (often despite a reduced appetite), lethargy, poor concentration and reduced cognitive function.
(3) Menstrual disturbances, e.g. amenorrhoea, oligomenorrhoea and infertility.
(4) Gastrointestinal disturbances, e.g. constipation.
(5) Voice changes.
(6) Depression.

Q: *What investigations other than thyroid function tests and thyroid autoantibodies are indicated in the management of this patient?*

A: Hypothyroidism may be associated with other autoimmune diseases and therefore the following investigations should be performed:

(1) Full blood count – anaemia is usually normochromic normocytic, but may be macrocytic particularly if there is an associated pernicious anaemia.
(2) Blood glucose to exclude diabetes mellitus.
(3) Urea and electrolytes – hyponatraemia secondary to Addison's disease.
(4) Liver function tests (primary biliary cirrhosis).
(5) Cholesterol and triglycerides (hypercholesterolaemia).

Q: *What ocular conditions are associated with hypothyroidism?*

A: Thyroid eye disease is almost exclusively the domain of Graves' disease, although rare cases have been reported in patients with primary hypothyroidism. A much more common clinical scenario is the development of thyroid eye disease in patients who have been rendered hypothyroid as a result of treatment for Graves' disease, e.g. following radioiodine therapy. Ophthalmologists and physicians should be aware of the importance of achieving and maintaining euthyroid status in patients with

Graves' disease, both to minimise the risk of developing thyroid eye disease and to limit the severity of established ocular involvement.

As primary hypothyroidism is often asso- ciated with other autoimmune diseases it is not uncommon to detect signs and symptoms of keratoconjunctivitis sicca secondary to Sjögren's disease.

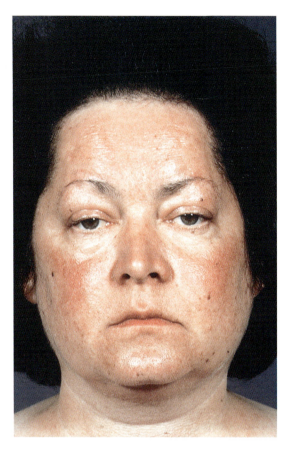 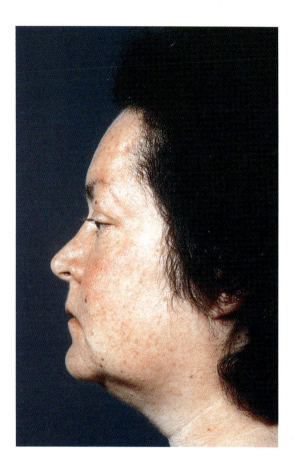

Fig. 5.4

Q: *What is the diagnosis? (see Fig. 5.4)*

A: This is the typical facies of a patient with Cushing's syndrome (hypercortisolism).

Q: *Aside from iatrogenic corticosteroid therapy what are the other causes of Cushing's syndrome?*

A: Cushing's syndrome can be separated into two categories:

(1) Corticotropin-dependent Cushing's syndrome (Cushing's disease):

(a) Cushing's disease is secondary to excessive secretion of corticotropin by a pituitary microadenoma and accounts for 70% of cases of Cushing's syndrome. Macroadenomas, corticotroph hyperplasia and carcinomas are extremely rare.

(b) Ectopic corticotropin syndrome is characterised by the rapid onset of hypertension, oedema, hypokalaemia and glucose intolerance. In the majority of cases it is secondary to small-cell lung carcinomas, although a more chronic syndrome is associated with less aggressive tumours such as bronchial or pancreatic carcinoids and phaeochromocytomas. This group accounts for approximately 10% of Cushing's syndrome cases.

(c) Ectopic corticotropin releasing hormone (CRH) syndrome is a rare sequelae of bronchial carcinoids and is clinically indistinguishable from the ectopic corticotropin syndrome.

(2) Corticotropin-independent Cushing's syndrome:

(a) Adrenocortical tumours are the most common cause of corticotropin-independent Cushing's syndrome. Adrenal adenomas and carcinomas make up 10 and 8%, respectively, of all cases of Cushing's syndrome.

(b) Bilateral micronodular adrenal hyperplasia may be a sporadic finding in patients under 30 years of age or may be inherited as part of an autosomal dominant syndrome. They account for 1% of all cases of Cushing's syndrome.

Q: *What initial screening test would you perform for this woman who had no history of corticosteroid treatment?*

A: Simple screening tests in cases of suspected Cushing's disease include:

(1) Urine free cortisol excretion – if this is normal it is highly unlikely that there is an abnormality of corticosteroid metabolism.

(2) Overnight dexamethasone suppression test– 1 mg of dexamethasone given at 10 p.m. should completely suppress the morning cortisol peak. This investigation has a high sensitivity but a low specificity.

(3) 9 a.m. and midnight cortisol levels – the normal diurnal pattern of corticosteroid production shows a trough at midnight and a peak first thing in the morning, loss of this variation is abnormal.

The above tests do not take into account the fact that in Cushing's disease (which accounts for the majority of cases of Cushing's syndrome) the abnormal pituitary–adrenal function blends imperceptibly into normal function, therefore the results from these screening tests may be ambiguous in borderline cases.

The most reliable and practical screening investigation for corticotropin hypersecretion is the 24-h urinary cortisol excretion. In cases of suspected Cushing's syndrome, two and preferably three 24-h samples should be collected, as cortisol excretion in these patients may vary from day to day or may be cyclical. The completeness of collection is determined by measuring the creatinine excretion, which should not vary by $>10\%$ from day to day. The upper limit of normal in many cortisol assays is 90–100 μg/ 24 h.

Q: *How would you proceed if the 24-h urinary cortisol excretion was just above the normal range in three consecutive samples?*

A: An elevated urinary cortisol excretion may be caused by any of the following:

(1) Cushing's syndrome.
(2) Pseudo-Cushing's syndrome.
(3) Major stress, e.g. trauma or infection.

The low-dose dexamethasone test may help distinguish cases of Cushing's syndrome from pseudo-Cushing's syndrome. This test will not provide any additional information if the 24-h urinary cortisol results are obviously abnormal. The dexamethasone suppression test involves the administration of 500 mg of dexamethasone q.d.s. over a 48-h period and measuring the urine free cortisol. Excess corticosteroid production secondary to alcoholic liver disease, depression or major stress will usually be suppressed by this test. Corticotropin-dependent and corticotropin-independent Cushing's syndrome will not be suppressed, with urinary cortisol values typically $>10\,\mu g/24\,h$. Physicians should bear in mind that if the urinary cortisol secretion is normal dexamethasone suppression is invariably normal and if urinary cortisol excretion is borderline, the dexamethasone suppression test may be only marginally elevated.

It may therefore be necessary to perform other investigations to differentiate pseudo–Cushing's syndrome from Cushing's syndrome:

(1) Midnight plasma cortisol – values >7.5 µg/dl are indicative of Cushing's syndrome, values <5 µg/dl exclude the diagnosis.
(2) CRH–dexamethasone are administered in sequence – in patients with pseudo-Cushing's plasma cortisol concentrations are low following dexamethasone administration and remain low after CRH is given. The pattern in Cushing's syndrome is a less profound lowering of plasma cortisol after dexamethasone followed by an increase with CRH administration.
(3) Naloxone test – this opioid antagonist stimulates the release of CRH. Less CRH is released in Cushing's syndrome patients (in whom normal secretion is already suppressed).

Q: *What are the ocular side effects of Cushing's disease?*

A: Visual field loss secondary to chiasmal compression is not a feature of Cushing's disease as this condition is secondary to a microadenoma (<1 cm in diameter) which is unlikely to produce any significant chiasmal compression. However, there is a high incidence of hypertension and diabetes in these patients and subsequent retinopathy may be a problem. Posterior subcapsular lens opacities secondary to hypercortisolism are common findings.

Recommended reading

Magiakou, M. A., Mastorakos, G., Oldfield, E. H., Gomez, M. T., Doppman, J. L., Cutler, G. B., Jr., *et al.* (1994) Cushing's syndrome in children and adolescents. Presentation, diagnosis and therapy. *N. Engl. J. Med.*, **331**, 629–636.

Orth, D. N. (1995) Cushing's syndrome [Review]. *N. Engl. J. Med.*, **332**, 791–803.

5.5

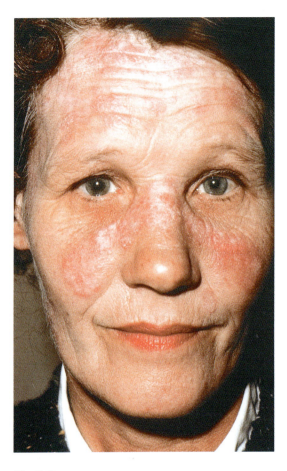

Fig. 5.5

Q: *Describe this facial photograph. What is the likely diagnosis? (see Fig. 5.5)*

A: There is diffuse erythema with maculopapular lesions over the nose and cheeks. This classical 'butterfly' distribution is characteristically seen in systemic lupus erythematosus (SLE). Similar lesions may also be found on the forehead, ears, and the dorsum of the hands. Approximately 80% of patients with SLE will have dermatological problems, such as non-specific erythema, urticaria, photosensitivity and alopecia.

Q: *What features of this patient's history may point to the diagnosis of SLE?*

A: SLE usually presents in women aged 20–40 years (90%), the following are common initial symptoms:

(1) Fever, weight loss and general malaise (80%).
(2) Migratory symmetrical polyarthralgia (90%).
(3) Pleuritic chest pain that may indicate pleurisy or a pericarditis (40%).
(4) Parasthesia secondary to a peripheral or cranial sensory neuropathy.
(5) Cognitive dysfunction, which is usually mild, is a feature in 30% of cases.

Q: *What are the criteria for making a diagnosis of SLE?*

A: The criteria devised by the American Rheumatism Society for the diagnosis of SLE (last revised in 1982) are as follows. Patients must have at least four of the criteria listed below during the course of their illness:

(1) Malar rash.
(2) Photosensitivity.
(3) Arthritis.
(4) Renal disorders.
(5) Haematological disorders.
(6) Discoid rash.
(7) Oral ulcers.
(8) Serositis.
(9) Neurological disorders.
(10) Immunological disorders.
(11) Positive antinuclear antibody titres.

Q: *What blood tests will help confirm the diagnosis and the extent of the systemic involvement?*

A:

(1) Antinuclear antibodies are positive in over 95% of cases. The positive predictive value of the test increases with higher titres:
  (a) Anti-double-stranded DNA is positive in 50% (very specific).
  (b) Anti-single-stranded DNA is positive in 60% (non-specific).
  The presence of either of these antibodies does not predict particular disease manifestations, although nephritis is more common in patients with antibodies to double-stranded DNA.
  (c) Anti-Sm (a ribonuclear protein (RNP) antigen) antibodies are associated with nephritis and CNS involvement.
  (d) Anti-RNP positivity is seen in mixed connective-tissue disease (arthritis, myositis and Raynaud's phenomenon).
  (e) Anti-Ro antibodies may be seen in another form of mixed connective-tissue disease characterised by photosensitivity, arthritis and Sjögren's syndrome.
  Antinuclear antibodies are not a specific test for SLE, they may be elevated in most other rheumatic diseases, autoimmune liver and thyroid disease, in some drug reactions and in a proportion of normal (particularly elderly) individuals. Physicians should therefore be aware that a positive test for antinuclear antibodies is of limited value in support of an uncertain clinical diagnosis.
(2) Anticardiolipin antibodies (may cause a falsely positive Venereal Disease Reserach Laboartoties (VDRL) test).
(3) Lupus anticoagulant (may cause a raised activated partial thromboplastin time).
(4) Serum complement titres will be reduced in the acute phases, especially the C3 and C4 fractions.
(5) The erythrocyte sedimentation rate (ESR) is raised in 90% of cases in the acute phase but conversely the C-reactive protein (CRP) is relatively normal.
(6) There may be thrombocytopaenia (30%), anaemia (partly haemolytic) and leucopaenia.
(7) Urea and electrolytes – 60% of patients will develop renal involvement, which is usually in the form of a nephrotic syndrome. An acute nephritic syndrome and chronic renal failure can also occur.

Q: *How may patients with SLE present to the ophthalmologist?*

A: There are a number of reasons why patients with SLE may present to the ophthalmologist:

(1) Red eyes:
  (a) Secondary Sjögren's syndrome and keratoconjunctivitis sicca.
  (b) Episcleritis.
  (c) Scleritis (rarely).
(2) Decreased visual acuity:
  (a) Branch or central retinal vein occlusions (especially if anticardiolipin positive).
  (b) Hypertensive retinopathy and choroidopathy secondary to renal involvement.
  (c) Retinal vasculitis/optic neuritis may complicate cerebral lupus.
(3) Diplopia:
  (a) Secondary to isolated microvascular IIIrd, IVth or VIth cranial nerve palsies
  (b) Secondary to brainstem cerebrovascular accidents (CVAs)
(4) Referral by rheumatologists to monitor the effects of hydroxychloroquine therapy. This is the most common reason for an ophthalmic opinion in the management of SLE!

Recommended reading

Boupas, D. T., Austin, H. A., III, Fessler, B. J., Balow, J. E., Klippel, J. H. and Lockshin, M. D. (1994) Systemic lupus erythematosus: emerging concepts. Part 1: Renal, neuropsychiatric, cardiovascular, pulmonary, and hematological disease [Review]. *Ann. Intern. Med.*, **122**, 940–950.

Boupas, D. T., Fessler, B. J., Austin, H. A. III, Balow, J. E., Klippel, J. H. and Lockshin, M. D. (1995) Systemic lupus erythematosus: emerging concepts. Part 2: Dermatological and joint disease, the anticardiolipin antibody syndrome, pregnancy and hormone therapy, morbidity and mortality, and pathogenesis [Review]. *Ann. Intern. Med.*, **123**, 42–53.

Mills, J. A. (1994) Systemic lupus erythematosus [Review]. *N. Engl. J. Med.*, **330**, 1871–1879.

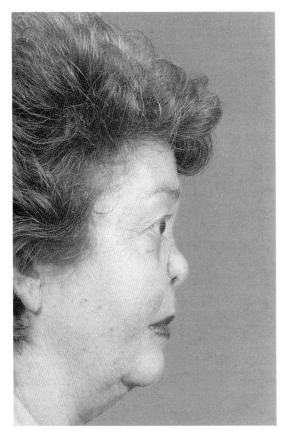

Fig. 5.6a

Q: *Describe the physical signs illustrated by this lateral facial photograph. What is the differential diagnosis? (see Fig. 5.6)*

A: This is an example of a saddle nose deformity. This appearance may be a feature of the following conditions:

(1) Wegener's granulomatosis.
(2) Midline granuloma (a variant of Wegener's granulomatosis with a poor prognosis).
(3) Syphilis.
(4) Leprosy.

This patient does in fact have Wegener's granulomatosis.

Q: *What are the usual presenting features of Wegener's granulomatosis?*

A: Wegener's granulomatosis is a necrotising vasculitis that has a peak incidence in the fifth decade. It is characterised by the triad of upper respiratory tract granulomas, lower respiratory tract granulomas and focal necrotising glomerulonephritis. All three features do not have to be present for the diagnosis to be made as there is often a considerable spectrum of disease severity and the disease may initially be localised.

The following are the most common presenting signs and symptoms of Wegener's granulomatosis:

(1) Pulmonary infiltrates (71%) – less than half of these patients will be symptomatic, e.g. cough, haemoptysis, dyspnoea or pleuritic chest pain.
(2) Sinusitis (67%) – frequently recurrent and only partially responsive to antibiotic therapy. Nasal crusting and epistaxis are typical features.
(3) Arthralgia and fever (44 and 34%, respectively).
(4) Ocular inflammation (16%).
(5) Renal failure (11%).

Q: *What are the ocular manifestations of Wegener's granulomatosis?*

A: Ocular involvement may be the presenting feature of Wegener's granulomatosis and will develop in almost 60% of patients at some point of their illness.

(1) Scleritis, which may be anterior (Fig. 5.6b) or posterior, is the most common ocular manifestation of Wegener's granulomatosis. It frequently occurs in patients who appear systemically well. Ophthalmologists

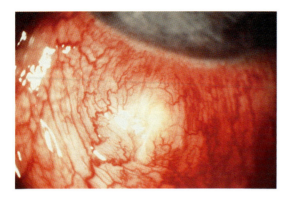

Fig. 5.6b

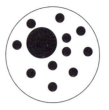

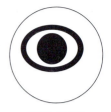

PR3-ANCA

- Coarsely granular and centrally accentuated pattern of IF
- Recognises proteinase 3/myeloblastin

MPO-ANCA

- Artifactual perinuclear staining
- Specific for myeloperoxidase
- Questionable clinical significance

Fig. 5.6c

should therefore have a high index of suspicion and directly question all scleritis patients about the symptoms listed above. The scleritis may progress to involve the cornea.

(2) Orbital involvement – a Tolosa–Hunt orbital apex syndrome with progressive proptosis, external ophthalmoplegia and optic nerve compression has been reported in 20% of patients.

(3) Nasolacrimal obstruction and dacryocystitis secondary to sinus involvement is common.

(4) Retinal vasculitis with or without a posterior uveitis has also been described.

(5) Isolated cranial neuropathies most commonly the VIth and VIIth cranial nerves

Q: *What is the role of antineutrophil cytoplasmic antibodies (ANCA) in the diagnosis and management of Wegener's granulomatosis?*

A: A diagnosis of Wegener's granulomatosis is primarily made on the clinical features and a positive biopsy (nasal mucosa, lung or renal).

ANCAs detected by granular staining of neutrophil on immunofluorescence (IF) microscopy were first shown to be associated with active Wegener's granulomatosis by Van der Woude in 1985. There are two characteristic patterns of immunofluorescence (Fig. 5.6c): cytoplasmic staining, proteinase 3-ANCA (originally described as C-ANCA) and perinuclear staining, myeloperoxidase-ANCA (previously P-ANCA)

PR3-ANCAs are a valuable test in the diagnosis of Wegener's granulomatosis, with a specificity of 90–99% (false-positives have been reported with other systemic vasculitides e.g. microscopic polyangiitis and Churg–Strauss syndrome) and a sensitivity of 80–99% in active classic Wegener's granulomatosis. The sensitivity falls to 60–70% in more limited forms of the disease.

Recently ELISA techniques have been introduced that offer a number of advantages over IF microscopy. They are reader independent, are quantitative and they detect changes more rapidly than IF, which may lag up to 8 weeks behind clinical improvement.

PR3-ANCAs are also helpful in monitoring treatment and detecting relapses. PR3-ANCA titres are raised in vasculitic relapses but not during infection, unlike the CRP, which is elevated in both relapse and infection. As rising titres precede relapses, there is a debate as to whether treatment should be commenced solely on the basis of a rising ANCA titre to prevent relapses.

The role of ANCAs in the pathogenesis of Wegener's granulomatosis remains an area of ongoing debate, theories postulated thus far include:

(1) ANCAs prevent inactivation of a serum protease.

(2) ANCAs alter the differentiation of neutro-
    phils.
(3) ANCAs stimulate unprimed neutrophils.
(4) ANCAs cross-react to initiate vasculitis.

Recommended reading

Fauci, A. S., Haynes, B.F. and Katz, P. (1983)
    Wegener's granulomatosis; clinical and therapeu-
    tic experience with 85 patients over 21 years. *Ann.
    Intern. Med.*, **98**, 76–85.
Ramirez, G. (1990) The ANCA test: its clinical
    revalence. *Ann. Rheumatic. Dis.*, **9**, 741–742.
Savage, C. O. S., Harper, L. and Adu, D. (1997)
    Primary systemic vasculitis. *Lancet*, **349**, 553–558.

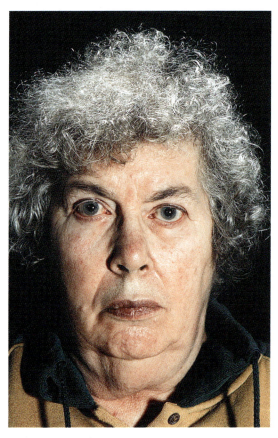

Fig. 5.7

monotonous speech. Progressive fatiguing and diminishing amplitude of repetitive alternating movements are other typical akinetic features.

(2) Rigidity – this may be predominantly unilateral and appears earliest in the neck musculature resulting in the typical 'flexed posture'. The hypertonus is uniform throughout the range of movement affecting agonists and antagonists alike. 'Cogwheeling' may also be demonstrable on passive limb movement.

(3) Tremor – the 'pill rolling' tremor that is present at rest and reduced by voluntary movement has a frequency of 3–5 Hz. It is absent in approximately 30% of Parkinsonian patients. It may be unilateral initially and may also manifest as a pronation-supination movement of the forearm. A faster 6–10 Hz postural tremor may be seen in addition to, or instead of, a classic rest tremor.

(4) Asking the patient to walk a short distance will demonstrate the bradykinesia mentioned above and the typical festinant (hurrying) gait. The blood pressure should also be measured lying and standing to rule out the postural hypotension found in the Shy–Drager syndrome.

Q: *What is the diagnosis? What are the characteristic features of this condition? (see Fig. 5.7)*

A: This is an example of a Parkinsonian facies, typified by the poverty of facial expression. Parkinson's disease is characterised by the triad of:

(1) Upper body akinesia – this is a symptom complex which is present in all cases of true Parkinson's disease, it is comprised of slowness in the initiation and execution of voluntary movements (manifest as the mask-like facies demonstrated above), reduced swinging of the arms while walking, and

Q: *What conditions may cause a pseudo-Parkinsonian state and how can they be distinguished from true Parkinsonism?*

A: A diagnosis of Parkinson's disease is often made erroneously in the following two conditions:

(1) Essential tremor – this differs from true Parkinsonism in a number of ways:
   (a) It is a monosymptomatic disorder with no accompanying akinesia.
   (b) The tremor is evident on posture but is not pill rolling in character. It may be

maximal on terminating a movement and for this reason can be mistaken for a cerebellar intention tremor. Alcohol and β-blockers dampen an essential tremor.

(c) Tremors in the arms, voice, or a tremor of the head on neck may be present. These are not usually seen in true Parkinsonism, although a tremor of the leg at rest or a slow vertical jaw tremor may be present in patients with true Parkinsonism.

(d) There is no lead pipe rigidity but secondary cog-wheeling may be a feature when tone is passively examined.

(2) Arteriosclerotic pseudo-Parkinsonism – this condition is characterised by:

(a) An absence of true Parkinsonism above the waist with an expressive face and voice, spontaneous use of the arms and lack of a rest tremor.

(b) A short stepped (marche à petit pas) wide based gait with postural instability.

(c) Poor or waning response to a trial of levodopa.

Physicians should be aware that some of these features such as atypical walking and balance problems may arise in true Parkinsonian patients with coexisting cerebrovascular disease.

Q: *What are the ocular manifestations of idiopathic Parkinson's disease and its treatment?*

A: The ocular manifestations may be secondary to the disease itself or anti-Parkinsonian medications.

(1) Reduced blink frequency and blepharoclonus are common ocular features.

(2) Oculogyric crises – upward deviation of the eyes often associated with facial flushing, tachycardia and hypertension. Oculogyric crises are more common in cases of drug-induced or postencephalitic Parkinson's disease.

(3) Brainstem lesions may manifest as pupillary abnormalities, ocular motility disturbances or vestibular nystagmus.

(4) Reduced convergence.

(5) Anticholinergic side effects of benzhexol and orphenadrine such as mydriasis, defective accommodation and precipitation of angle-closure glaucoma (in patients with narrowed angles).

(6) Visual hallucinations with or without insight.

Q: *What are the dyskinetic side effects of anti-Parkinsonian medications and how should they be managed?*

A: There are three types of dyskinetic levodopa side effects:

(1) Peak-dose dyskinesia – painless choreic or mobile dystonic movements, usually of the limbs, which occur as an overshoot phenomenon at the peak of effect. This may progress to such an extent that the patient is either off and immobile or on and dyskinetic. It is not a feature of dopamine agonist monotherapy, but may be exacerbated by concomitant anticholinergic medications. Partial replacement with a dopamine agonist such as pergolide may be helpful.

(2) Diphasic dyskinesia – is more common in younger patients, it occurs at the beginning and/or end of the dose, and results in often violent ballistic movements. Again, partial replacement with dopamine agonists may be helpful but patients often resort to taking levodopa three times daily to improve the predictability of these episodes.

(3) Off-period dystonia characterised by fixed and frequently painful dystonic spasms of the feet can be helped by taking the first dose of levodopa (preferably fast acting) on waking. Other alternatives include using a night time controlled-release levodopa or agonist, an anticholinergic or apomorphine injection to turn on rapidly in the morning, or an antispasmodic.

Q: *What drugs have been implicated in drug-induced Parkinsonism?*

A: A number of classes of drugs are known to produce Parkinsonian side effects:

(1) Neuroleptic drugs, such as phenothiazines (chlorpromazine), butyrophenones (haloperidol) and thioxanthines (flupenthixol). These drugs are commonly used as major tranquillisers in psychiatric disorders. The absence of arm swinging and facial amimia are not uncommon findings in many psychiatric patients. However, the development of additional Parkinsonian signs such as truncal akinesia, rigidity and tremor should alert psychiatrists to the potential side effects of these medications. Other pointers to the development of neuroleptic-related Parkinsonism are the presence of akasthesia (motor restlessness), stereotypies and the seemingly paradoxical finding of orofacial dyskinesia in a patient with untreated Parkinsonism. Neuroleptic agents may also be found in combination with antidepressants in preparations such as Motival, Motipress and Parstelin. Prescibing physicians may be unaware of the neuroleptic component of these preparations which are listed as anxiolytics or antidepressants.

(2) Prochlorperazine and metoclopramide may cause acute dystonia.

(3) Cinnarizine (an atypical calcium channel blocker).

There is usually a fairly rapid resolution of these Parkinsonian side effects on discontinuing the causative medication, although in the case of depot neuroleptics the timescale for improvement is months rather than weeks.

Recommended reading

Quinn, N. (1995) Parkinsonism recognition and differential diagnosis [Review]. *Br. Med. J.*, **310**, 447–452.

Quinn, N. (1995) Drug treatment of Parkinson's disease [Review]. *Br. Med. J.*, **310**, 575–579.

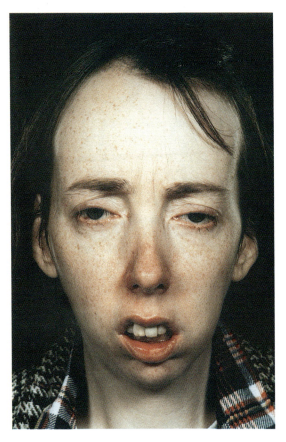

Fig. 5.8a

Q: *Describe the physical signs illustrated in this photograph. What is the diagnosis? (see Fig. 5.8a)*

A: The most striking facial features of this 25-year-old woman are the 'droopy' facial expression with a degree of bilateral ptosis and an unusually high hairline. These features are characteristic of myotonic dystrophy (dystrophia myotonica).

Q: *Clinically how might you confirm the diagnosis of myotonic dystrophy?*

A: In myotonic dystrophy percussion of the thenar eminence will demonstrate delayed relaxation of the muscles and prolonged wrinkling. This phenomenon may also be seen occasionally in patients with polymyositis, polyneuropathy and spinal muscular atrophy. Shaking the patient's hand may reveal the characteristic tonic grip although this is not invariably present and may also be a feature of hypothyroidism. A positive family history in conjunction with the pathognomonic EMG findings of myotonic discharges evoked by movement of the exploring electrode, and myopathic potentials from weakened and wasting muscles during volition, will confirm the diagnosis.

Q: *What are the ocular features of myotonic dystrophy?*

A: Ocular manifestations include:

(1) Presenile cataracts which are predominantly stellate or posterior subcapsular.
(2) Pigmentary retinopathy.
(3) Myotonic ptosis with reduced levator function, and a degree of orbicularis and frontalis weakness in the more severely affected individuals. Surgeons should adopt a conservative approach to ptosis surgery in patients with orbicularis weakness and a reduced Bell's phenomenon if postoperative exposure problems are to be avoided.
(4) Extraocular muscle weakness.

Q: *Clinically how does myotonic dystrophy differ from the non-dystrophic myotonias?*

A: The non-dystrophic myotonias are a heterogeneous group of conditions which include, hyperkalaemic periodic paralysis, paramyotonia congenita and myotonia congenita. Table 5.1 outlines how they differ from myotonic dystrophy.

Table 5.1

Feature	Hyperkalaemic periodic paralysis	Paramyotonia congenita	Myotonia congenita/Thomsen's Becker's	Myotonic dystrophy
Periodic paralysis	Yes	Yes	No/Yes	No
K$^+$-induced weakness	Yes	In some families	No/No	No
Cold-induced weakness	No	Yes	No/No	No
Paradoxical myotonia	Occasional	Yes	No/No	No
Progressive weakness	Variable	Variable	No/Rare	Usual
Multisystem involvement	No	No	No/No	Yes

Q: *What are the genetic features of myotonic dystrophy?*

A: Myotonic dystrophy is inherited as an autosomal dominant trait (as are all the non-dystrophic myotonias with the exception of Becker's) with variable expression. The gene for myotonic dystrophy has been tracked to the long arm of chromosome 19. This gene encodes for a cyclic AMP-dependent protein kinase that is involved with the regulation of ion channels in cell membranes. The more severe congenital form that accounts for 10–15% of cases is invariably inherited through the maternal line. This genomic imprinting is thought to be secondary to the differential expression of maternally and paternally transmitted DNA. The disease phenotype is frequently manifest in a more severe form and at an earlier age in successive generations. This genetic phenomenon is known as anticipation. It is linked to the expression of increasing triplet repeats (adenine–guanine–cytosine (AGC)) in the DNA of patients from successive generations, there being a positive correlation between repeat size and clinical severity. Direct testing for the mutation and the AGC repeat size is now available as a diagnostic tool in difficult cases and for prenatal counselling.

Q: *If this patient was about to have a cataract extraction under general anaesthesia what features of her illness would be of interest to an anaesthetist?*

A: Patients with myotonic dystrophy pose a number of problems for the anaesthetist:

(1) Cardiomyopathy and conduction defects, e.g. 2:1 heart block.
(2) Hypokalaemia or hyperkalaemia.
(3) Glucose intolerance or frank diabetes mellitus.
(4) Myotonic weakness that may manifest as respiratory difficulties following a general anaesthetic.

Testicular atrophy, ataxia and dementia are other features of myotonic dystrophy.

Recommended reading

Pizzuti, A., Friedman, D. L. and Caskey, C. T. (1993) The myotonic dystrophy gene [Review]. *Arch. Neurol.*, **50**, 1173–1179.
Ptacek, L. J., Johnson, K. J. and Griggs, R. C. (1993) Genetics and physiology of the myotonic muscle disorders [Review]. *N. Engl. J. Med.*, **328**, 482–489.

Section 6
Hands

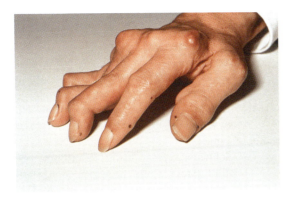

Fig. 6.1a

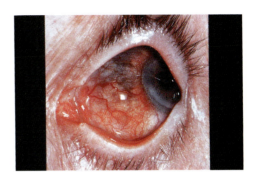

Fig. 6.1b

Q: *What physical signs are demonstrated in this photograph? What is the diagnosis? (see Fig. 6.1a)*

A: This photograph illustrates several features typical of rheumatoid arthritis.

(1) Spindling of the fingers with involvement of the metacarpophalangeal joints. Note that the terminal interphalangeal joints are spared.

(2) There are swan neck deformities of the fourth and fifth digits.

(3) There is a rheumatoid nodule overlying the second metacarpophalangeal joint and five splinter haemorrhages are visible on the first three digits.

Q: *What ocular conditions are associated with rheumatoid arthritis?*

A: The ocular conditions associated with rheumatoid arthritis predominantly involve the anterior segment and include:

(1) Keratoconjunctivitis sicca as part of a secondary Sjögren's syndrome. Dry eye symptoms and/or xerostomia are reported by 20% of patients with rheumatoid arthritis.

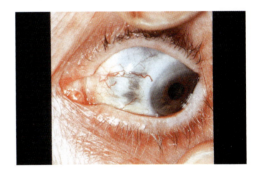

Fig. 6.1c

(2) Episcleritis – this may be nodular or diffuse and normally responds well to topical steroids and/or oral non-steroidal anti-inflammatory drugs (NSAIDs), e.g. froben.

(3) Scleritis – this may be a diffuse or nodular non-necrotising scleritis (Fig. 6.1b), or a necrotising scleritis without inflammation. Most cases of non-necrotising scleritis respond well to NSAIDs or oral prednisolone (Fig. 6.1c). Cases that are unresponsive to corticosteroid monotherapy often require treatment with second-line immunosuppressive agents, such as cyclophosphamide.

Necrotising scleritis (scleromalacia perforans) without inflammation is a painless

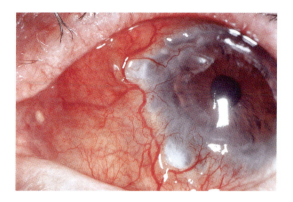

Fig. **6.1d**

condition that results in progressive scleral thinning with marked ischaemia (Fig. 6.1d), although actual perforation is in fact rare.

(4) Peripheral corneal ulcers which tend to be painless and mimic other forms of marginal corneal degenerations.

(5) Keratomalacia is characterised by a central corneal melt and accompanying xerosis. It is most commonly seen in third world children suffering from vitamin A deficiency (with or without measles). Ulceration and perforation may occur.

(6) Iatrogenic effects of treatment:
    (a) Cataracts secondary to corticosteroid therapy.
    (b) Hydroxychloroquine retinopathy (see Question 1.29).

Q: *What are the features of the ocular examination that are of particular relevance in patients with 'dry eyes'?*

A: The tear film is a bi-layered structure consisting of an outer lipid layer produced by the meibomian glands and a much thicker mucin/aqueous layer produced by conjunctival goblet cells and by the main and accessory lacrimal glands, respectively. Patients with 'dry eye' symptoms may have an abnormality of one or a combination of these tear film constituents. Their symptoms may reflect an insufficiency of tear production or an abnormality in the distribution or retention of tears covering the ocular surface. It is therefore essential that all compo-

nents of the tear film are assessed during the ocular examination.

(1) The lipid layer may be affected by meibomian gland dysfunction (inspissated secretions, chalazia, acne rosacea) and blepharitis. When this layer is deficient there is increased evaporation of the aqueous layer.

(2) The aqueous component may be assessed in a number of ways:
    (a) Height of the marginal tear strip between the globe and lower lid (normally 1 mm).
    (b) Schirmer's tests using Whatman #41 filter paper 5 mm in width, placed at the junction of the lateral and middle third of the lower lid. With topical anaesthesia wetting of <5 mm in 5 min is suggestive of aqueous tear insufficiency, <3 mm of wetting is thought to be specific. Without topical anaesthesia wetting of >15 mm in 5 min is considered normal. It should be noted that excess illumination and poor technique are factors that adversely affect the reliability and reproducibility of these tests, the results of which should be interpreted with caution.

The tear film break-up time is assessed by lightly touching the inferior tarsal conjunctiva with a fluorescein strip. After a few blinks the cornea is inspected with a slit-lamp using the cobalt-blue filter and the time from a blink to the appearance of the first corneal dry spot is measured. A tear film break-up time of <10 s is considered abnormal and may be secondary to a deficient mucin or aqueous layer.

(3) The corneal and conjunctival epithelium should also be inspected closely with the aid of fluorescein and Rose Bengal dye. The former will stain areas devoid of epithelium, whilst the latter stains dead and degenerating epithelial cells, mucous threads, plaques, and filaments. As devitalised rather than denuded epithelial cells are characteristic of keratoconjunctivitis sicca,

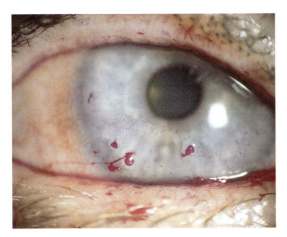

Fig. 6.1e

Rose Bengal demonstrates these epithelial abnormalities more clearly than fluorescein. Figure 6.1e illustrates the pathognomonic interpalpebral zone staining, corneal filaments and mucous plaques seen in keratoconjunctivitis sicca.

(4) Lid margin abnormalities, inadequate lid closure (e.g. VIIth nerve palsy), cicatricial conjunctival disease and reduced corneal sensation are other causes of secondary dry eye.

Q: *What are the treatment strategies for patients with keratoconjunctivitis sicca?*

A: The primary pathology in patients with keratoconjunctivitis sicca is aqueous tear insufficiency. Management options include the following:

(1) Supplementation of the tear film:
  (a) Artificial tear substitutes, e.g. hypromellose, liquifilm, Sno Tears, etc. The half-life in the conjunctival sac is short and frequent applications may therefore be required. Unfortunately sensitivity to preservatives such as benzylkonium chloride and chlorhexidine are common place, and in such cases non-preserved preparations are preferable.
  (b) Hydrogel preparations, e.g. viscotears. This is a gel consisting of the 940 carbomer, which slowly liquefies on contact with the tarsal conjunctiva giving it a half-life in the conjunctival sac seven times that of conventional artificial tear preparations.
  (c) Ointments, e.g. lacrilube or simple ointment, are relatively long acting but cause blurring of vision.

(2) Improving meibomian gland dysfunction with adequate lid hygiene measures, e.g. lid scrubs with dilute solutions of baby shampoo or sodium bicarbonate.

(3) Mechanical removal of mucous filaments and plaques and/or the use of a mucolytic agent such as acetylcysteine.

(4) Reducing nasolacrimal drainage:
  (a) Insertion of silicone lacrimal plugs into the upper and lower cannaliculi.
  (b) Cautery or suturing of the cannaliculi. In cases of severe tear insufficiency this option may be considered after a successful trial of occlusion with lacrimal plugs.

It is important to explain to the patient that chronic tear insufficiency is not curable and that treatment is aimed at controlling rather than eradicating the condition.

Q: *If the patient in Fig. 6.1a were to develop keratoconjunctivitis sicca, what would be the main obstacle to successful treatment?*

A: The treatment of keratoconjunctivitis sicca more than any of the ocular conditions mentioned above requires the frequent and prolonged application of topical medications. Ophthalmologists must take into account the degree of physical deformity and the resultant functional impairment caused by this arthropathy before prescribing a treatment regime that requires a considerable degree of manual dexterity to be carried out successfully!

Q: *What are the extraglandular manifestations of primary Sjögren's syndrome?*

A: Systemic manifestations are commonly seen in patients with primary Sjögren's syndrome. They include the following:

(1) Arthritis/arthralgia – articular signs and symptoms including arthralgias, morning stiffness, intermittent synovitis and chronic polyarthritis occur in 50% of patients. The arthritis, unlike that of rheumatoid arthritis, is non-erosive.

(2) Raynaud's phenomenon (35–40%) – unlike scleroderma, telangiectasias and digital ulcers are uncommon.

(3) Pulmonary involvement (10–20%) – although common is rarely of clinical importance. The spectrum of pulmonary disease varies from a mild lymphocytic infiltrate of the interstitium to severe interstitial fibrosis.

(4) Renal involvement (10–15%) – most patients present with hyposthenuria and hypokalaemia. The distal renal tubular acidosis reflects interstitial lymphocytic infiltration and destruction. If left untreated this may lead to renal calculi, nephrocalcinosis and compromised renal function.

(5) Hepatic involvement (5–10%) – hepatomegaly and/or an elevated alkaline phosphatase is typical, as are the biopsy findings of chronic inflammation of the intrahepatic bile ducts. Sicca manifestations (secondary Sjögren's syndrome) are found in 50% of patients with primary biliary cirrhosis.

(6) Lymphoma (5–8%) – patients with primary Sjögren's syndrome have a 44 times greater risk of developing lymphoma compared with an age-, sex- and race-matched control population. These tend to be primarily of B cell origin and range from the highly undifferentiated to the well differentiated (immunocytomas).

Recommended reading

Foster, H. E., Gilroy, J. J., Kelly, C. A., Howe, F. and Griffiths, I. D. (1994) The treatment of sicca features in Sjögrens syndrome: a clinical review [Review]. *Br. J. Rheumatol.*, **33**, 278–282.

Moutsopoulos, H. M. and Tzioufas, A. (1994) Sjögrens syndrome. In *Rheumatology* (J. H. Klippel and P. Dieppe ed.), pp. 6:27.1–6:27.12. Mosby, St Louis, MO.

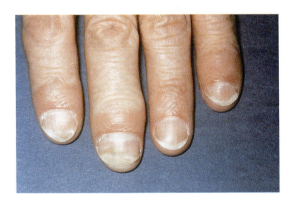

Fig. 6.2

Q: *Describe these digits. What is the most likely diagnosis? (see Fig. 6.2)*

A: The second, third and fifth distal interphalangeal joints are swollen and erythematous. There is evidence of onycholysis (separation of the distal edge of the nail from its vascular bed) and early nail pitting. These findings are typical of psoriatic arthropathy. Other nail changes that may be present in psoriasis are a red/brown or pink discoloration over the nail proximal to the onycholysis and/or nail ridges or furrows.

Q: *What would be the significance of these nail changes in the absence of any dermatological or articular involvement?*

A: These changes may occur in isolation with no evidence of dermatological involvement, although there may be a family history of psoriasis. The significance of these findings lies in their close association with psoriatic arthritis. Nail involvement will be present in 85% of patients with joint disease and in some cases may predate the arthritis. The incidence of nail changes in uncomplicated psoriasis is approximately 20%.

Q: *What are the characteristic features of psoriatic arthritis?*

A: Psoriatic arthritis is a seronegative arthritis that develops in approximately 5–7% of patients with psoriasis. Dermatological involvement may be minimal and a careful inspection of the scalp, natal cleft, feet, tongue and genitalia for signs of psoriasis should be performed. There are several different patterns of arthropathy, these include:

(1) Asymmetrical polyarthritis affecting the small joints of the hands including the distal interphalangeal joints (giving a 'drum-stick' pattern). This is the most common and benign pattern of arthropathy. Approximately 90% of patients with nail changes present with distal interphalangeal arthritis.
(2) Bilateral symmetrical arthritis similar to rheumatoid arthritis.
(3) Rapidly progressive destructive variant (arthritis mutilans).
(4) There is an increased incidence of ankylosing spondylitis.

Q: *What are the treatment options for patients with psoriatic arthritis?*

A: NSAIDs are the treatment of choice for spinal stiffness, pain and persistent synovitis. In recent years methotrexate and sulphasalazine have become the mainstays of treatment for persistent, aggressive joint disease. Although the former is also effective in treating skin disease. Methotrexate is usually administered as a once-weekly oral or parenteral regime (7.5–15 increasing to 25–30 mg); minor side effects such as nausea and stomatitis are common. More serious side effects include bone marrow toxicity, alveolitis and hepatic fibrosis, although the latter has rarely been reported with these intermittent low doses. Some authorities recommend folic acid supplements for all patients on methotrexate. Sulphasalazine is usually given in combination with a NSAID. A starting dose of 0.5–1 g daily is increased over 3–4 weeks to a maintenance dose of 2.0 g daily. Minor side effects include nausea, headache and abdominal discomfort. Bone marrow toxicity and hepatitis are more common in the initial 6 months of treatment; a full blood count and liver function tests should be performed prior to treatment, monthly for 3 months, and then 3- to 6-monthly thereafter.

Gold preparations are more effective in the polyarticular subtype of psoriatic arthritis, rather than the spondylitic or oligoarticular forms. The efficacy of other agents such as colchicine, cyclosporin, bromocriptine and etretinate has yet to be proven in large double-blind trials. There are very few indications for the use of corticosteroids in psoriatic arthritis as the disease usually relapses despite continued treatment.

Q: *What is the significance of these nail changes to the ophthalmologist?*

A: Approximately one-third of patients with psoriatic arthritis will have ocular involvement.

This is usually in the form of conjunctivitis (20%) or anterior uveitis (7%). When confronted with a uveitic patient these nail changes (which may coexist with or predate psoriatic arthropathy) should alert the ophthalmologist to the possible aetiology of the uveitis. As the arthropathy is associated with an increased incidence of HLA B27, the uveitis tends to mimic the pattern seen in ankylosing spondylitis, i.e. predominantly an acute anterior uveitis with fine keratic precipitates. The association of intermediate uveitis, with or without anterior uveitis, and psoriasis is also well recognised.

Recommended reading

Espinoza, L. R. and CuÕllar, M. L. (1994) Psoriatic arthritis: management. In *Rheumatology* (J. H. Klippel and P. Dieppe ed.) pp. 3 33.1–34.4. Mosby, St Loius, MO.

Helliwell, P. S. and Wright, V. (1994) Psoriatic arthritis: clinical features. In *Rheumatology* (J. H. Klippel and P. Dieppe, ed.), pp. 3 31.1–31.8. Mosby, St Loius, MO.

Veys, E. M. and Mielants, H. (1994) Current concepts in psoriatic arthritis [Review]. *Dermatology*, **189**, 35–41.

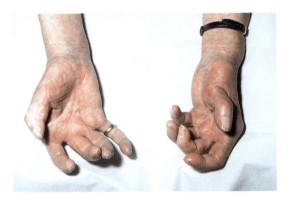

Fig. 6.3

Q: *Describe the physical signs illustrated in this photograph? What condition is this appearance typical of? What features of the history and examination may help confirm this diagnosis? (see Fig. 6.3)*

A: The most striking features are the tight shiny skin, the tapering digits and flexion contractures. This is a severe example of sclerodactyly.

These changes are typical of those found in limited cutaneous scleroderma, formerly known as CR(E)ST syndrome. This condition is a variant of systemic sclerosis.

Limited cutaneous scleroderma consists of:

(1) **C**alcinosis.
(2) **R**aynaud's syndrome is characterised by attacks of bilateral pallor of the extremities (i.e. fingers and toes) precipitated by cold which is followed by cyanosis and finally hyperaemia. Patients often complain of numbness or pain in these areas especially during the re-warming phase.
(3) **O**esophageal motility disturbances may cause dyspepsia, dysphagia, or aspiration pneumonitis.
(4) **S**clerodactyly.
(5) **T**elangiectasia.

(6) Pulmonary hypertension.
(7) Small bowel malabsorption.
(8) Unsightly puckering, wrinkling and thickening of the skin around the mouth. The early phase of the disease (within 10 years of diagnosis) is dominated by the Raynaud's phenomenon and oesophageal symptoms, the other manifestations tending to become apparent in the latter stages of the disease.

Q: *How does diffuse scleroderma differ from the limited cutaneous form?*

A: Diffuse scleroderma accounts for two-thirds of all cases of systemic sclerosis. The history is usually shorter than that of the limited cutaneous form with an abrupt onset of Raynaud's phenomenon associated with fatigue and weight loss. Arthritis, myositis and tendon involvement are common. A fibrotic phase is characterised by extensive skin involvement (with hyper- or hypopigmentation), renal failure, pulmonary fibrosis, and early cardiac and gastrointestinal disease. In the late phase (5 years after diagnosis) constitutional symptoms usually subside although existing visceral disease may continue to progress. Antibodies to scleroderma-70 (topoisomerase-1), although found in 25% of patients overall, are more characteristic of diffuse cutaneous scleroderma. Positive antinucleolar and anticentromere antibody titres are more common in limited cutaneous scleroderma, having a prevalence of 70–80%.

Q: *How can one predict which patients with Raynaud's phenomenon will go on to develop clinical features of scleroderma or other autoimmune rheumatic diseases?*

A: The incidence of Raynaud's disease is 1–5% in women and 0.1% in men. However, only 5% of patients presenting with this condition will develop an autoimmune rheumatic disease or scleroderma. Predictive factors for such a development include:

(1) Biphasic (pallor, cyanosis) or triphasic (pallor, cyanosis, red flush) Raynaud's phenomenon.
(2) Positive antinuclear antibody titres.
(3) An abnormal nailfold capillary bed (detectable by capillaroscopy), tortuous dilated capillaries and areas of atrophy and scarring.

Q: *What could be the relevance of her systemic condition if this lady was found to have bilateral disc cupping, progressive arcuate field defects, 'normal' intraocular pressures (measured over a 24-h period) and normal imaging of the optic nerves and chiasm?*

A: The findings described above are very suggestive of normal tension glaucoma. Factors that predispose to visual field loss in this condition may differ from those found in patients with a raised intraocular pressure. A number of hypotheses linking normal-tension glaucoma with other systemic conditions have been proposed:

(1) Vasospastic syndromes:
   (a) Raynaud's syndrome.
   (b) Migraine.
   The degree of vasospasticity may be quantitatively assessed using laser Doppler techniques to measure alterations in finger-tip blood flow induced by temperature change.

(2) Hypotensive episodes:
   (a) Acute hypotensive crises secondary to haemorrhagic hypovolaemia.
   (b) Nocturnal hypotension in patients currently taking antihypertensive therapy. This has also been implicated in high-pressure glaucoma as a cause of progressive field loss.

Q: *What are the ocular complications of scleroderma?*

A: Approximately 70% of patients with scleroderma will have secondary Sjögren's syndrome manifest in the form of keratoconjunctivitis sicca. Keratitis, conjunctival shrinkage and corneal furrows unrelated to areas of keratitis have also been reported.

Other rare associations include choroidal vasculitis and extraocular myositis.

Recommended reading

Isenberg, D. A. and Black, C. (1995) ABC of Rheumatology. Raynaud's phenomenon, scleroderma and overlap syndromes [Review]. *Br. Med. J.*, **310**, 795–798.
Systemic Sclerosis: Current Pathogenetic Concepts and Future Prospects for Targeted Therapy (1996) Grand Round Report of a Meeting of Physicians and Scientists, Royal Free Hospital School of Medicine London. *Lancet*, **347**, 1453–1458.

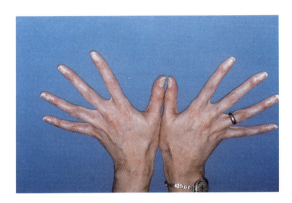

Fig. 6.4a

Q: *Describe these hands. What is the likely diagnosis? What features of the systemic examination would confirm this diagnosis? (see Fig. 6.4a)*

A: These long slender digits are an example of arachnodactyly. The most common association of arachnodactyly is Marfan syndrome. The diagnosis of Marfan syndrome is based on typical clinical features and a positive family history when available:

(1) Tall, thin body habitus with pectus excavatum or carinatum. It should be noted that although disproportionately long limbs are a feature of patients with Marfan syndrome, span exceeds height in 59–78% of normal adult white males and is not therefore a reliable indicator of Marfan syndrome.

(2) Cardiac signs – aortic and mitral regurgitation, aortic aneurysm and dissection, aortic root dilatation, and congestive cardiac failure.

(3) Spine – scoliosis, kyphoscoliosis or thoracic lordosis.

(4) Ocular signs (see below).

(5) Respiratory signs – pneumothorax, pulmonary blebs, and emphysema.

(6) Abdominal signs – inguinal and femoral hernias.

(7) Joints – mild to moderate joint laxity is a common feature. However, signs such as the ability to make a fist around the thumb, which will protrude medial to the little finger, or an overlap between the thumb and index finger when placed around the wrist (Fig. 6.4b), are not specific to Marfan syndrome and are present in many normal individuals.

(8) Narrow highly arched palate with crowding of the teeth.

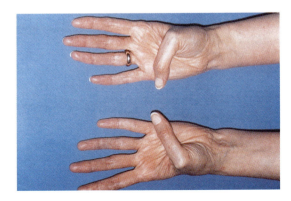

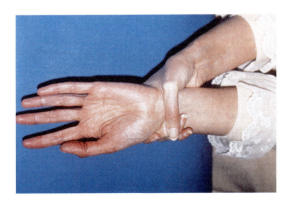

Fig. 6.4b

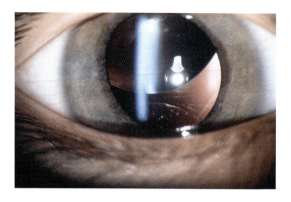

Fig. 6.4c

Typical involvement of at least two of the following systems should be present for the diagnosis to be made: skeletal, ocular and cardiovascular.

Q: *What are the ocular manifestations of Marfan syndrome?*

A: The ocular manifestations of Marfan syndrome include:

(1) Corneal disorders:
   (a) Keratoconus.
   (b) Cornea plana.
(2) Lenticular disorders:
   (a) Classically superotemporal lens subluxation (ectopia lentis) (Fig. 6.4c). Some patients retain excellent vision despite quite dramatic lens subluxation. This may be progressive or non-progressive and accommodation may be maintained.
   (b) Lens opacities.
(3) Glaucoma – secondary to angle anomalies or angle closure due to anterior lens subluxation causing pupil block.
(4) Hypoplastic dilator pupillae muscles, which may compromise the fundal view during retinal detachment surgery.

(5) Axial myopia, vitreoretinal degeneration and retinal detachment.

An ophthalmological opinion is often invaluable in making the diagnosis of Marfan syndrome.

Q: *What is the mode of inheritance and underlying biochemical defect in Marfan syndrome?*

A: Marfan syndrome is inherited as an autosomal dominant trait, variable expression is the rule, but non-penetrance is rare. Approximately one-quarter of affected individuals arise as new mutations. A paternal age effect may be present in sporadic cases. Heterozygosity is the norm but homozygotes have been described.

Fibrillin was discovered in 1986; its presence in the suspensory ligament, aorta and periosteum suggested it may be involved in the pathogenesis of Marfan syndrome. When the majority of patients with Marfan syndrome were found to have a defect in the synthesis, secretion, or incorporation of fibrillin into the extracellular matrix it was proposed as the major candidate protein responsible for the condition. Mapping studies have shown that the gene responsible for Marfan syndrome is an autosomal dominant fibrillin gene mutation located on chromosome 15q (15-q21.3).

Recommended reading

Maslen, C. L. and Glanville, R. W. (1993) The molecular basis of Marfan syndrome. [Review]. *DNA Cell Biol.*, **12**, 561–572.

Wheatley, H. M., Traboulsi, E. I., Flowers, B. E., Maumenee, I. H., Azar, D., Pyeritz, R. E. and Whittum-Hudson, J. A. (1995) Immunohistochemical localization of fibrillin in human ocular tissues. Relevance to the Marfan syndrome. *Arch. Ophthalmol.*, **113**, 103–109.

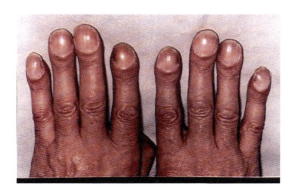

Fig. 6.5a

Q: *What is the physical sign illustrated above? What are the cardinal features of this condition? (see Fig. 6.5a)*

A: This is an example of finger clubbing. A diagnosis of finger clubbing can be made when the following features are present:

(1) Fluctuant nail bed noted on palpation, this is secondary to an increase in the nail bed vascularity.
(2) Loss of the normal angle between the base of the nail and the nail fold. This is the first and most universal sign of clubbing.

(3) Increased curvature of the nail in all directions.

Q: *What conditions causing clubbing are of interest to the ophthalmologist?*

A: Clubbing is most commonly seen in association with suppurative lung disease or cyanotic heart disease, neither of which are of particular relevance to the ophthalmologist. However, there are a number of conditions causing clubbing that may have associated ocular signs, these include:

(1) Subacute infective endocarditis – Roth spots, cranial nerve palsies and retinal embolic episodes.
(2) Inflammatory bowel disease – anterior uveitis associated with Crohn's disease or ulcerative colitis.

Bronchial carcinoma (squamous cell) may in theory produce a Horner's syndrome.

Q: *Describe these changes. How do they differ from the clubbing illustrated above? What is the relevance of this appearance to the ophthalmologist? (see Fig. 6.5b)*

A: There is swelling of the terminal phalanges and increased curvature of the nails in all direc-

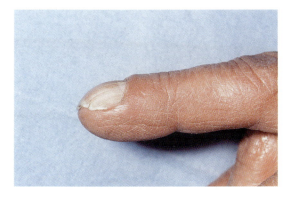

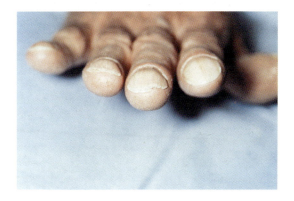

Fig. 6.5b

tions. These changes are secondary to thyroid acropachy. This may be distinguished from 'true' clubbing by the preservation of the normal angulation between the base of the nail and the nail bed. Thyroid acropachy, like pretibial myxoedema, is only seen in association with Graves' disease. Both are associated with the more severe forms of thyroid eye disease.

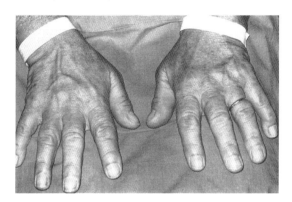

Fig. 6.6a

Q: *Describe the hands of this 56-year-old woman. What is the diagnosis? When taking a history from this patient what questions may help confirm the diagnosis? (see Fig. 6.6a)*

A: The most striking features are the broad fingers and the tight fitting ring. These are the characteristic 'spade-like' hands seen in acromegaly. When shaking the patient's hand they have what is described as a 'doughy' handshake.

The following questions may help confirm the diagnosis of acromegaly:

(1) Have rings become tighter?
(2) Has her shoe size increased?
(3) Has she or her family noted any change in her facial features (old photographs are often invaluable)?
(4) Is there a history of headaches or visual loss?
(5) Lethargy, weight gain, breathlessness and joint pains are all symptoms associated with acromegaly.
(6) Is there a history of polyuria and polydipsia; diabetes may be the initial presentation of acromegaly.

Q: *Once the diagnosis of acromegaly has been confirmed what are the treatment options?*

A: The aims of treatment in acromegaly are symptomatic relief and the restoration of biochemical normality. The large surgical series define 'cure' as growth hormone (GH) levels of <5 µg/l. However, some patients at these levels will still have an elevated insulin-like growth factor (ILGF)-I and there is debate as to whether a level of <2.5 µg/l should be the gold standard for treatment.

Surgery remains the mainstay of treatment and the majority of patients with microadenomas will have GH levels of <2.5 µg/l postoperatively. The success rate for larger intrasellar tumours is lower, with a remission rate of <20% being reported in cases of extrasellar spread. Surgery for these more extensive tumours also carries a 30% risk of postoperative hypopituitarism.

Radiotherapy achieves a satisfactory reduction in GH levels in 90% of patients and prevents recurrence in 99%. However, the response to radiotherapy is slow, with the biggest fall in GH levels occurring in the first 2 years and a slow continuing decline over the following 15 years. Medical suppression of GH should be used in the initial period until GH concentrations fall to a satisfactory level. Up to 50% of patients will develop hypopituitarism and an annual or biannual assessment of pituitary function is recommended. There is also the theoretical risk of long-term radiation damage to the optic nerves and chiasm. Radiotherapy is commonly used postoperatively when GH levels remain >2.5 µg/l and there is an increased concentration of ILGF-1.

The advent of octreotide, a somatostatin analogue, has added a third therapeutic option for the treatment of acromegaly. Variable suppression of GH and ILGF-1 is seen in 90% of patients, with GH levels <5 µg/l achieved in 50% of cases. Octreotide is faster acting than bromocriptine and has proved particularly effective in eliminating headache, and reducing symptoms from joint and cardiac involvement. The disadvantages of this treatment are that it must be given as a three times daily subcutaneous regime and costs £6000 per year. Approximately 20% of octreotide-treated patients will develop gallstones or sludge after 2 years, although these are usually asymptomatic and require no treatment.

Q: *If this patient presented with a sudden history of severe headache followed by a collapse and impaired consciousness, what is the likely underlying pathology and how should she be managed?*

A: In patients with symptomatic or asymptomatic pituitary adenomas the above scenario may be indicative of a haemorrhage into, or an infarct of, the pituitary tumour. This is known as pituitary apoplexy and often results in life threatening hypopituitarism. The clinical presentation of pituitary apoplexy is dependent on the direction of the swelling in the necrotic/haemorrhagic pituitary gland. The MRI in

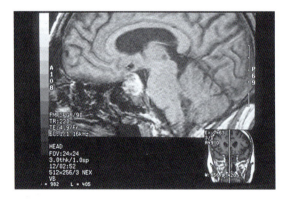

Fig. 6.6b

Fig. 6.6b illustrates haemorrhage within a pituitary adenoma.

A severe headache evolving over a 24- to 48-h period is typical. Chiasmal and cavernous sinus compression may cause rapid visual loss and/or ophthalmoplegia. A reduced level of consciousness is suggestive of diencephalon and midbrain involvement. In rare cases this may be secondary to lateral expansion causing compressing of the carotid arteries, with resultant cerebral infarction.

Initial treatment consists of high-dose corticosteroids, followed by hormonal replacement (panhypopituitarism is the norm) and restoration of normotension. Surgical resection of the tumour should be performed as soon as the patient's medical condition is stable.

Q: *What is the empty sella syndrome?*

A: The empty sella syndrome describes a condition characterised by a sella turcica that is apparently devoid of pituitary tissue this may be due to:

(1) Cisternal herniation caused by a defect in the diaphragma sellae and extension of the subarachnoid space. The pituitary in these cases is usually eccentrically placed or pressed against the floor or roof of the pituitary fossa.
(2) Following infarction of a pituitary tumour (this event may also be asymptomatic). The surprising feature of this condition is that pituitary function is usually normal.

Recommended reading

Acromegaly Therapy Consensus Development Panel (1994) Consensus statement: benefits versus risks of medical therapy for acromegaly [Review]. *Am. J. Med.*, **97**, 468–473.

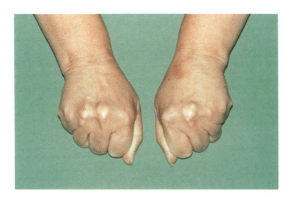

Fig. 6.7a

Q: *What are these lesions and with what condition are they associated? (see Fig. 6.7a)*

A: These firm raised nodules over the metacarpophalangeal joints are tendon xanthomata, note that the skin overlying them is a normal colour and does not appear yellow. They represent localised infiltrates of lipid-containing histiocytic foam cells and collagen deep within the tendons. Along with the Achilles tendon the knuckles are the most common site for tendon xanthomata. These lesions are the diagnostic hallmark of familial hypercholesterolaemia (WHO classification: Primary hyperlipoproteinaemia in which there is hypercholesterolaemia (type IIa)). This occurs in heterozygotes in the third decade and during childhood in homozygotes.

Tendon xanthomata are also associated with two rare metabolic disorders, cerebrotendinous xanthomatosis and phytosterolaemia. They are not found in patients with secondary hypercholesterolaemia.

Q: *What are the causes of secondary hypercholesterolaemia?*

A: Many factors have been implicated in the development of secondary hypercholesterolaemia:

(1) Diet:
    (a) Alcohol.
    (b) Obesity.
(2) Endocrine disease:
    (a) Hypothyroidism.
    (b) Diabetes mellitus.
    (c) Pituitary disease.
(3) Liver disease:
    (a) Primary biliary cirrhosis.
    (b) Porphyria.
(4) Renal disease:
    (a) Nephrotic syndrome.
    (b) Chronic renal failure.
(5) Drugs.

Q: *What are the other ocular sequelae of hyperlipidaemia?*

A: Xanthelasmata are yellowish plaques which commonly involve the skin of the upper and lower eyelids in the medial canthal area. They represent collections of lipid material found in foam cells of the superficial dermis and are usually an idiopathic finding. Occasionally they may be associated with congenital or acquired disorders of cholesterol metabolism.

Lipaemia retinalis (Fig. 6.7b) is a rare ocular association of hyperlipidaemia in which the retinal vessels exhibit a striking sheathed appearance. This may be mistaken for a retinal

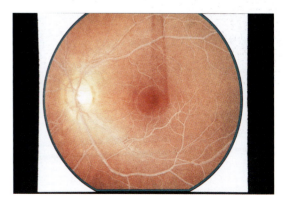

Fig. 6.7b

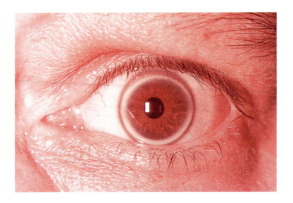

Fig. 6.7c

vasculitis by the inexperienced observer. Hyper-lipidaemia is also a risk factor for the development of retinal vascular disease.

Arcus senilis is characterised by deposition of lipids in the limbal corneal stroma, these first appear at 6 and then 12 o'clock but eventually coalesce to encircle the peripheral cornea (Fig 6.7c).

Unlike the anterior border, the posterior edge of the arcus is well defined and is separated from the limbus by an area of clear cornea. Arcus senilis is almost a universal finding in patients >70 years of age and is not associated with hyperlipidaemia nor hypercholesterolae-mia. Arcus senilis is uncommon in healthy patients <40 years of age and is an independent risk factor for ischaemic heart disease in these patients.

6.8

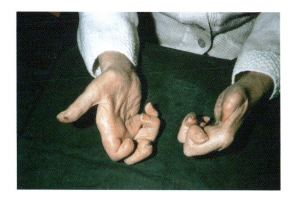

Fig. 6.8a

Q: *Describe the hands of this 65-year-old woman. This patient originally presented aged 30-years-old with pain in her arms that was exacerbated by coughing and exertion. What is the most likely diagnosis? (see Fig. 6.8a)*

A: This photograph illustrates gross claw like contractures of all the fingers and left thumb, with bilateral wasting of the small muscles of the hands. These long-standing deformities may be secondary to:

(1) Bilateral cervical ribs.
(2) Bilateral ulnar nerve palsies (mononeuritis multiplex).
(3) Syringomyelia.

The latter is the most likely diagnosis given that there was a history of upper limb pain exacerbated by exertion. This is the typical presenting complaint of patients with syringomyelia.

Q: *What is the underlying pathology in this condition and what other neurological signs may be present on examining the limbs?*

A: Syringomyelia arises in the presence of an anatomical abnormality at the foramen magnum, which is often associated with birth trauma, spina bifida, Arnold–Chiari malformation or hydrocephalus. This allows the normal CSF pressure waves to be transmitted to the cervical cord and brainstem resulting in cavity formation. The cavity or syrinx thus formed is anterior to, and in continuity with the central canal of the spinal cord. As the cavity slowly expands it gradually impinges on the following:

(1) The spinothalamic tracts in the cervical cord; this produces loss of pain and temperature sensation in the upper limbs. Areas of dissociated sensory loss may also be found over the trunk and upper limbs.
(2) The anterior horn cells resulting in hyporeflexia of the upper limbs.
(3) The lateral corticospinal tracts resulting in a spastic paraparesis which may initially be asymptomatic.

Q: *What symptoms and signs would point to extension of the cavity through the foramen magnum?*

A: Extension of the cavity through the foramen magnum (syringobulbia), may damage the following structures:

(1) Vestibular nuclei causing nystagmus – central vestibular nystagmus may be uni-directional or bi-directional, and is usually purely horizontal. The direction of this jerk nystagmus may change direction with a change in the direction of gaze. Downbeat nystagmus is indicative of extension to the lower brainstem and the foramen magnum.
(2) The XIIth cranial nerve nuclei producing atrophy and fasiculation of the tongue.
(3) The caudal regions of the trigeminal nuclei producing facial parasthesia.
(4) The VIIIth cranial nerve nuclei and tracts resulting in hearing loss.
(5) The sympathetic tracts producing a central Horner's syndrome.

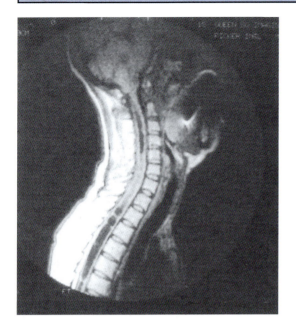

Fig. 6.8b

The investigation of choice in syringomyelia is MRI (Fig. 6.8b) as myelography may cause the cavity to expand resulting in clinical deterioration. Unfortunately there is no curative treatment, although surgical decompression or aspiration of the cysts may be attempted.

6.9

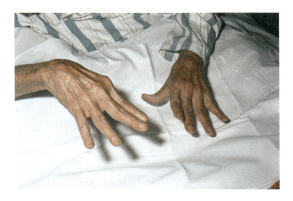

Fig. 6.9

Q: *Describe the physical signs illustrated below. This 70-year-old man had a spastic gait. What is the most likely diagnosis? (see Fig. 6.9)*

A: There is evidence of bilateral wasting of the intrinsic muscles of the hands. This combination of atrophy and weakness in the hands and the upper limbs (plus fasciculation) in combination with hyper-reflexia and spasticity of the lower limbs (in the absence of sensory signs), is highly suggestive of motor neurone disease.

Q: *What are the common patterns of sporadic motor neurone disease?*

A: There are several well-recognised patterns of sporadic motor neurone disease:

(1) Amyotrophic lateral sclerosis (ALS) – this is the most common type (65%) and is characterised by upper motor neurone signs in the lower limbs and lower motor neurone signs in the upper limbs.
(2) Primary bulbar palsy (PBP) 25% – this may be spastic, flaccid or mixed.
(3) Progressive muscular atrophy (PMA) 10% – predominantly lower motor neurone changes.

(4) Familial motor neurone disease – this has been linked to a defect on chromosone 21.

Q: *What are the causes of limb fasciculation other than motor neurone disease?*

A: Fasciculation over a limited area may be seen in the following conditions:

(1) Cervical spondylosis.
(2) Syringomyelia.
(3) Acute stages of poliomyelitis.
(4) Thyroid myopathy.
(5) Polymyositis.

Q: *What is the natural history and treatment of motor neurone disease?*

A: The prognosis for patients with motor neurone disease is poor. The natural history is one of an unrelenting decline with a 50% mortality 3 years from the time of diagnosis. The exact pattern of disease progression is dependent on a number of factors:

(1) Disease subtype – in order of increasing survival: PBP < ALS < PMA.
(2) Age of onset – survival in patients with disease onset before 40 years may be 3.5–4.0 times longer than in those with onset after 60 years.
(3) Pulmonary function – the majority of deaths are secondary to respiratory failure. Until recently no treatment had been shown to alter the natural history of motor neurone disease. A controlled trial of riluzole, an agent that decreases the release of glutamate from nerve terminals, showed significant slowing of loss of muscle strength and a decreased 1-year mortality (especially in the PBP group). Follow-up studies have shown an average increased survival of 3 months and a higher proportion of survivors at 18 months in patients receiving riluzole compared with placebo. Although neurotrophic factors prolong sur-

vival of motor neurones in cell culture, clinical trials have shown that they are only moderately tolerated with no proven benefit in preventing loss of muscle function.

Q: *What are ocular features of motor neurone disease?*

A: Ocular motor function is generally spared in motor neurone disease. The occasional appearance of ocular motor dysfunction in the form of impaired pursuit and saccadic eye movements, probably reflects the incidence of secondary abnormalities such as Parkinsonism.

Recommended reading

Tandan. R. (1994) Clinical features and differential diagnosis of classical motor neuron disease. In *Motor Neuron Disease* (A. C. Williams ed.), pp. 327. Chapman & Hall, London.

Section 7
Skin lesions

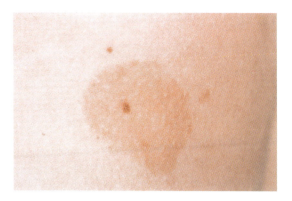

Fig. 7.1a

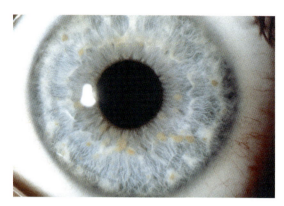

Fig. 7.1b

Q: *What are these skin lesions? (see Fig. 7.1a)*

A: These are examples of café au lait spots. These flat pigmented lesions may range in size from 1–2 mm to >50 cm in diameter. They are usually present at birth or develop in the first year of life.

Q: *How many of these lesions must be present for a diagnosis of neurofibromatosis to be considered? What other pigmented skin lesions may be present in neurofibromatosis?*

A: In a prepubertal person six or more café au lait spots with a diameter of >5 mm (or >15 mm in postpubertal patients) are one of the diagnostic criteria for neurofibromatosis. They are present in 99% of neurofibromatosis patients and may be as large as 50 cm in diameter.

Other pigmentary skin lesions include:

(1) Axillary and inguinal freckles.
(2) Diffuse skin hyperpigmentation.
(3) Large café au lait type lesions overlying a plexiform neuroma.

Q: *What are the ocular pigmentary lesions that may be found in association with neurofibromatosis?*

A:
(1) Lisch nodules are melanotic iris hamartomas (Fig. 7.1b), they are the most common ocular lesions associated with neurofibromatosis. Although they may be detectable at birth their prevalence in neurofibromatosis type 1 (NF1) steadily increases from 50% of 5 year olds to 95% of adults over 25 years old. The presence of two or more Lisch nodules in conjunction with neurofibromata or café au lait spots confirms the diagnosis of neurofibromatosis.
(2) Combined retinal–retinal pigment epithelial hamartomas (Fig. 7.1 c) are more common in neurofibromatosis type 2 (NF2), they are usually solitary grey juxtapapillary lesions with variable pigment and vascularity.
(3) There is an increased incidence of choroidal naevi and possibly of uveal melanomas.

Q: *What are these lesions? (see Fig. 7.1d)*

A: These are examples of neurofibromatas. These lesions may be lobulated or sessile, and either soft or firm. The finding of two or more neurofibromata of any type, or a single plexiform neuroma in combination with café au

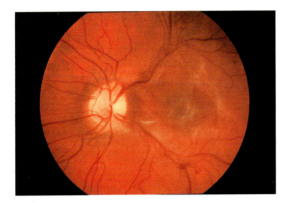

Fig. 7.1c

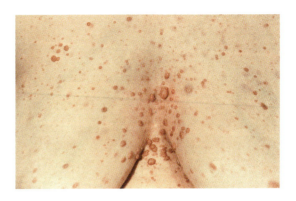

Fig. 7.1d

lait spots or Lisch nodules, is diagnostic of neurofibromatosis.

Eyelid neurofibromatas are usually well-circumscribed lesions, which typically become manifest just before puberty. Plexiform neurofibromata of the lid may be nodular or diffuse. The latter have a characteristic 'bag of worms' texture and are of particular interest to the ophthalmologist as 50% will be associated with glaucoma in the involved eye.

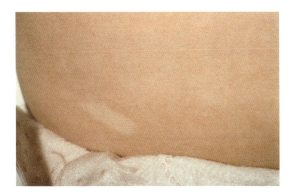

Fig. 7.2a

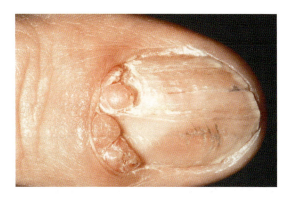

Fig. 7.2b

Q: *What is this lesion? With what condition is it associated? (see Fig. 7.2a)*

A: This is an example of an ash leaf spot. These flat depigmented skin lesions are best visualised with a Woods ultraviolet light. They are pathognomonic of tuberous sclerosis (occurring in 80% of cases) and are the feature most likely to be present in the first year of life.

Q: *What is the classical presenting triad of features associated with tuberous sclerosis? What other lesions are considered to be pathognomonic of this condition?*

A: Tuberous sclerosis or Bournville's disease is a condition that presents in childhood with seizures, mental retardation and specific skin lesions. The following features are thought to be pathognomonic of tuberous sclerosis:

(1) Facial angiofibromas (adenoma sebaceum) in a butterfly distribution over the nose and cheeks. Angiofibromas are rarely present before 2 years of age and may not develop until late adolescence.
(2) Multiple cortical tubers.
(3) Subependymal glial nodules.
(4) Bilateral renal angiomyolipomas.

(5) Ungual fibromas (Fig 7.2b).
(6) Retinal astrocytomas (two or more). See Question 1.27.

If a first degree relative is affected the condition can be diagnosed if any of the following are found:

(1) Shagreen patch or forehead fibrous plaque.
(2) Multiple cardiac rhabdomyomas.
(3) An isolated cortical tuber or retinal astrocytoma.

Q: *What are the genetic features of tuberous sclerosis?*

A: Tuberous sclerosis is a member of the phakomatoses group and is inherited as an irregular autosomal dominant trait. However, approximately two-thirds of cases arise as a result of spontaneous mutations (the risk of normal parents having a second affected child is 25%).

Collaborative studies have established that there is considerable genetic heterogeneity, although a linkage with chromosome 9 and a weaker linkage to chromosome 11 have been proven.

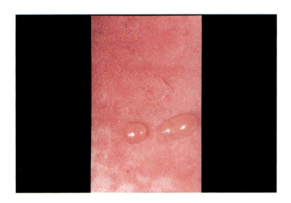

Fig. 7.3a

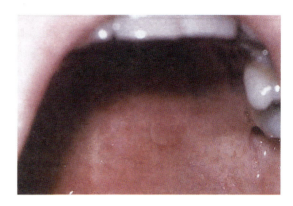

Fig. 7.3b

Q: *What is the diagnosis? (see Fig. 7.3a)*

A: The tense blisters of varying sizes with surrounding areas of erythema and urticaria are characteristic of bullous pemphigoid.

Q: *What are the histological features of these blisters and what is the pathophysiology of their formation?*

A: The tense blisters of bullous pemphigoid arise in the subepithelial layer between the epidermis and the dermis (at the level of the lamina lucida). Immunoflourescence studies demonstrate IgG, IgM, IgA and C3 aggregating at the level of the basement membrane. The basement membrane is thought to be damaged by a type II hypersensitivity reaction mediated by the above immunoglobulins and complement. Anti-basement membrane antibodies are found circulating in 70% of these patients but their exact role in this cytotoxic reaction is unclear. The flaccid thin-roofed blisters of pemphigus arise in the epidermis. Frusemide, clonidine and PUVA have all been associated with the development of bullous pemphigoid.

Q: *What is the association of ocular cicatricial pemphigoid (OCP) with bullous pemphigoid? What are the features of OCP?*

A: OCP is a vesicobullous disease of the mucous membranes. Although the underlying pathology is identical to that of bullous pemphigoid, i.e. subepithelial bullae secondary to cytotoxic destruction of basement membranes, skin involvement is only found in 15% of cases. Other mucosal sites such as the nose, mouth, pharynx, larynx, anus, vagina and urethra may also be involved. There is no significant correlation between the degree of systemic involvement and the visual acuity. In studies of OCP up to 50% of patients had involvement of the oral mucosa (Fig. 7.3b). OCP may also be drug induced; many topical medications have been implicated. Prolonged treatment with propine is the most common cause of drug-induced OCP.

The primary ocular lesion is a chronic cicatrizing conjunctivitis. Transient conjunctival bullae result in subepithelial fibrosis and scarring with destruction of goblet cells, shortening of the inferior fornices (Fig. 7.3c) and symblepharon formation (Fig. 7.3d).

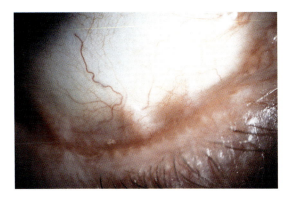

Fig. 7.3c

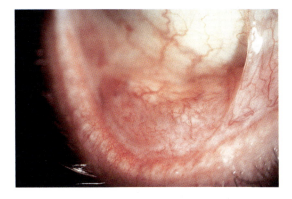

Fig. 7.3d

If this cycle of bullae formation and cicatricial changes continues the lacrimal ductules may become involved resulting in an aqueous and mucinous tear insufficiency with subsequent conjunctival keratinization. Persistent epithelial defects, limbal inflammation and ongoing conjunctival inflammation are important factors that lead to keratopathy. End-stage disease is characterised by entropion formation, trichiasis with corneal scarring and ulceration. The visual prognosis even with treatment is poor, approximately one-third of patients becomes legally blind.

Q: *What investigations may help you confirm the diagnosis of OCP?*

A: Inferior forniceal shortening, with fine gossamer-like white linear opacities in the deep conjunctiva, and associated oral mucosal lesions are very suggestive of OCP. Scraping of the conjunctiva may reveal eosinophils so helping to confirm the diagnosis. Biopsies should be avoided if possible as surgical manipulations and trauma can promote conjunctival scarring. Before considering conjunctival biopsy the ophthalmologist should be aware that the absence of immunoglobulin and/or complement deposition at the epithelial basement membrane does not rule out OCP, and that these changes may be seen in the active phase of other conjunctival diseases of other causes.

Q: *What are the treatment options for patients with OCP?*

A: If untreated the visual prognosis for patients with OCP is dismal. The principles of treatment for OCP are as follows:

(1) Copious preservative free lubrication with or without punctal occlusion in cases of severe tear insufficiency.
(2) High water content contact lenses may be useful in patients with persistent epithelial defects and trichiasis.
(3) Conjunctival sparing lid surgery for entropion, e.g. Jones procedure for inferior entropion. Electrolysis to eliminate distichiasis and trichiasis.
(4) Aggressive treatment of any staphylococcal lid disease with topical antibiotics or ointments and lid hygiene measures.
(5) Topical steroids alone are ineffective in preventing disease progression.
(6) Systemic immunosuppression – approximately 75% of cases will require immunosuppressive therapy, agents used include:
    (a) Prednisolone – used in approximately 30% of cases.
    (b) Dapsone – the current drug of choice for moderate to marked ocular inflammation. Partial or complete

improvement of ocular inflammation has been reported in 70% of cases, but long-term control (>3 years) is only achieved in 45% of cases.

(c) Sulphapyridine – a 50–56% success rate in preventing progression of cicatrisation in moderate to marked OCP has been reported.

(d) Cyclophosphamide is usually reserved for severe OCP.

Q: *What is the mechanism of action of dapsone? What are the side effects of dapsone and how should patients be monitored?*

A: Dapsone is a sulphone that inhibits the myeloperoxidase enzyme system of neutrophils, so inhibiting their migration. It also stabilises lysosomal membranes. The clinical response in OCP is mainly due to this suppressive effect on neutrophil migration. The most significant side effect is chronic haemolysis with 95% of patients having a 1.0–3.4 g/dl decrease in haemoglobin. Nausea (20%), abdominal pain (10%), peripheral neuropathy (5%) and hepatitis (5%) have also been reported. Monitoring for patients taking dapsone should include monthly:

(1) Full blood count with differential.
(2) Liver function tests.

Recomended reading

Elder, M. J., Leonard, J. and Dart, J. K. (1996) Sulphapyridine – a new agent for the treatment of ocular cicatricial pemphigoid. *Br. J. Ophthalmol.*, **80**, 549–552.

Elder, M. J., Bernauer, W., Leonard, J. and Dart, J. K. (1996) Progression of disease in ocular cicatricial pemphigoid. *Br. J. Ophthalmol.*, **80**, 292–296.

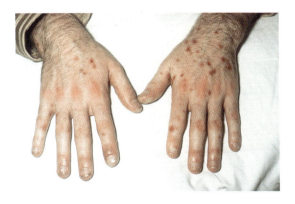

Fig. 7.4a

Q: *Describe the lesions on the wrists and hands of this 45-year-old man. What is the most likely diagnosis? (see Fig. 7.4a)*

A: There are numerous concentric target lesions with central erythema surrounded by a pale ring and then a red ring, a few frank bullae are also present. These lesions are the classical ones seen in erythema multiforme.

Q: *What are the other clinical features of erythema multiforme?*

A: Erythema multiforme is an immune complex-mediated vasculitis that predominantly affects children, teenagers and young adults. The clinical manifestations of this condition are extremely variable. Initial symptoms include fever, malaise, arthralgia and upper or lower respiratory tract infections. Skin involvement occurs 2–3 days later (if the condition is confined to the skin it is known as erythema multiforme minor), and this may be followed by mucous membrane involvement including the mouth, eyes and genitalia (this is known as erythema multiforme major or Stevens–Johnson syndrome). The acute phase lasts 2–3 weeks in the minor type and 5–6 weeks in the major variant. In the latter, ocular involvement is frequently severe. A mucopurulent conjunc-

tivitis with associated membrane formation is seen in the acute phase during which adhesions between the lids and bulbar conjunctiva may form. Secondary bacterial infection and late scarring lead to lid margin abnormalities, trichiasis and chronic tear insufficiency. All of which contribute to corneal epithelial breakdown, ulceration and scarring.

Q: *How should patients with the Stevens–Johnson syndrome be managed?*

A: Stevens–Johnson syndrome is a potentially fatal condition and all patients should be admitted to hospital for supportive care during the acute phase of the illness. Careful monitoring of fluid balance, respiratory function and nutritional requirements are essential. The role of corticosteroids remains controversial. Some studies suggest that systemic corticosteroids arrest the necrolysis, whilst others show no beneficial effect. Antibiotics are in the main reserved for cases where there is culture-positive sepsis.

The mainstays of ocular treatment in the acute phase are copious preservative free lubricants and topical steroids. Preservative-free topical antibiotics should be administered to prevent secondary infection and cycloplegics to alleviate ciliary spasm. Separation of conjunctival adhesions with a glass rod in an effort to prevent symblepharon formation is commonly performed but is rarely effective.

Q: *What factors have been implicated in the development of erythema multiforme?*

A: The exact aetiology of erythema multiforme is unknown, possible predisposing factors include:

(1) Infections:
 (a) Type 1 Herpes simplex (30% of cases).
 (b) Streptococcal infection.
 (c) *Mycoplasma pneumoniae*.

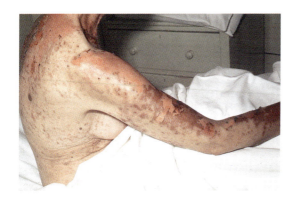

Fig. 7.4b

(d) Tuberculosis, yersiniosis and histoplas-
    mosis are rare associations.
(2) Drugs:
    (a) Sulphonamides are the most commonly
        implicated medications.
    (b) Sulphonylurea derivatives, e.g. chlor-
        propamide.

(c) Penicillin, ampicillin and isoniazid.
(d) Anticonvulsants.

Q: *What other conditions can produce similar
skin lesions?*

A: The differential diagnosis for these skin
lesions should include:

(1) Toxic epidermal necrolysis (TEN) – this
    condition is characterised by interepithelial
    bullae and extensive sloughing of the epi-
    dermis (Fig. 7.4b). Hence the inflammation
    is more superficial and produces less scar-
    ring, although conjunctival scarring does
    occur. Target lesions may be present at
    the margins of necrotic lesions.
(2) Scalded skin syndrome – this is a subgroup
    of toxic epidermal necrolysis believed to be
    caused by an exfoliative toxin produced by
    Staphylococcus aureus (phage group II type
    71).

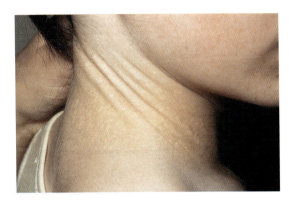

Fig. 7.5a

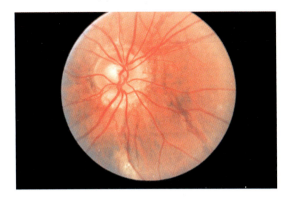

Fig. 7.5b

Q: *What is the underlying disorder?*
(see Fig. 7.5a)

A: The skin of the neck has the typical 'chicken-skin' appearance of pseudoxanthoma elasticum. A similar appearance, along with redundant folds of skin, may also be present in the axillae, groin and antecubital fossae. Pseudoxanthoma elasticum is a disorder of elastin that may be inherited as an autosomal dominant or recessive trait.

Q: *What are the other systemic associations of pseudoxanthoma elasticum? What simple investigations should be performed in the clinic?*

A: Cardiovascular and musculoskeletal anomalies are commonly found in patients with pseudoxanthoma elasticum.

(1) Cardiovascular examination:
  (a) Blood pressure; 50% of these patients will have renovascular hypertension.
  (b) Peripheral pulses may be weak or absent as a result of peripheral vascular disease.
  (c) Pansystolic murmur of mitral incompotence.
(2) Musculo-skeletal examination:

(a) Joint hyperextensibility.
(3) Investigations:
  (a) ECG – ischaemic heart disease is a common association.
  (b) Faecal occult bloods to detect gastro-intestinal haemorrhage.
  (c) Urine testing to check for evidence of genitourinary haemorrhage (pulmonary haemorrhage may also occur).

Q: *What are the ocular associations of pseudoxanthoma elasticum?*

A:

(1) Angioid streaks represent breaks in a thickened and calcified Bruch's membrane. They are visible as irregular dark red or brown streaks that radiate from the optic nerve head (Fig. 7.5b).
(2) Angioid streaks are present in 60% of patients with pseudoxanthoma elasticum, this association is known as the Grönblad–Strandberg syndrome. The major sight threatening complication of these lesions is choroidal neovascularisation and subretinal neovascularisation, via the breaks in Bruch's membrane. Unfortunately laser photocoagulation either as a prophylactic measure or to treat established

neovascular membranes is in the main unsuccessful. The risk of neovascularisation may be increased following relatively minor blunt ocular trauma, which can produce an extension of the breaks in Bruch's membrane.

(3) 'Peau d'orange' appearance of the peripheral fundus describes the stippled appearance often seen in pseudoxanthoma elasticum.

(4) Peripapillary choroidal atrophy.

(5) Optic disc drusen – if buried these may cause the appearance of pseudopapilloedema. Rarely neovascular membranes may be associated with these drusen.

Q: *What other conditions are associated with angioid streaks?*

A: Although pseudoxanthoma elasticum is the most common association of angioid streaks they may also be found in the following conditions:

(1) Ehlers–Danlos and Marfan syndromes.
(2) Sickle cell disease and thalassaemia.
(3) Paget's disease.

It should be noted that 50% of patients with angioid streaks will have no associated systemic disorders.

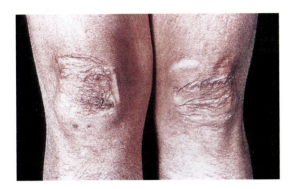

Fig. 7.6a

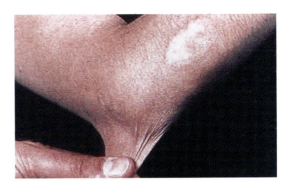

Fig. 7.6b

Q: *What is the diagnosis? What features of the musculoskeletal examination will help you confirm this diagnosis? (see Fig. 7.6a)*

A: This is an example of the 'cigarette paper' skin. seen in the Ehlers–Danlos syndrome. This syndrome arises as a result of a defect in type III collagen production. There are at least nine distinct subtypes of Ehlers–Danlos syndrome, the severity of which varies as does the mode of inheritance. Autosomal dominant, recessive and X-linked recessive pedigrees have all been reported.

A prominent feature of this condition is joint hyperextensibility, which often results in recurrent dislocations of the shoulders, hips and patellae. Kyphoscoliosis and genu recurvatum are other common features. A hypochromic microcytic anaemia, secondary to gastrointestinal haemorrhage from friable telangiectatic mucosal vessels, is also well described.

Q: *What features of the skin involvement in Ehlers–Danlos syndrome distinguish it from those seen in cutis laxa?*

A: In both of these conditions the skin is hyperextensible (Fig. 7.6b). However, in Ehlers–Danlos the elasticity of the skin is preserved, whereas in cutis laxa this elasticity is lost and the skin tends to hang in folds. In the former condition there may also be evidence of thin scars over the knees and elbows caused by relatively minor trauma. Pseudotumours produced by calcification of organised haematomas may also be present. Joint hyperextensibility is not a feature of cutis laxa.

Q: *What are the ocular features of Ehlers–Danlos syndrome?*

A:

(1) Lid signs:
   (a) Epicanthic folds.
   (b) Easy lid inversion (Metenier's sign).
(2) Corneal signs:
   (a) Microcornea.
   (b) Keratoconus.
   (c) Myopia.
(3) Blue sclera.
(4) Ectopia lentis.
(5) Retinal detachments.
(6) Angioid streaks.

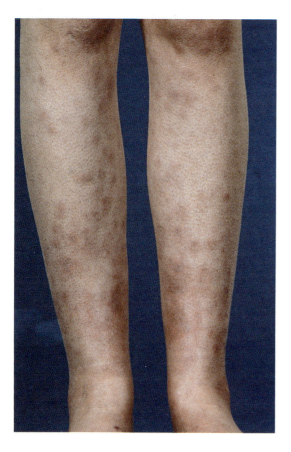

Fig. 7.7a

(1) Infectious conditions:
   (a) Haemolytic streptococcal upper respiratory tract infection is the most common cause of erythema nodosum in the UK.
   (b) Mycobacterial infections, e.g. tuberculosis and leprosy are the most common causes in developing countries.
   (c) Chlamydial infections, e.g. lymphogranuloma venereum and psittacosis.
   (d) Other infectious conditions associated with erythema nodosum include tuleraemia, cat-scratch disease and coccidioidomycosis.
(2) Sarcoidosis – 24–34% of Caucasian patients with sarcoidosis present with erythema nodosum.
(3) Inflammatory bowel disease – approximately 5–10% of patients will develop erythema nodosum.
(4) Drugs:
   (a) Sulphonamides.
   (b) Oral contraceptive pill.
(5) Idiopathic – in 50% of cases no underlying cause is found.

This patient had a recent history of a swinging fever and polyarthralgia, she was found to have bilateral hilar lympadenopathy and a presumptive diagnosis of sarcoidosis was made.

Q: *What is the diagnosis? What are the possible aetiologies of this condition? (see Fig. 7.7a)*

A: The nodules and plaques on the skin over the shins are the typical findings of erythema nodosum. This is an acute painful panniculitis in which the nodules or plaques appear in crops over 12 weeks and slowly fade leaving a mottled staining of the skin. There is often a concurrent malaise, fever and arthralgia. Erythema nodosum may also be found on the thighs and arms. It has a number of well-recognised associations:

Q: *In cases of suspected sarcoidosis what further investigations are indicated if the history, clinical and radiological findings are not as characteristic as in the above case?*

A: In cases where the diagnosis of sarcoidosis is in doubt because of atypical clinical/radiological features and/or in patients for whom corticosteroid therapy is being considered, corroborative histological evidence should be sought.

Lung parenchymal involvement may be confirmed by the following investigations:

(1) Transbronchial biopsy – mononuclear (T cell) infiltration of alveolar walls and the interstitial spaces with or without non-caeseating granulomas. This will be positive in 90% of cases even if the chest X-ray is normal. It has replaced the less specific and less sensitive Kveim test as the investigation of choice in sarcoidosis.

(2) Broncho-alveolar lavage – increased numbers of CD4 lymphocytes and reduced alveolar macrophages and B lymphocytes are found in cases of active pulmonary sarcoidosis. This lymphocyte cell profile although characteristic of sarcoidosis is not diagnostic, as pulmonary lymphocytosis may be demonstrated in active pulmonary tuberculosis and extrinsic allergic alveolitis.

Skin, conjunctival lesions, and superficial lymph nodes that show clinical signs of involvement are also convenient sites for biopsy.

Other investigations in cases of suspected sarcoidosis include:

(1) Serum angiotensin-converting enzyme (ACE) – elevation of the serum ACE two standard deviations above the mean value is seen in 75% of patients with sarcoidosis. It is seldom elevated in early subacute sarcoidosis but levels tend to rise in clinically active disease. However, the test is not specific to sarcoidosis as less elevated titres may also be seen in atypical mycobacterial infections, asbestosis, silicosis and lymphoma. An elevated serum ACE has also been reported in association with alcoholic liver disease, diabetes mellitus and hyperthyroidism.

(2) Serum calcium and a 24-h urine collection to measure urinary calcium excretion should be performed.

(3) The tuberculin test series up to a concentration of 1:100 will be negative in two-thirds of patients with sarcoidosis.

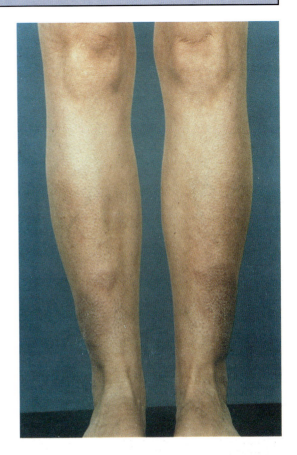

Fig. 7.7b

Q: *Describe the skin changes illustrated above. What is the diagnosis? (see Fig. 7.7b)*

A: There are bilateral raised, symmetrical lesions over the shins. The overlying skin is shiny and has an orange peel appearance. These changes are typical of pretibial myxoedema. This condition is only found in association with Graves' disease (5% of cases) and is secondary to the deposition of mucopolysaccharide and hyaluronic acid in the superficial layers of the skin by dermal fibroblasts. It is associated with smoking and with more severe forms of thyroid eye disease.

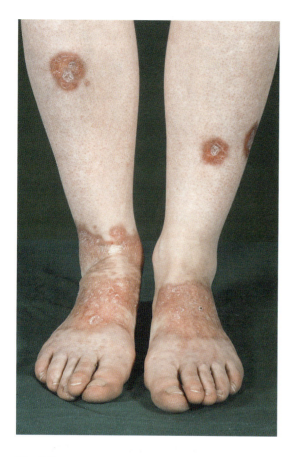

Fig. 7.8a

Q: *Describe this lesion. What is the diagnosis? (see Fig. 7.8a)*

A: There are pigmentary changes over the shin with areas of fibrosis and scarring, the blood vessels of the skin are also clearly visible.

These are the characteristic changes of necrobiosis lipoidica. These painless lesions are typically found on the anterior aspects of the lower leg, vary from 2–8 cm in length and are most commonly seen in insulin-dependent diabetics between the ages of 15–40 years.

Q: *What is the underlying pathophysiology of this condition and how does it correlate with the degree of diabetic retinopathy?*

A: A microangiopathy is thought to be the underlying pathological change in this condition. Occlusion of the small vessels to the dermis results in partial necrosis of the dermal collagen and connective tissues with subsequent macrophagic infiltration. Necrobiosis lipoidica is a relatively uncommon complication of diabetes and its presence does not appear to correlate with the development of small vessel disease elsewhere such as retinopathy or nephropathy.

Q: *What is illustrated in Fig. 7.8b*

A: This is an example of diabetic dermopathy which is commonly found over the shins of diabetic patients. Although the lesions are initially erythematous and papular they eventually flatten with time, becoming pigmented and atrophic. Unlike necrobiosis lipoidica these changes are associated with microangiopathy elsewhere.

The hyperpigmentation seen over the shins in chronic venous insufficiency (which may coexist with diabetes) may mimic the changes illustrated above, although fibrosis and scarring will not be present.

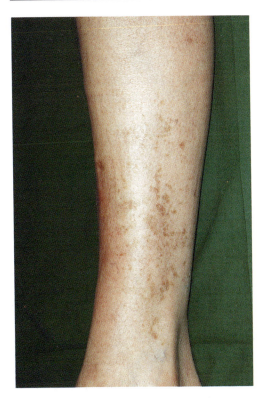

Fig. 7.8b

Q: *Describe these feet. (see Fig. 7.8c)*

A: Three toes have been amputated from the right foot, there is also evidence of critical ischaemia of the third toe on the left foot. These findings are typical of diabetic foot disease.

Q: *What pathological factors will contribute to the development of diabetic foot disease.*

A: Diabetic foot disease arises due to a combination of the following factors:

(1) Neuropathy – loss of sensation to light touch, pinprick and vibration in a stocking distribution.
(2) Microvascular disease – this will contribute to the poor local perfusion of tissue caused by large vessel disease. It is also in part responsible for the development of the neuropathy. Autonomic neuropathy may also contribute to a disturbed pattern of blood flow.

(3) Macrovascular disease – large vessel disease is an important factor in critical limb ischaemia. The absence of the pedal pulses is a bad prognostic sign.
(4) Trauma and friction caused by foot deformities and ill-fitting footwear.
(5) Glycosaemia – this provides an ideal environment for replicating microbes.

Q: *What features will distinguish a neuropathic from an ischaemic foot?*

A: Although most diabetic foot disease is due to a combination of the above factors some cases are predominantly neuropathic and others predominantly vascular in origin. Features that will help differentiate the two include:

(1) History:
  (a) Claudication and rest pain suggest a vascular aetiology.
  (b) If a neuropathic foot is painful, this discomfort is not exercise dependent.
(2) Examination:
  (a) Cold pulseless feet versus warm feet with bounding pulses.
  (b) High arches and clawing of the toes is suggestive of a neuropathic problem.
  (c) Painful ulcers over the heels and toes are more common in ischaemic cases, painless plantar ulcers are more typical of neurotrophic feet.

Q: *What are the other causes of a painful peripheral neuropathy?*

A:

(1) Subacute combined degeneration of the cord secondary to vitamin B12 deficiency and alcohol. Pain in the calves (not related to exercise) and burning feet are common symptoms.
(2) Hereditary sensory neuropathy is characterised by mutilating ulcers on the extremities.
(3) Arsenic.
(4) Cryoglobulinaemia.
(5) Lyme disease – 30% of these patients will develop a reversible peripheral nerve disorder, e.g. Bell's palsy and painful radiculopathies.

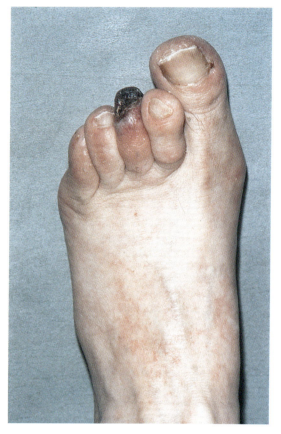

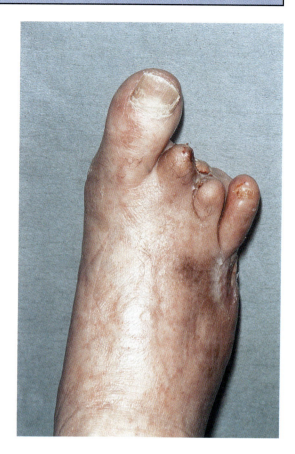

Fig. 7.8c

Q: *Describe the ankle of this diabetic patient. What would you expect to find on examination of this joint? (see Fig. 7.8d)*

A: There is gross deformity and swelling of the ankle joint; on examination one would expect to find an abnormal range of movement associated

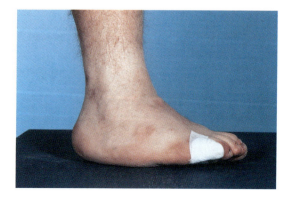

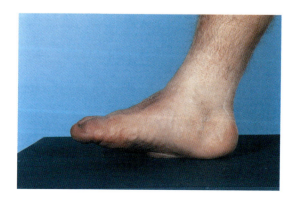

Fig. 7.8d

with painless crepitus. This is a typical example of a Charcot's joint (neuropathic arthropathy).

Q: *What condition characteristically produces Charcot's joints in the upper limbs?*

A: In theory any condition that reduces the sensation of a joint could predispose it to develop a neurotrophic arthropathy. Charcot's joints are usually found in the lower limbs (e.g. diabetes and tabes dorsalis); joints of the upper limbs, i.e. the shoulders and elbows, are characteristically involved in syringomyelia.

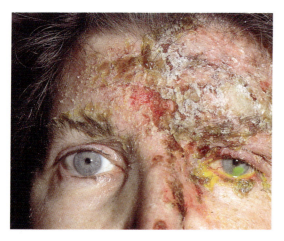

Fig. 7.9

Q: *What is the diagnosis? What features of this rash are of particular interest to the ophthalmologist? (see Fig. 7.9)*

A: This is the characteristic crusting rash of Herpes zoster (shingles) involving the ophthalmic division of the trigeminal nerve. This dermatome is affected in 7–17% of all cases of Herpes zoster. Lesions of the skin on the lateral aspect of the nose signals external nasal nerve and therefore anterior ethmoidal and nasociliary nerve involvement. The nasociliary nerve supplies a large proportion of the sensory innervation to the eye and hence a rash in the external nasal distribution (Hutchinson's sign) may point to potential ocular involvement with Herpes zoster.

Q: *What is the role of systemic antivirals in the treatment of Herpes zoster ophthalmicus (HZO)?*

A: The underlying pathology in both the dermatological and ocular manifestations of shingles is characterised by a pervasculitis and perineuritis. There is little evidence to suggest that actively replicating virus is responsible for the damage to the ocular tissues. There are therefore few indications for systemic antiviral agents such as acyclovir or famciclovir; however, systemic treatment is indicated in the following situations:

(1) If a patient presents within 48–72 h of developing discomfort and parasthesia in the area of the rash, there is some evidence that a 7-day course of antiviral therapy will reduce the incidence of post herpetic neuralgia (famciclovir may be given as a single daily dose in Herpes zoster). However, if the rash is well established with visible crusting antiviral treatment is unlikely to be beneficial.

(2) Optic nerve involvement is an indication for treatment with high-dose prednisolone (80 mg/day decreasing rapidly over 1 week) with intravenous acyclovir. Involvement of the oculomotor nerves (e.g. IIIrd, IVth or VIth nerve palsies) are not uncommon but usually resolve spontaneously and do not require corticosteroid treatment. Aberrant regeneration following a IIIrd nerve palsy secondary to Herpes zoster has been reported.

Q: *What are the common causes of a red eye in a patient presenting with acute HZO?*

A: The following are the most common causes of a red eye in association with acute Herpes zoster ophthalmicus:

(1) Conjunctivitis – treat with topical antibiotic for one week to prevent secondary bacterial infection.

(2) Keratitis – the raised pseudo-dendritic lesions are easily distinguished from true dendritic ulcers secondary to Herpes simplex infection. They are usually self-limiting and require no treatment. Nummular keratitis is more common in young people and may require treatment with low dose topi-

cal steroids when active. Mucous plaque, neurotrophic, stromal and disciform keratitis are late corneal complications of HZO.

(3) Episcleritis – this is a common association with HZO and is in general self-limiting although oral flurbiprofen may be beneficial.

(4) Iritis (with or without raised intraocular pressure, with or without sectorial iris atrophy) – this condition may be self-limiting but in the more severe cases topical steroids and cycloplegics without acyclovir cover are the treatment of choice.

Once topical steroid therapy is commenced, be it for corneal disease or iritis, it may be difficult to wean patients off treatment. Long-term low-dose topical therapy may be necessary. In some patients one drop of predsol weekly may be enough to maintain corneal disease in remission. There is no evidence that the use of topical acyclovir influences the natural history of the acute or chronic sequelae of HZO mentioned above.

Q: *How would your management change if the above patient were a 30-year-old man?*

A: Shingles is a condition that predominantly occurs in elderly patients, although it is not uncommon in healthy young adults and children. However, in such cases the physician should consider the possibility of underlying immunosuppression. In these patients a full current and past medical history should be attained with the emphasis on the following features:

(1) HIV risk factors, e.g. intravenous drug abuse, homosexuality, haemophilia or blood transfusions. The pros and cons of HIV testing should be discussed with such patients.

(2) Recent weight loss, lethargy or infections that may point to an underlying haematological disorder such as lymphoma. A full blood count is probably advisable even if there is no significant history to suggest the above.

(3) Iatrogenic immunosuppression, e.g. chemotherapy or transplant patients.

(4) Immunocompromised patients with HZO should receive a full 7-day course of oral acyclovir 800 mg 5 times a day. Recurrent Herpes zoster in immunocompromised patients should be treated with intravenous acyclovir 5–10 mg/kg t.d.s. for at least 10 days.

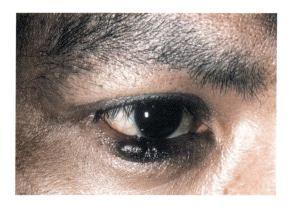

Fig. 7.10

Q: *What is the diagnosis? (see Fig. 7.10)*

A: This is an example of a Kaposi's sarcoma, a malignant vascular tumour that in this case involves the lower eyelid. The distinctive purple hue helps to distinguish it from other innocent lid lesions such as a chalazion.

Q: *Where else may Kaposi's sarcoma be found?*

A: This tumour was first described as a chronic slow growing cutaneous lesion found on the legs of elderly Mediterranean fishermen (classical form). However, a more aggressive variant is now frequently seen in immunosuppressed patients, especially those who are HIV-positive. The condition is usually a multifocal one with multiple sarcomas found over the face, trunk and to a lesser extent the limbs. These tumours often begin as small flat red or violet patches that gradually become more raised and nodular. Up to 40% of patients will also have gastrointestinal or pulmonary involvement, this is usually asymptomatic but can cause gastrointestinal haemorrhage/obstruction or dyspnoea. Palatal involvement is common; the initial lesions are typically found on the hard palate adjacent to the second molar.

Q: *At what stage of their illness do patients with HIV infection develop Kaposi's sarcoma? What are the treatment options?*

A: Kaposi's sarcoma is second only to pneumocystis pneumonia as the most common presenting AIDS defining illness (25% of patients). It is more prevalent in homosexual men with AIDS than those infected by other routes.

Treatment of Kaposi's sarcoma is dependent on the site and the extent of the disease:

(1) Local excision – should only be used for small isolated lesions.
(2) Irradiation – is the treatment of choice for enlarging lesions that are cosmetically disfiguring. A single dose of 800 cGy is usually sufficient. Electron beam therapy may be used for multiple lesions.
(3) Intralesional chemotherapy – vinblastine (0.10.2mg/ml) injections are painful and are no more effective than irradiation.

If the sarcoma is widespread and/or rapidly growing systemic treatment may be necessary:

(4) Chemotherapy – a 30–80% response rate has been reported with agents such as vinblastine, VP16, and vincristine alone or in combination with bleomycin.
(5) Immunotherapy – interferon-α, unlike chemotherapy, does not cause neutropaenia; however, the high doses used (3–10 MIU subcutaneously on alternate days) inevitably cause shivering, fevers and malaise.

Unfortunately Kaposi's sarcoma frequently recurs when treatment is stopped and with improved treatment of opportunistic infections it is an increasing cause of death in AIDS patients.

Section 8

Biochemistry and haematology

Addenbrooke's NHS Trust : Pathology Report

| Cons : **CULANK L S** | | | Hospital No.: **A0026793** |
| Ward : **Biochemistry Department** | **MUNCHAUSEN Baron** | | D.O.B. : |

Spec : 0307:C00750R			Rec'd : 03/07/97-1414	
Test	Result	Abn	Reference	Units
U/E				
Sodium	133	L	135-145	mmol/l
Potassium	7.7	*H	3.4-5.0	mmol/l
Glucose	9.2	H	3.5-9	mmol/l
Urea	49.5	H	0.0-7.5	mmol/l
Creatinine	471	H	35-125	umol/l

Fig. 8.1a

Q: *What do these urea and electrolytes indicate? (see Fig. 8.1)*

A: The most striking features are the hyperkalaemia, the profound uraemia and the elevated creatinine. These all point to the diagnosis of acute renal failure. The serum calcium may also be low secondary to renal phosphate retention, or acquired vitamin D resistance, if there has been pre-existent renal failure.

Q: *Why may a patient with the above biochemistry complain of deteriorating vision?*

A: Patients with acute or chronic renal failure may present with reduced visual acuity for a variety of reasons:

(1) Sequelae of poorly controlled hypertension:
  (a) Retinal venous occlusions (also common in systemic lupus erythematosus).
  (b) Multifocal serous retinal detachments and choroidal infarcts (in acute hypertensive/uraemic crises).
(2) Diabetic retinopathy.
(3) Presenile cataract secondary to corticosteroid treatment, e.g. renal transplant patients.
(4) Scleritis – Wegener's granulomatosis.

Intraocular pressure rises following haemodialysis have been reported, but patients are rarely symptomatic.

Q: *Why is there a correlation between the development of diabetic nephropathy and diabetic retinopathy?*

A: The underlying pathology in both diabetic nephropathy and retinopathy is a microvascular angiopathy. The main features of these angiopathies are the loss of pericytes, endothelial dysfunction and capillary closure with resultant ischaemia. The vast majority of patients with proliferative diabetic retinopathy will have a degree of proteinuria indicating compromised renal function.

Q: *What is the significance of microalbuminuria in the diabetic patient?*

A: Approximately 45% of all diabetics will develop some degree of nephropathy. However, clinical proteinuria (albumin excretion rate (AER) of >300 mg/24 h), which can be detected by conventional dipstick testing, takes from 10 to 20 years to develop. Attempts to tighten diabetic control and the aggressive management of hypertension once proteinuria has developed are usually too late to prevent the progression of both retinopathy and nephropathy. Micro-albuminuria and an AER of 30–300 mg/24 h are early warning signs of microangiopathy; tightening diabetic control and treatment of hypertension at this stage are more likely to arrest or retard the development of retinopathy and neuropathy.

8.2

Addenbrooke's NHS Trust : Pathology Report

| Cons : **CULANK L S** | | Hospital No.: **A0026793** |
| Ward : **Biochemistry Department** | **MUNCHAUSEN Baron** | D.O.B. : |

Spec : 0307:C00760R   Rec'd : 03/07/97-1417

Test	Result	Abn	Reference	Units
U/E				
Sodium	115	*L	135-145	mmol/l
Potassium	5.8	H	3.4-5.0	mmol/l
Glucose	7.7		3.5-9	mmol/l
Urea	3.3		0.0-7.5	mmol/l
Creatinine	79		35-125	umol/l

Fig. 8.2

Q: *A 55-year-old woman collapsed after presenting to an Accident & Emergency department with a history of nausea, vomiting, epigastric pain and listlessness. She was hypotensive and appeared dehydrated. Her urea and electrolytes were as above. What is the most likely diagnosis? (see Fig. 8.2)*

A: The most obvious abnormalities are the profound hyponatraemia and moderate hyperkalaemia. Hyponatraemia with the history and signs described above is indicative of an Addisonian crisis. In such a crisis the mineralocorticoid (aldosterone) deficiency results in sodium and water depletion, eventually the circulating volume is depleted to such a degree that antidiuretic hormone (ADH) secretion is stimulated. Water is then reabsorbed in excess of sodium and hyponatraemia develops.

Q: *How would you manage this patient in the acute situation?*

A: Acute adrenal insufficiency is a medical emergency and treatment should not be delayed while waiting for definitive proof of the diagnosis. Having said this, it should be possible to take samples for plasma cortisol and (ACTH) measurement prior to treatment. Resuscitation involves the following measures:

(1) Intravenous hydrocortisone 100 mg stat and then 6-hourly.
(2) Correction of hypovolaemia with dextrose saline (because of possible hypoglycaemia). One litre over the first hour with subsequent replacement titrated against the patient's condition and biochemical status.
(3) Recognise and treat any associated condition that may have precipitated the crisis.

Q: *What are the causes of Addison's disease (primary hypoadrenalism)?*

A: The most common causes of Addison's disease are:

(1) Autoimmune.
(2) Tuberculosis.
(3) Intra-adrenal haemorrhage following meningococcal septicaemia.

(4) Metastatic tumour or lymphoma.
(5) Bilateral adrenalectomy.
(6) Haemachromatosis.

With the exception of autoimmune adrenal insufficiency and tuberculosis other causes of primary hypoadrenalism are rare.

Q: *How may an ophthalmologist/physician inadvertently precipitate hypoadrenalism?*

A: The most common cause of secondary hypoadrenalism is the sudden cessation of exogenous glucocorticoid therapy or a failure to give glucocorticoid cover for intercurrent stress in a patient who is on long-term glucocorticoid therapy. Glucocorticoid therapy suppresses the hypothalamic–pituitary–adrenal axis with consequent adrenal atrophy and it is therefore imperative that such therapy should be tapered slowly. The degree of adrenal suppression is dependent not only on the dose of glucocorticoid, but also on the circadian timing of the doses. Larger evening doses are known to suppress the morning surge of ACTH, whereas a similar dose given in the morning will have a minimal effect on ACTH secretion.

Although the adrenals may recover relatively quickly with exogenous ACTH therapy, suppression of the pituitary and hypothalamus may last for many months.

Q: *What is the normal maintenance therapy for a patient with primary adrenal insufficiency? What precautions should be taken with such a patient who is about to undergo cataract extraction under local anaesthetic?*

A: The commonly used maintenance regime for patients with primary adrenal insufficiency is:

(1) Hydrocortisone 20 mg on waking and 10 mg at 18.00 h. These doses will be titrated against the urea and electolytes and the clinical status of the patient. This dose should be doubled in the event of a febrile illness, accident or mental stress.
(2) Fludrocortisone 0.1 mg daily. Not all patients with primary adrenal insufficiency require mineralocorticoid replacement, patients with secondary adrenal insufficiency require glucocorticoid alone. Indications for mineralocorticoid replacement therapy include postural hypotension, hyperkalaemia and an elevated plasma renin activity. The dose is adjusted according to the lying and standing blood pressure.

Cataract extraction under local anaesthesia may be regarded as a minor procedure and therefore a covering dose of 100 mg hydrocortisone hemisuccinate intramuscularly immediately prior to the operation will be sufficient to prevent any relapses caused by the stress of surgery.

8.3

| Cons : **CULANK L S** | | | Hospital No.: **A0026793** |
| Ward : **Biochemistry Department** | **MUNCHAUSEN Baron** | | D.O.B. : |

Spec : 0307:C00746R   Rec'd : 03/07/97-1411

Test	Result	Abn	Reference	Units
LFT				
Albumin	28	L	30-51	g/l
Calcium	2.20		2.2-2.6	mmol/l
Cor Calcium	2.40			mmol/l
	supine : 2.2 - 2.6 mmol/l			
	upright : 2.0 - 2.4 mmol/l			
I.Phosphate	1.25		0.8-1.4	mmol/l
T.Bilirubin	43	H	0-17	umol/l
Alk Phos	244	H	30-135	U/L
ALT	181	H	0-50	U/L
Gamma gt	268	H	0-51	U/L

Fig. 8.3a

Q: *Comment on these liver function tests of a 21-year-old non-drinker who presented with an insidious onset of tremor and dysarthria. (see Fig. 8.3a)*

A: The features of note are:

(1) An elevated bilirubin and alkaline phosphatase indicative of cholestasis.

(2) A raised alanine transaminase (ALT) pointing to damage to the cytoplasmic membranes of the hepatocytes.

(3) An elevated γ-glutamyltransferase (γ-GT). γ-GT is derived from the endoplasmic reticulum of the cells of the hepatobiliary tract, however elevated levels do not always indicate hepatocellular damage.

(4) A slightly reduced albumin.

These liver function tests are indicative of chronic active hepatitis. In the absence of a history of alcohol abuse or hepatitis B exposure, the presence of chronic active hepatitis accompanied by tremor and dysarthria in a young person is suggestive of Wilson's disease.

In 90% of patients the disease presents with juvenile hepatic disease or with neurological/ psychiatric manifestations. Approximately 40% of patients with Wilson's disease present with a spectrum of liver disease from acute to chronic hepatitis. A minority of patients present with fulminant hepatitis and encephalopathy, although the most common clinical scenario is one of chronic active hepatitis that progresses to cirrhosis.

Wilson's disease is a disorder of copper metabolism, which like most inborn errors of metabolism is inherited as an autosomal recessive trait. It has a prevalence of 1/30 000 and a carrier frequency of 1/90.

Q: *What further investigations may confirm the diagnosis?*

A: Screening investigations for patients suspected of having Wilson's disease include:

(1) Full blood count – to detect anaemia and haemolysis.

(2) Serum caeroplasmin – the activity and concentration of this glycoprotein is reduced or absent in 95% of patients with Wilson's disease.

(3) Urine copper – 24-h urinary excretion of copper is always increased in Wilson's disease (>70–$100\,\mu g$/day). This abnormality may also be present in primary biliary cirrhosis and other forms of chronic active hepatitis.

Q: *Why may an ophthalmological opinion be sought in patients with suspected Wilson's disease?*

A: An ophthalmological opinion is always helpful in cases of suspected Wilson's disease as the majority of patients with Wilson's disease will have Kayser–Fleischer rings (Fig. 8.3b).

These greenish brown rings represent deposition of copper at the level of Descemet's membrane and are said to be the single most important diagnostic sign of Wilson's disease. It is invariably present in patients with overt neurological disease. The ring typically appears first between 10 and 2 o'clock, then inferiorly between 5 and 7 o'clock. It begins at the limbus

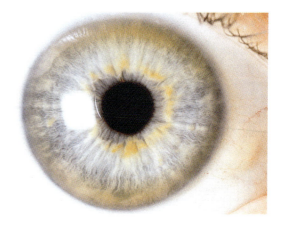

Fig. 8.3b

and then extends centrally and circumferentially. Gonioscopy will often reveal pigment in peripheral Descemet's membrane not visible by slit lamp biomicroscopy alone. The Kayser-Fleischer rings will slowly disappear with effective treatment. Similar changes may occasionally be seen in cryptogenic cirrhosis and prolonged cholestasis.

A sunflower cataract is a less universal manifestation of Wilson's disease.

8.4

Addenbrooke's NHS Trust : Pathology Report

Cons : CULANK L S			Hospital No.: A0026793
Ward : Biochemistry Department	MUNCHAUSEN Baron		D.O.B. :

Spec : 3006:C00104R — Rec'd : 30/06/97-1043

Test	Result	Abn	Reference	Units
TSH	Less than 0.03	L	0.4-4	mU/l
Free T4	29.2	H	9.0-20.0	pmol/l

Fig. 8.4a

Addenbrooke's NHS Trust : Pathology Report

Cons : CULANK L S			Hospital No.: A0026793
Ward : Biochemistry Department	MUNCHAUSEN Baron		D.O.B. :

Spec : 3006:C00110R — Rec'd : 30/06/97-1050

Test	Result	Abn	Reference	Units
TSH	0.03	L	0.4-4	mU/l
Free T4	21.2	H	9.0-20.0	pmol/l
Free T3	10.6	H	3.0-7.5	pmol/l

Fig. 8.4b

Q: ***What do these thyroid function tests signify? What is the differential diagnosis? (see Fig. 8.4a)***

A: The undetectable TSH is highly suggestive of hyperthyroidism. With third-generation immunometric assays, symptomatic hyperthyroidism is almost invariably present when TSH levels are <0.03 mU/l. Hyperthyroidism in this case is confirmed by the elevated Free T4.

The differential diagnosis for hyperthyroidism should include:

(1) Graves' disease.
(2) Solitary toxic nodule.
(3) Toxic multinodular goitre.
(4) Acute thyroiditis (viral, autoimmune).
(5) Iatrogenic (secret consumption of thyroxine).
(6) Hyperthyroid phase of Hashimoto's thyroiditis.
(7) Amioderone toxicity.
(8) Differentiated metastatic thyroid carcinoma.

The first two conditions listed above account for 95% of cases of hyperthyroidism.

Q: ***What do these thyroid function tests signify? (see Fig. 8.4b)***

A: The TSH is just detectable and the Free T4 is marginally above the normal range.

In this situation the laboratory should perform a Free T3 assay, which in this case confirms the diagnosis of mild thyrotoxicosis.

Although plasma concentrations of T3 and T4 are both usually elevated in hyperthyroidism, as T3 is secreted directly by the thyroid, the increase in plasma levels is greater and may be evident earlier, than that of T4. Rarely the T3 alone remains elevated with a barely recordable TSH, this is known as T3 toxicosis.

Q: *In what situations is the serum TSH level an inaccurate indicator of the thyroid status?*

A: With the advent of modern assays the TSH levels can now be accurately measured to <0.03 mU/l (normal range 0.3–5.0 mU/l), this has rendered the thyroid hormone uptake tests and the TRH test almost redundant. However, there are a number of situations in which the serum TSH may be misleading:

(1) During the early stages of thyrotoxicosis treatment.
(2) The 'sick euthyroid' syndrome, in which systemically ill patients have an apparently low total T4 and T3 with a normal or slightly low TSH.
(3) The first trimester of pregnancy.
(4) Hypothyroidism secondary to pituitary dysfunction, in 50% of such cases the TSH will be normal but the Free T4 is low (the TRH test would then be useful).

(5) Concurrent medication, e.g. lithium and amioderone.

Although TSH is the most sensitive single test of thyroid function it is preferable to interpret it alongside the Free T4 and T3 whose normal ranges are approximately 9–25 and 3–9 pmol/l, respectively.

Q: *What is the correlation between thyroid status and the activity of thyroid eye disease?*

A: Thyroid eye disease may become manifest prior to the onset of thyrotoxicosis or long after the initial thyrotoxic presentation. Although thyroid status does not correlate directly with the activity of thyroid eye disease, fluctuations in the control of thyroid function predisposes to the development of ophthalmopathy and worsens pre-existing eye disease. Swings from hyperthyroidism to hypothyroidism following radioiodine therapy may explain the increased incidence of ophthalmopathy in this group of patients. It is therefore essential that all patients with Graves' disease especially those with ocular involvement should have their thyroid status closely monitored. Both the Free T4 and TSH should be requested, as the latter may remain suppressed for many months in patients on medical treatment for Graves' disease, despite a Free T4 within the normal range.

8.5

Cons : **CULANK L S** Ward : **Biochemistry Department**	**MUNCHAUSEN Baron**	Hospital No.: **A0026793** D.O.B. :

Spec : 3006:C00115R		Rec'd : 30/06/97-1058

Test	Result	Abn	Reference	Units
TSH	Greater than 100.00	H	0.4-4	mU/l
Free T4	3.4	L	9.0-20.0	pmol/l

Fig. 8.5a

Addenbrooke's NHS Trust : Pathology Report

Cons : **CULANK L S** Ward : **Biochemistry Department**	**MUNCHAUSEN Baron**	Hospital No.: **A0026793** D.O.B. :

Spec : 3006:C00626R		Rec'd : 30/06/97-1510

Test	Result	Abn	Reference	Units
TSH	20.10	H	0.4-4	mU/l
Free T4	8.2	L	9.0-20.0	pmol/l

Fig. 8.5b

Q: *What do these thyroid function tests signify? What is the differential diagnosis? (see Fig. 8.5a)*

A: The marked TSH elevation is indicative of primary hypothyroidism, the low Free T4 confirms this. The most common causes of primary hypothyroidism are:

(1) Autoimmune (atrophic) hypothyroidism.
(2) Hashimoto's thyroiditis.
(3) Iatrogenic hypothyroidism:
   (a) Post-thyroidectomy.
   (b) Antithyroid medications.
   (c) Post-radioiodine therapy.
(4) Defects in hormone synthesis.
(5) Iodine deficiency.

Q: *What do these thyroid function tests signify? (see Fig. 8.5b)*

A: The TSH is moderately elevated and the Free T4 just falls within the normal range. This is an example of mild or 'compensated' hypothyroidism in which the TSH raised by negative feedback maintains the Free T4 in the normal range.

Q: *What other thyroid investigations are indicated in cases of hypothyroidism?*

A: The presence of a multinodular goitre associated with hypothyroidism is suggestive of Hashimoto's thyroiditis (although patients may be euthyroid). Thyroid microsomal antibodies are often grossly elevated in such patients; several antibodies have been identified, the most common is that against thyroid peroxidase. Microsomal antibody titres may also be elevated in atrophic hypothyroidism.

8.6

Q: *What do these results signify?*
Random plasma glucose – 12 mmol/l
Fasting plasma glucose – 8 mmol/l

A: The diagnosis of diabetes mellitus is confirmed if:

(1) The fasting plasma glucose level is 7.8 mmol/l or more, *on two occasions*; or
(2) The random plasma glucose is 11.1 mmol/l or more, *on two occasions*; or
(3) *Both* a fasting level of more than 7.8 mmol/l and a random level of more than 11.1 mmol/l are found.

Therefore these results confirm the diagnosis of diabetes mellitus.

It should be noted that if the glucose concentrations are measured in whole blood, levels will be approximately 1 mmol/l lower.

Q: *What are the indications for performing an oral glucose tolerance test? How should this test be performed?*

A: The indications for performing an oral glucose tolerance test are:

(1) Fasting plasma glucose values of between 5.5 and 7.8 mmol/l.
(2) Random plasma glucose values of between 7.8 and 11.1 mmol/l.
(3) If there is a high clinical index of suspicion.

Although details of the glucose tolerance test may vary slightly with individual laboratories the following guidelines are broadly applicable.

Patients should be resting and may not smoke during the test.

(1) The patient fasts overnight (10–16 h), only water being allowed during this period.
(2) A venous sample is withdrawn for plasma glucose estimation and a double-voided urine specimen collected.

(3) The equivalent of 75 mg of anhydrous glucose (or 1.75 mg/kg body weight for children), usually in the form of 353 ml of 'Lucozade' is given. This must be drunk within 5 min.
(4) Further blood and urine samples are taken 2 h after the dose.
(5) Diabetes is confirmed if fasting glucose levels are 7.8 mmol/l or more or if 2 h levels are 11.1 mmol/l or more.

Q: *What is the first line of treatment in non-insulin-dependent diabetes mellitus (NIDDM)?*

A: The first line treatment in any patient recently diagnosed as a non-insulin dependent diabetic is dietary. The ideal diet should consist of the following:

(1) Adequate energy – 1000–1600 kcal/day for obese patients and 2500 kcal/day for lean patients.
(2) Fats should provide 30–35% of the total energy.
(3) Protein should provide 10–15% of the total energy (this is reduced in the presence of proteinuria).
(4) Carbohydrate should be in the form of unrefined high complex carbohydrates to prevent rapid swings in blood glucose levels. They should provide the remaining 50% of the total calories. In the past the diabetic diet was low in carbohydrate and high in fats which actually caused a deterioration in glucose tolerance and predisposed to macrovascular disease!

Hypoglycaemic agents should only be added after the patient's dietary knowledge and compliance has been adequately assessed.

Q: *Comment on the diabetic control of this 25-year-old woman.*
Home blood glucose monitoring: average over the previous 6 weeks – 8.4 mmol/l
HbA_{1C} 14%

A: The average blood glucose level of 8.4 mmol/l, as recorded by home blood glucose monitoring, suggests that this patient's diabetic control has been reasonably good over this 6-week period. However, the grossly elevated HbA_{1C} level contradicts this. The average post-prandial blood glucose level should ideally be <8.6 mmol/l (as recommended by the (DCCT)). However, the values attained by self-monitoring are still dependent on the accuracy/honesty of the patient's daily recordings. Glycosylated haemoglobin (HbA_{1C}) is formed by the covalent linkage of a glucose molecule to the terminal valine of the β-chain of the haem moiety. It is expressed as a percentage of the total haemoglobin and is an accurate indicator of the glycaemic control over the preceding 6–8 weeks. The target HbA_{1C} set by the DCCT was 6.5%, but in practice a more realistic level is 8.0%.

When there is such a large disparity between the blood glucose levels as recorded by the patient and the HbA_{1C} the validity of the former should be questioned.

Q: *In what circumstances may the HbA_{1C} be misleading?*

A: The HbA_{1C} will only provide an accurate measurement of diabetic control if the red blood cells have a 'normal' life-span. If there is coexistent haemolytic anaemia, chronic sepsis, rheumatoid arthritis or chronic blood loss, the red blood cell life is shortened and the percentage of glycosylated haemoglobin may be unduly low.

In colorimetric assays an elevated urea (which carbamylates the valine amino groups of amino acids on the side chains of haemoglobin) or an elevated acetaldehyde (derived from ethanol) may cause a spurious high HbA_{1C}. Acetaldehyde is only likely to be raised in patients consuming 30 or more units of alcohol per week.

Q: *How does the incidence and severity of diabetic retinopathy differ between type I and type II diabetes: (1) at the time of diagnosis and (2) after 15 years of known diabetes.*

A: The Wisconsin study has provided valuable information regarding the incidence and severity of retinopathy in patients diagnosed as being diabetic before (type I or IDDM) and after (type II or NIDDM) the age of 30 years. The baseline results from this study are outlined in Fig. 8.7a and 8.7b.

(1) At the time of diagnosis no insulin-dependent diabetic was found to have any retinopathy. However, 20–25% of patients with type II diabetes were found to have some degree of retinopathy at this time.
(2) After 15 years 97.5% of patients with type I diabetes had some degree of retinopathy, 25% had proliferative changes. The incidence of retinopathy in the type II diabetes was 77.8% in those receiving insulin and 55% in those patients not receiving insulin. Only 15.5% had proliferative disease.

The 10-year incidence and progression of diabetic retinopathy in the Wisconsin study has now been reported. Table 8.1 summarises some of the data from this study.

Although the duration of diabetes is known to be a significant risk factor for the development of diabetic retinopathy, there did not appear to be a linear relationship between it and the rate of development or progression of retinopathy, in the Wisconsin study. The 10-year risk of progression declined in the younger-onset cohort who had been diabetic

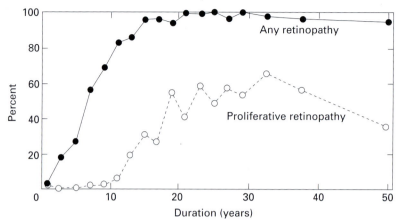

Fig. 8.7a Frequency of diabetic retinopathy in subjects with type I diabetes as a function of the duration of diabetes in years.

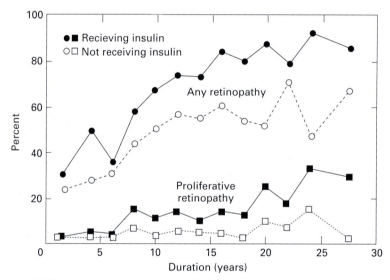

Fig. 8.7b Frequency of diabetic retinopathy in subjects with type II diabetes as function of the duration of diabetes in years.

for >20 years, while rates of improvement increased.

Q: *When should screening for diabetic retinopathy be carried out in the following patients: (1) children or young adults with type I diabetes (IDDM) and (2) adults with type II diabetes (NIDDM)?*

A:

(1) Significant diabetic retinopathy rarely develops within 5 years of the diagnosis of IDDM. Furthermore, although minimal retinopathy in children is not rare prepoliferative or proliferative retinopathy does not occur in prepubertal children irrespective of the duration of their diabetes. After adjusting for the duration of the diabetes and sex, the relative odds of having retinopathy (of any form) in post-pubescent patients relative to pubescent or prepubescent patients is 4.8. The following guidelines for screening are based on the above information:

Table 8.1

Ten-year progression of retinopathy	Younger onset group (%)	Older onset group taking insulin (%)	Older onset group not taking insulin (%)
No retinopathy at baseline to any grade of retinopathy	89	79	67
Progression of two or more steps (EDTRS severity scheme)	76	69	53
Progression to proliferative retinopathy	30	24	10

(a) Children with IDDM need only be screened when they reach puberty irrespective of the duration of their diabetes.

(b) Adolescents diagnosed as diabetic at the time of puberty and young adults should be screened 5 years after the diagnosis of diabetes mellitus.

(2) The Wisconsin study demonstrated that unlike patients with IDDM a high proportion of patients with NIDDM have significant retinopathy at the time of diagnosis. It is therefore advisable that all patients with newly diagnosed NIDDM are screened within 3 months if unnecessary visual loss is to be prevented.

Recommended reading

Klein, R., Klein, B. E., Moss, S. E., Davis, M. D. and DeMets, D. L. (1984) The Wisconsin epidemiological study of diabetic retinopathy. III. Prevalence and risk of diabetic retinopathy when age at diagnosis is less than 30 years. *Arch. Ophthalmol.*, **102**, 520–506.

Klein, R., Klein, B. E., Moss, S. E., Davis, M. D. and DeMets, D. L. (1984) The Wisconsin epidemiological study of diabetic retinopathy. III. Prevalence and risk of diabetic retinopathy when age at diagnosis is 30 or more years. *Arch. Ophthalmol.*, **102**, 527–532.

Klein, R., Klein, B. E., Moss, S. E. and Cruickshanks, K. J. (1994) The Wisconsin epidemiological study of diabetic retinopathy. XIV. Ten-year incidence and progression of diabetic retinopathy. *Arch. Ophthalmol.*, **112**, 1217–1228.

8.8

Q: *A 35-year-old woman with a 15-year history of IDDM had the following findings at a routine clinic follow-up.*
HbA$_{1C}$ 15%
Urine dipstix – sugar ++, no protein
Urea 6 mmol/l, creatinine 110 mmol/l
Preproliferative diabetic retinopathy
Blood pressure 160/95 mmHg (on three separate visits to clinic and GP). Comment on the above results. What other investigation may be helpful in the management of this patient?

A: The elevated HbA$_{1C}$ indicates poor glycaemic control over the preceding 6–8 weeks and it is therefore not surprising that there is ++ of sugar on testing the urine. There was no albuminuria that could be detected with conventional 'stix' methods and the urea and creatinine are within the normal range. However, the presence of preproliferative retinopathy and hypertension (noted on three consecutive visits) suggests that already there is a degree of microvasculopathy affecting the retinal and renal circulations. The initial warning sign of diabetic nephropathy other than hypertension is the development of microalbuminuria. This should only be diagnosed if, during a period of 6 months, three independent measurements confirm albumin excretion between 20 and 200 µg/min in morning urine specimens (approximately equivalent to 30–300 mg/24 h).

Q: *What is the link between hypertension and nephropathy in patients with diabetes mellitus?*

A: The relationship between hypertension and nephropathy appears to be different for IDDM and NIDDM.

(1) Patients with IDDM tend to be normotensive until microalbuminuria has supervened, at this point blood pressure begins to rise. The close relationship between elevated blood pressure and evidence of renal damage in these patients suggests that the hypertension is a consequence of renal parenchymal changes. Other factors that may contribute to hypertension in patients with IDDM are renal sodium retention and increased responsiveness to pressor agents.

(2) The majority of patients with NIDDM have been hypertensive for a variable period prior to the onset of overt diabetes, with 70–80% of patients being hypertensive at the time of diagnosis. The development of nephropathy will contribute to blood pressure elevation as will an increased pulse pressure secondary to diminished aortic elasticity. Increased peripheral vascular resistance and decreased baroreceptor sensitivity will also predispose to hypertension in these patients. Isolated systolic hypertension in elderly diabetic patients is linked to a higher cardiovascular mortality, even when the mean arterial pressure is normal.

Q: *What is the first line treatment for hypertension in patients with diabetes? What is the threshold for treating hypertension associated with diabetes?*

A: The choice of antihypertensive drugs in diabetes remains a controversial area as there is conflicting evidence from several large randomised trials. However, most physicians would agree that angiotensin-converting enzyme (ACE) inhibitors, such as captopril, are a reasonable first-line therapy for hypertensive diabetic patients. Although captopril has been shown to have a similar antihypertensive effect as atenolol in type 2 diabetics it tends to be better tolerated than atenolol. It is also hypothesised that ACE inhibitors have a specific renoprotective action; they have been shown to reduce albuminuria more markedly and to attenuate the decrease in glomerular filtration rate more effectively, than do β-blockers at a given level of blood pressure. They may also reduce retinal blood flow via vascular endothelial ACE receptors.

Calcium channel blockers were associated with an excess cardiac morbidity in The Appropriate Blood Pressure Control in Diabetes Study (ABCD) and the Fosinopril versus Amlodipine Cardiovascular Events randomised Trial (FACET). However, results from the Hypertension Optimum Treatment randomised trial (HOT) suggested that calcuim antagonists reduced cardiovascular mortality.

Second- (and third-) line treatment may be required in 60% of patients with type 2 diabetes. In patients with advanced renal disease combination therapy is almost always necessary. Calcium channel blockers and α-adrenergic agonists can be used, although a diuretic may be preferred if there is a degree of peripheral oedema. Thiazide diuretics should be avoided as they tend to impair glucose tolerance as well as elevate blood lipids. β-Blockers also raise lipid levels and impair insulin secretion, but may still be of benefit in those diabetics with ischaemic heart disease.

The early and aggressive management of hypertension has been shown in controlled prospective trials to attenuate or even prevent the reduction of glomerular filtration rate and to reduce albuminuria in patients with diabetic nephropathy. The UK Prospective Diabetes Study has also proven that tight blood pressure control reduces the risk of developing retinopathy and retards progression of established retinopathy.

The recent Joint British Societies' recommendations for the treatment of hypertension in diabetes are as follows:

Type 1 diabetes

Threshold ≥130 systolic or ≥80 diastolic
Target <130 systolic and ≤80 diastolic
<120 systolic and <75 diastolic if proteinuria.

Type 2 diabetes

Threshold ≥160 systolic or ≥90 diastolic
≥140 systolic or ≥90 diastolic if target organ damage, microvascular or macrovascular complications or absolute coronary risk
Target <130 systolic and ≤80 diastolic.

Recommended reading

Gillow, J. T., Gibson, J. M. and Dodson, P. M. (1999) Hypertension and diabetic retinopathy what's the story? *Br. J. Ophthalmol.*, **83**, 1083–1087.

HB	5.2 (10.5–13.5)	WBC	210.0 (6.0–18.0)	PLT	11 (140–500)
HCT	.161 (0.36–0.44)	LYMPH	12.6 (3.5–9.0)	VIS	1.69 (1.50–1.72)
MCV	77.0 (70.0–86.0)	MONO	2.10 (0.7–1.5)		
MCH	24.9 (23.0–30.0)	NEUT	4.20 (2.0–6.0)		
MCHC	32.3 (31.0–35.5)	EOS	0.00 (0.2–1)		
RBC	2.09 (3.60–5.20)	BASOS	0.00 (0.01–0.1)		
		BLAST	191		
NRBC	0.00			K1	
				DA	
				DA	

```
Severe THROMBOCYTOPAENIA.
Polychromasia +
Due to high white cell count corrected HB = 4.6 g/dl.
Some of the blast show block PAS positivity.
```

Fig. 8.9a

Q: *Comment on the full blood count of this 5-year-old girl. What signs would you specifically look for on a systemic examination? What further investigations are indicated? (see Fig. 8.9a)*

A: There is a severe normochromic normocytic anaemia, the white blood count is grossly elevated and there is a marked thrombocytopaenia. This haematological picture is suggestive of a haematological malignancy, the most common condition producing such a picture in childhood is acute lymphoblastic leukaemia (ALL). Evidence of lymphadenopathy, splenomegaly, hepatomegaly, bruising, petechial haemorrhages and gingival bleeding or hypertrophy should be looked for specifically.

The diagnosis may be confirmed by a bone marrow examination. This will reveal a hypercellular marrow with numerous leukaemic blast cells that account for over 50% of the marrow cell total. Immunophenotyping, chromosome and gene rearrangement studies may be used to distinguish ALL from acute myeloid leukaemia (AML), and then to subclassify them.

X-rays may reveal lytic bone lesions in children with ALL; an enlarged thymus and mediastinal nodes are characteristic of T cell-ALL. Liver function tests and urea and electrolytes should also be performed prior to treatment.

Q: *What are the other ophthalmic manifestations of acute and/or chronic leukaemia?*

A: In general ophthalmic manifestations are more common in acute leukaemias. Ophthalmic involvement has been reported in 60% of newly diagnosed cases of acute leukaemia. Autopsy series show that 75% of patients with chronic leukaemia and 82% of patients with acute leukaemias have intraocular involvement at the time of death. The ophthalmic manifestations of leukaemia include:

(1) Retinal abnormalities:
   (a) Roth spots (see Question 1.14).
   (b) Cotton wool spots secondary to anaemia induced ischaemia.

(c) Venous tortuosity and/or retinal venous occlusions secondary to hyperviscosity (see Question 1.12).

(d) A low platelet count is also an important risk factor for the development of retinal haemorrhages.

(e) Hyperviscosity may also cause peripheral capillary non-perfusion resulting in retinal neovascularisation.

(f) Retinal or preretinal infiltrates are relatively rare manifestations of more advanced disease.

(g) Vitreous infiltrates and/or haemorrhage.

(2) Apart from retinal infiltrates, the presence and degree of leukaemic retinopathy does not appear to correlate with the general prognosis.

(3) Uveal abnormalities:
  (a) Creamy choroidal infiltrates with or without overlying serous retinal detachment are the most common infiltrative manifestations of leukaemia.
  (b) Hypopyons that arise in painless relatively 'quiet' eyes should alert the ophthalmologist to the possibility of an underlying haematological malignancy. In children <3 years of age there may be an alternative explanation for a similar presentation. Retinoblastoma most commonly presents with a leucocoria (white pupil); however, it may also cause a painless hypopyon. Both haematological malignancy and retinoblastoma are part of a group of conditions known as the Masquerade syndromes, which mimic intraocular inflammatory conditions.

(4) Disc abnormalities:
  (a) Unilateral disc swelling suggests direct infiltration of the optic nerve.
  (b) Bilateral disc swelling is more likely to be caused by raised intracranial pressure.

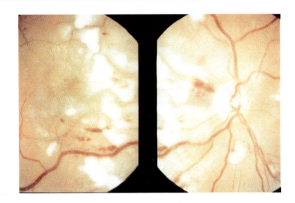

Fig. 8.9b

(5) Central nervous system involvement:
  (a) Visual field loss secondary to chiasmal or intracranial optic nerve infiltration.
  (b) Brainstem involvement may result in IIIrd, IVth or VIth nerve palsies.

(6) Orbital masses secondary to infiltrative disease.

(7) Opportunistic ocular infections:
  (a) *Candida albicans* endophthalmitis is a well-described complication of intravenous lines in immunosuppressed patients.
  (b) Herpes zoster ophthalmicus.
  (c) Toxoplasma retinochoroiditis.
  (d) CMV and herpetic retinitis.

(8) Graft versus host disease:
  (a) Keratoconjunctivitis sicca secondary to lacrimal gland involvement is the most common ocular manifestation of graft versus host disease.
  (b) Retinal haemorrhages and cottonwool spots (Fig. 8.9b).

Recommended reading

Kincaid, M. C. and Green, W. R. (1983) Ocular and orbital involvement in leukaemia. *Surv. Ophthalmol.*, **27**, 211–232.

```
HB        8.6 (11.5-16.5)     WBC      8.5 (4.0-12.0)      PLT       110 (140-500)

HCT      .239 (0.37-0.47)     LYMPH    1.02 (1.0-4.0)      VIS       1.67 (1.50-1.72)
MCV     121.9 (80.0-98.0)     MONO     0.00 (0.2-0.8)
MCH      43.9 (26.0-31.0)     NEUT     7.48 (2.0-8.0)
MCHC     36.0 (31.0-35.5)     EOS      0.00 (0.1-0.4)
RBC      1.96 (3.80-5.80)     BASOS    0.00 (0.01-0.1)
NRBC     0.00                                                               NE8
                                                                            DA
                                                                            JR


Slight thrombocytopaenia.
Macrocytosis ++
Schistocytes +
Tear drop cells +
Neutrophils show moderate hypersegmentation.
```

Fig. 8.10

Q: *Comment on the full blood count of this 75-year-old lady who is known to have vitiligo and dry eyes. What other initial investigations may be appropriate? (see Fig. 8.10)*

A: The low haemoglobin in combination with a raised MCV (121.9) is indicative of a macrocytic anaemia. There is also evidence of a slight thrombocytopaenia and examination of a peripheral blood film revealed a number of polymorphs with abnormal segmented nuclei.

The most likely causes of a macrocytic anaemia in an elderly woman are vitamin B12 or folic acid deficiency. Pernicious anaemia affects 1/8000 of the population >60 years old (in Western countries). It is frequently associated with other autoimmune conditions such as vitiligo, myxoedema, Hashimoto's disease, Addison's disease and hypoparathyroidism.

In this age group initial investigations should include:

(1) Serum vitamin B12 < 160 ng/l.

(2) Serum folate and serum iron levels will be normal or slightly raised, but the red cell folate will be low. Liver function tests a raised serum bilirubin (secondary to haemolysis) is responsible for these patient's characteristic 'lemon tinged' pallor. An autoimmune screen may also be advisable.

Q: *Having confirmed vitamin B12 deficiency what additional investigations are indicated?*

A: The first step in investigating the cause of vitamin B12 deficiency is to take a detailed dietary history, e.g. veganism which is common in Hindu Indians. Absorption tests will help to distinguish malabsorption from an inadequate diet:

(1) An oral dose of radioactive cobalt (^{57}Co)-labelled cyanocobalamin is given and absorption is then measured indirectly by the urinary excretion (Schilling) technique in

which labelled B12 is flushed into a 24-h urine sample by a large (1000 µg) dose given simultaneously with the oral dose. Alternatively whole-body counting, faecal excretion, or plasma counting (following an oral dose of radioactive B12) may be used.

(2) The test is then repeated with an activated intrinsic factor (IF) preparation. In pernicious anaemia and other gastric lesions IF will correct B12 absorption, but it will not increase absorption in other gastrointestinal diseases.

In all cases of pernicious anaemia X-ray or endoscopic studies should be performed to confirm the presence of gastric atrophy and to exclude gastric carcinoma.

Q: *Why may this patient have dry eyes? What are the ocular manifestations of severe anaemia?*

A: As mentioned above, pernicious anaemia is often associated with other autoimmune diseases and it is therefore not uncommon for such patients to present with dry eye symptoms, secondary to the aqueous tear insufficiency of keratoconjunctivitis sicca. Ocular manifestations of severe anaemia may include the following:

(1) Retinal haemorrhages with or without Roth spots.
(2) Nutritional optic neuropathy (see Question 3.1), although this condition is more characteristically seen in the B12-deficient alcoholic patient it may arise in severe cases of pernicious anaemia.

Q: *A 65-year-old man with a prosthetic mitral valve is found to have an International Normalised Ratio (INR) of 4.2 when he attends for cataract surgery under local anaesthesia. What does the INR represent and how is it measured?*

A: The INR is the ratio of the patient's prothrombin time (PT) to the PT of a normal population. The PT is measured by adding thromboplastin (an activator of factor VII) to citrated plasma which is then incubated for one minute. Calcium is added and the time to clot is noted, this is normally in the range of 12–16 s.

Q: *What part of the clotting cascade does the PT assess? What conditions or drugs other than warfarin will cause it to be prolonged?*

A: The PT is a test of the extrinsic clotting system and the whole of the final common pathway. It will be prolonged in liver disease, consumptive coagulopathies, factor VII deficiency (rare) and heparin therapy.

Q: *What is the mechanism of action of warfarin? Why may there be an increased risk of thrombosis in the first 24 h of warfarin therapy?*

A: Warfarin is a competitive inhibitor of vitamin K, which is involved in the post ribosomal production of calcium binding sites on factors II, VII, IX and X. Factor II has the longest half-life of the above factors, approximately 100 h, therefore the onset of action of warfarin is 2–3 days.

Warfarin is also known to inhibit antithrombin III which may lead to a seemingly paradoxical thrombotic tendency in the first 24 h of warfarin therapy.

Q: *How may concurrent medications affect the INR of a patient taking warfarin?*

A: The actions of warfarin may be potentiated or inhibited by concurrent medications, these include:

(1) Drugs that will potentiate the effect of warfarin:
   (a) Aspirin, sulphonamides and chlorpromazine displace warfarin from albumin.
   (b) Cimetidine, allopurinol, tricyclic antidepressants, metronidazole and sulphonamides will inhibit hepatic microsomal degradation of warfarin.
   (c) Some cephalosporins may reduce absorption of vitamin K.
(2) Drugs that will inhibit the effect of warfarin:
   (a) Barbiturates, thiazides and rifampicin are known to potentiate the microsomal breakdown of warfarin in the liver.
   (b) Oral contraceptives may enhance synthesis of clotting factors.

Q: *What is the normal range for the INR in a patient with: (1) a prosthetic heart valve and (2) a pulmonary embolus?*

A: The INR recommended by the British Society of Haematology for a range of conditions is as follows.

INR	Clinical state
2.0–2.5	Prophylaxis of deep vein thrombosis (DVT), including high-risk surgery
2.0-3.0	Treatment of DVT, *pulmonary embolism*, systemic embolism, treatment of venous thromboembolism after myocardial infarction, mitral stenosis with embolism, atrial fibrillation, transient ischaemic attacks.
3.0–4.5	Recurrent DVT or pulmonary embolism, *prosthetic valves*, arterial grafts, arterial disease including myocardial infarction.

Q: *Is an INR of 4.2 a contraindication to cataract surgery under local anaesthetic?*

A: An INR of 4.2 will actually be within the therapeutic range for certain patients (see above guidelines) and therefore lowering the INR preoperatively may compromise the efficacy of the anticoagulation regime. Ideally peribulbar or retrobulbar local anaesthesia should be avoided in all patients taking warfarin irrespective of the INR. Subtenon's anaesthesia with a blunt cannula is less traumatic than the above techniques and carries a lower risk of retrobulbar haemorrhage. The Royal College of Ophthalmology Guidelines recommend that the INR should ideally be 2.5 or less at the time of cataract surgery. If it is not possible to lower the INR, phacoemulsification may be safely performed. Phacoemulsification may be performed via a clear corneal incision under topical anaesthesia.

8.12

Q: *Comment on the clotting screen of this 25-year-old man. How is the activated partial thromboplastin time (APTT) performed? What is the most likely diagnosis?*
APTT 120 s
PT 14 s
TT 12 s

A: The prothrombin and the thrombin times are within the normal range. The activated partial thromboplastin time, which is a measure of the intrinsic clotting system, is grossly elevated (normal range 35-45 s).

The APTT is measured by adding kaolin, an activator of factor XII, to citrated plasma and incubating it for 10 min. Phospholipid is then added and the plasma is incubated for a further minute before adding calcium and measuring the time to clot. An elevated APTT in the presence of a normal PT and TT is invariably secondary to haemophilia A or haemophilia B (factor IX deficiency).

Q: *What is the molecular basis of the coagulation defect in haemophilia A? What preoperative work-up would be required if the above patient was due to undergo squint surgery?*

A: The defective gene located on the X chromosome codes for the coagulant activity of factor VIII. Factor VIIIc acts as a coenzyme for factor XIa in the intrinsic pathway which along with calcium and platelet factor 3 catalyses the conversion of factor X to Xa.

A clotting screen should be performed for all haemophiliacs embarking on any form of surgical treatment. If the APTT is prolonged, as in the above case, the factor VIII levels should also be measured. The severity of the deficiency in haemophilia is expressed as a percentage of a normal range of factor VIII.

Severe	<1%
Moderate	<15%
Mild	<5–25%

For all forms of major surgery where there is a risk of haemorrhage the factor VIII levels should ideally be elevated to 100% and then maintained above 60% for the immediate postoperative period.

The number of units of factor VIII needed (X), can be calculated as follows:

$$X = \% \text{ rise in factor VIII} \times \text{weight (kg)}/1.5$$

Section 9

Radiology

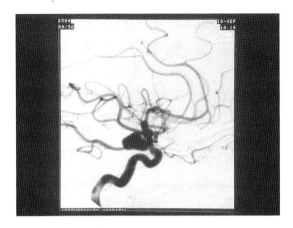

Fig. 9.1a

Q: *What is the lesion illustrated by this carotid angiogram? (see Fig. 9.1a)*

A: The lesion illustrated by this carotid angiogram is a right posterior communicating artery aneurysm.

Q: *What are the common sites of saccular ('berry') aneurysms? What conditions are associated with an increased incidence of these aneurysms?*

A: Saccular aneurysms may arise at numerous sites in the circle of Willis:

(1) Anterior communicating artery (47%).
(2) Internal carotid artery (17% – one-third of which arise in the cavernous sinus).
(3) Middle cerebral artery (15%).
(4) Posterior communicating artery (15%).
(5) Others include the posterior cerebral, vertebrobasilar and the superior cerebellar arteries.

Aneurysmal subarachnoid haemorrhage has an incidence of 1/10 000 people. Intracranial aneurysms are present in 0.5–1.0% of the population, with multiple sites being involved in 20–30% of cases.

An increased incidence of saccular aneurysms is reported in Marfan syndrome, Ehlers–Danlos syndrome type IV, polycystic kidneys and neurofibromatosis type 1. Other risk factors for aneurysmal subarachnoid haemorrhage are a positive family history (4-fold risk), smoking (3- to 10-fold risk) and hypertension.

Q: *What are the presenting signs and symptoms of intracranial aneurysms other than subarachnoid haemorrhage?*

A: Intracranial aneurysms may produce a variety of signs and symptoms by virtue of a compressive effect on neighbouring structures:

(1) Posterior communicating artery aneurysms:
 (a) Painful IIIrd nerve palsy with pupillary involvement is a feature of 70% of symptomatic aneurysms.
 (b) Aberrant regeneration may follow the resolution of such IIIrd nerve palsies.
(2) Anterior communicating and ophthalmic artery aneurysms:
 (a) Reduced visual acuity and visual field loss secondary to optic nerve compression.
 (b) Headaches (often persistent and severe).
(3) Internal carotid artery aneurysms:
 (a) Aneurysms arising within the cavernous sinus may result in a progressive external ophthalmoplegia with involvement of the IIIrd, IVth and VIth cranial nerves.
 (b) Ophthalmic and maxillary divisions of the Vth cranial nerve may be involved causing trigeminal neuralgia.
 (c) Sympathetic fibres associated with the carotid artery may be disrupted resulting in a Horner's syndrome. Carotid-cavernous sinus fistula formation result

in a pulsatile proptosis with an associated bruit, venous engorgement and
an external ophthalmoplegia.
(d) Compressive optic neuropathy.
(e) Hypothalamic-pituitary dysfunction.
(4) Vertebrobasilar artery aneurysms:
(a) These may occasionally cause a Pari-
naud's syndrome or skew deviations.

Q: *What is the role of screening for asymptomatic intracranial aneurysms?*

A: Screening for asymptomatic intracranial aneurysms remains a contentious area for a number of reasons. Firstly, the natural history of intracranial aneurysms is not known, many aneurysms will develop over a relatively short period of time and may rupture immediately, while others may develop slowly and never rupture. Secondly, the morbidity ($<5\%$) and mortality ($<2\%$) of intervention is not insignificant. Magnetic resonance angiography will detect all aneurysms >5 mm and most >2–3 mm making it a relatively sensitive screening investigation. The two groups of patients most commonly screened are those with a positive family history and those with autosomal dominant polycystic kidney disease.

Q: *What are the treatment options for symptomatic intracranial aneurysms?*

A: Symptomatic intracranial aneurysms may be treated surgically or by endovascular therapy.

(1) Surgery – the placement of a clip across the neck of an aneurysm is the most definitive treatment and with the introduction of microsurgical techniques and other surgical advances, the risk directly attributable to the surgery is low. Some aneurysms will not be suitable for direct clipping and other

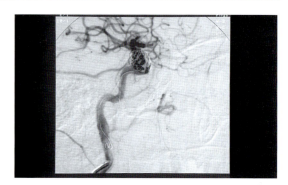

Fig. 9.1b

techniques such as vascular bypass grafting or surgical occlusion of the proximal vessel may be employed.
(2) Endovascular therapy – this involves the insertion of soft metallic coils within the lumen of the aneurysm. A local thrombus is then formed around these detached coils by a process of electrothrombosis leading to complete obliteration of the aneurysmal sac. Figure 9.1b illustrates the appearance of an intracavernous carotid aneurysm following the insertion of metallic coils into the aneursymal sac.

The most important factor for successful treatment is the ratio of the neck of the aneurysm to the fundus. Incomplete treatment is more common in aneurysms with wide necks in which coils have become impacted in the dome of the aneurysm resulting in an aneurysm remnant. Although the long-term results of this relatively low risk procedure are not yet known, the proportion of patients with intracranial aneurysms treated with endovascular coiling (alone or in combination with surgery), is likely to increase.

Recommended reading

Schievink, W. I. (1997) Intracranial aneurysms [Review]. *N. Engl. J. Med.*, **336**, 28–40.

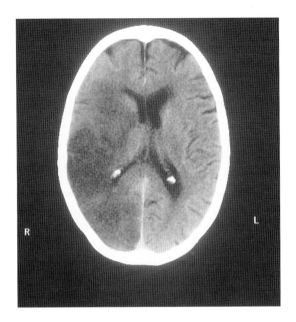

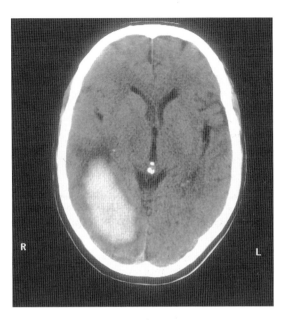

Fig. 9.2a

Fig. 9.2 b

Q: *What do these CT scans demonstrate? (see Fig. 9.2a and 9.2b)*

A: These CT scans both demonstrate right sided occipito-parietal lesions. The low-density lesion in Fig. 9.2a represents an ischaemic stroke, whereas the high-density lesion in Fig. 9.2b is indicative of an intracerebral haemorrhage.

Q: *How may the acute management of these two patients differ from one another?*

A: Over recent years there have been numerous trials that have investigated the role of thrombolysis in the management of acute ischaemic stroke.

- Multicentre Acute Stroke Trial-Europe (MAST-E)
- Multicentre Acute Stroke Trial-Italy (MAST-I)
- Australian Streptokinase Trial (ASK)
- European Cooperative Acute Stroke Study (ECASS)
- National Institute of Neurological Disorders and Stroke r-TPA Stroke Study (NINDS study)
- International Stroke Trial Collaborative Group (IST)

The results of these trials are summarised below.

The three trials of streptokinase, MAST-E, MAST-I and ASK, were all stopped early because of an increased risk of death, largely due to intracerebral haemorrhage. In MAST-E death due to intracerebral haemorrhage was 16 times more frequent in the streptokinase group. None of these trials showed a significant reduction in the likelihood of death or disability at 6 months after treatment with streptokinase.

The effect of intravenous r-TPA (tissue plasminogen activator) was studied in the ECASS and NINDS study. In both studies there was a significant increase in symptomatic intracerebral haemorrhage in all r-TPA groups compared with controls, although in the NINDS Study this was lower than in the ECASS (6.4 versus 19.8%). In the ECASS a significant increase in deaths due to intracerebral haemorrhage was also reported, 65% of which occurred within 72 h of stroke onset.

The NINDS Study was the only trial to report a net benefit for intravenous thrombolysis, with an 11–13% absolute increase in favourable outcomes at 90 days among patients treated within 3 h with intravenous r-TPA.

The IST study examined antithrombotic therapy (aspirin and heparin) given within 24 h of ischaemic stroke. Aspirin therapy was associated with about 10 fewer deaths or recurrent strokes in the first 4 weeks per 1000 patients treated, but with slightly more haemorrhagic strokes. There was no benefit from subcutaneous heparin given with or without aspirin.

The current recommendations from the Stroke Council of the American Heart Association for the treatment of ischaemic stroke are as follows:

(1) Intravenous r-TPA (0.9 mg/kg, maximum 90 mg) with 10% of the dose given as a bolus followed by an infusion over 60 min is the recommended treatment within 3 h of ischaemic stroke. Intravenous r-TPA is not recommended when the time of onset of stroke cannot be ascertained reliably, including strokes recognised upon awakening.

(2) Intravenous streptokinase administration is not indicated for ischaemic stroke outside the setting of a clinical investigation.

(3) Thrombolytic therapy is not recommended unless the diagnosis is established by a physician with expertise in the diagnosis of stroke and CT of the brain assessed by physicians with expertise in reading this imaging study. Thrombolysis should be avoided if there is CT evidence of a recent major infarction, such as sulcal effacement, mass effect, oedema or possible haemorrhage.

(4) Thrombolytic therapy cannot be recommended for persons excluded from the NINDS study for one of the following reasons:

(a) Current use of oral anticoagulants or an INR >1.7.

(b) Use of heparin within the previous 48 h and a prolonged partial thromboplastin time.

(c) A platelet count <100 000/mm^3.

(d) Another stroke or previous head injury in the previous 3 months.

(e) Major surgery within the previous 14 days.

(f) Pre-treatment systolic blood pressure >185 mmHg or a diastolic blood pressure >110 mmHg.

(g) Rapidly improving neurological signs.

(h) Isolated mild neurological deficits such as ataxia alone, sensory loss alone, dysarthria alone or minimal weakness.

(i) Blood glucose <50 or >400 mg/dl.

(j) Seizures at the onset of stroke.

(k) Gastrointestinal or urinary bleeding within the preceding 21 days.

(l) Recent myocardial infarction.

(5) Thrombolytic therapy should not be given unless there are the facilities immediately available to manage bleeding complications.

(6) Caution is advised before giving r-TPA to persons with severe stroke (NIH stroke score scale >22).

(7) Persons receiving r-TPA should not receive aspirin, heparin, warfarin or other antiplatelet aggregating or antithrombotic drugs within 24 h of treatment.

(8) Whenever possible the risks of potential benefits of r-TPA should be discussed with the patient and their family prior to treatment being initiated.

Recommended reading

Adams, H. P., Brott, T. G., Furlan, A. J., Gomez, C. R., Grotta, J., Helgason, C. M., *et al.* (1996) Guidelines for thrombolytic therapy for acute stroke: a supplement to the guidelines for the management of patients with acute ischaemic stroke. *Circulation*, **94**, 1167–1174.

Furlan, A. J. and Kanoti, G. (1997) When is thrombolysis justified in patients with acute ischaemic stroke? A bioethical perspective. *Stroke*, **28**, 214–218.

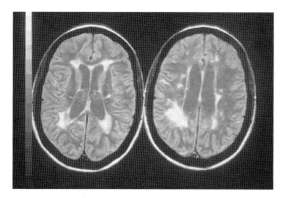

Fig. 9.3a

Q: *This 32-year-old woman presented with a 4-day history of unilateral progressive visual loss. Describe this MRI scan. What is the most likely cause of her reduced vision? (see Fig. 9.3a)*

A: There are multiple discrete and confluent high signal lesions in the cerebral white matter, these are predominantly in the deep white matter in a periventricular distribution. These T_2-weighted MRI lesions are typical of demyelination and the most likely cause of this patient's visual loss is a demyelinating optic neuritis.

Q: *Is there a correlation between MRI appearance and disability in multiple sclerosis (MS)?*

A: Relapsing-remitting MS (RRMS) is characterised by unpredictable attacks resulting in neurological deficits, separated by periods of remission of variable duration. Serial cranial MRI studies have shown that in contrast to its clinical profile RRMS is almost always active with new and recurrent MRI lesions appearing and disappearing during periods of clinical remission. However, the majority of these new lesions are neurologically silent. Several cross-sectional studies have demonstrated that disability correlates with MRI lesion burden although the strength of this correlation is variable. One study has reported a strong correlation between the magnitude of MRI lesion burden at the beginning of clinical symptoms, and subsequent disability at 5 years. There was also a correlation between initial lesion burden and lesion burden at 5 years. Other studies have concluded that cranial MRIs do not correlate well with clinical status as measured by standard impairment scales. An explanation for these variable results may be that progression is incompletely reflected by T_2-weighted MRI activity and that progressive disability in multiple sclerosis may result from axonal loss.

Q: *What treatments may reduce the number of relapses in patients with MS?*

A: There have been a number of clinical trials that have studied the effects of interferon (IFN)-β on the natural history of RRMS. The results of these trials are summarised below.

(1) Subcutaneous alternate day IFN-β1b:
  (a) Patients treated with 8 MIU of IFN-β1b avoided one in three relapses by the end of the second year and had an average of 1.5 relapses over 5 years.
  (b) The total mean area of abnormality on T_2-weighted MR scans had increased by 20% in the placebo group but decreased by 0.1% in the high-dose group.
  (c) Confirmed disease progression occurred in 35% of patients in the 8 MIU treatment arm compared with 46% in the placebo arm. However, this difference in disability as measured by the Kurtzke expanded disability

status scale was not statistically significant.

(2) Once-weekly intramuscular IFN-β1a:

    (a) The primary end point for this trial that recruited 301 patients with relapsing and remitting multiple sclerosis was the time to progression from baseline by 1 unit on the expanded disability status scale. A significant delay in deterioration, as demonstrated by Kaplan–Meier survival curve analysis was found in the treatment group.

    (b) Relapse rates were also lower in the treatment group.

    (c) Gadolinium-enhanced MR scans showed a 50% reduction of active lesions in the treated group at 2 years.

In view of the uncertainty over the long-term results of treatment and the cost of therapy (£10 000 per person per year), the Association of British Neurologists are of the opinion that 'the widespread use of β-interferon can not yet be recommended'. The results of larger scale studies with disability as the primary end point are awaited with interest.

Recommended reading

INFβ Multiple Sclerosis Study Group and the University of British Columbia MS/MRI Analysis Group (1995) Interferon beta-1b in the treatment of multiple sclerosis: final outcome of the randomised controlled trial. *Neurology*, **45**, 1277–1285.

Jacobs, L. D., Cookfair, D. L., Rudick, R. A., Herndon, R. M., Richert, J. R. and Salazar, A. M. (1996) Intramuscular interferon beta1a for disease progression in relapsing multiple sclerosis. *Ann. Neurol.*, **39**, 285–294.

Paty, D. W. and Li, D. K. B. (1993) The UBC MS/MRI Study Group and the INFβ Multiple Sclerosis Study Group. Interferon beta-1b is effective in relapsing-remitting multiple sclerosis. II. MRI results of a multicentre, randomised, double-blind, placebo-controlled trial. *Neurology*, **43**, 662–667.

9.4

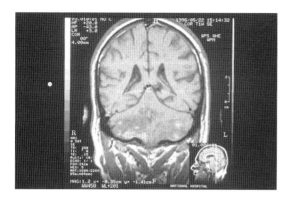

Fig. 9.4

Q: *Describe this MRI. What neurological signs may be present on examining this patient? (see Fig. 9.5)*

A: The widespread heterogeneous cerebellar lesions seen on this T$_1$-weighted MRI are consistent with extensive cerebellar infarcts.

Most acquired cerebellar disease falls into four categories:

(1) Infiltrative – cerebellar tumours account for 65% of intracranial tumours in children.
(2) Inflammatory – most commonly due to demyelination.
(3) Ischaemic.
(4) Degenerative.

Neurological signs of cerebellar disease include the following:

(1) Truncal ataxia – this is a feature of midline vermal lesions and is best demonstrated by asking the patient to walk. The gait is broad based and particularly unsteady when turning or when attempting heel/toe walking. Unlike sensory ataxia, it is not exacerbated by closing the eyes. Unilateral hemispheric cerebellar lesions will cause deviation or falling to the ipsilateral side.

(2) Limb dysmetria – this is manifest as past-pointing with the finger-nose test or inability to place the heel on the opposite knee-cap.
(3) Dysdiadochokinesia – this describes an inability to perform rapid, smooth repetitive movements. This is best demonstrated by asking the patient to tap your hand or a table rapidly, regularly and gently with their fingers.
(4) Intention tremor – this describes a tremor which is augmented throughout a movement from inception to completion. It is a term that is often used erroneously to describe postural tremors that are positionally dependent and should be avoided if there are no other signs of cerebellar disease.
(5) Cerebellar dysarthria – this may simply manifest as slurred speech. Scanning or explosive speech is caused by an inability to modulate the rate, rhythm or force appropriately. Dysarthria is a feature of vermal or global cerebellar disease, but may be absent in unilateral lateral hemispheric lesions.
(6) Pendular knee jerks.
(7) 'Rebound phenomenon' – this is caused by impaired damping of limbs when a load is removed suddenly.

Q: *What are the ocular features of cerebellar disease?*

A: The ocular signs associated with cerebellar disease are dependent on both the nature and the extent of the underlying pathology.

Non-localising signs of cerebellar disease:

(1) Papilloedema – increased intracranial pressure commonly occurs in patients with cerebellar tumours secondary to the obstruction of cerebrospinal fluid flow at the cerebral aqueduct, fourth ventricle or the

foramina of Lushka or Magendie. Not all children with hydrocephalus will develop papilloedema. However, all patients irrespective of their age, who present initially with headaches and vomiting secondary to raised intracranial pressure will have papilloedema.

(2) Visual field defects are related to papilloedema and post papillodema optic atrophy.

(3) Strabismus is a relatively common finding in patients with cerebellar tumours; this is typically an esotropia associated with a unilateral or bilateral abducens nerve paresis related to raised intracranial pressure. Less common forms of strabismus such as divergence paralysis and skew deviations have also been reported.

The following are localising eye signs that although not pathognomonic, are more specific of cerebellar dysfunction.

(1) Gaze-evoked nystagmus – pulse neurones initiate an eccentric eye movement which is then maintained by the activity of step neurones. The activity of these two classes of neurones is controlled by a neural 'integrator'. Gaze-evoked nystagmus is caused by a failure of this 'integrator'; on attempting eccentric gaze the eyes drift towards the centre with an exponentially decreasing slow phase velocity, a nystagmus beat then returns the eyes to the eccentric position. Anticonvulsant medication or sedatives are the most common cause of bilateral gaze-evoked nystagmus. In the absence of drugs it indicates bilateral brainstem and/or cerebellar dysfunction. Asymmetric but conjugate gaze-evoked nystagmus is almost always secondary to unilateral cerebellar disease and occurs on looking to the side of the lesion. In cerebellar disease persistent eccentric gaze may cause the gaze-evoked nystagmus to decrease in amplitude or even to reverse (rebound nystagmus), this is more indicative of chronic cerebellar disease. Gaze-paretic nystagmus is characterised by a slow rate

and large amplitude gaze-evoked nystagmus that is elicited by attempted eccentric gaze into the field of action of a paretic muscle. It is commonly seen in cases of abducens nerve paresis that have partially recovered or in patients with ocular myasthenia, it should not be confused with gaze-evoked nystagmus secondary to cerebellar disease. Bilateral gaze-evoked nystagmus may also be elicited in normal subjects in the extremes of gaze (end-point nystagmus), it tends to be of lower amplitude, is of equal amplitude in right and left gaze and is not associated with other oculomotor abnormalities.

(2) Saccadic pursuits – saccadic movements when attempting to perform smooth pursuits are typical of cerebellar disease. The presence of saccadic pursuits will help differentiate gaze-evoked from end-point nystagmus.

(3) Downbeat nystagmus – although present in the primary position it is more marked in down gaze, it is characterised by upward drifts and downward quick phases. It is most commonly associated with disorders of the craniocervical junction. Cerebellar lesions producing downbeat nystagmus include cerebellar ectopias such as Chiari malformation, demyelination and acquired and familial cerebellar degenerations.

Inappropriate saccades that mimic nystagmus:

(1) Saccadic dysmetria – this is the ocular equivalent of past-pointing. During voluntary change of gaze there is a conjugate overshoot (hypermetria) followed by several oscillations about the new fixation point before the eyes come to rest. As there is often coexistent gaze-evoked nystagmus saccadic dysmetria is best demonstrated on attempted refixation to the primary position. The exact nature of saccadic dysmetria will vary according to the site of the cerebellar lesion. Hypometric saccades are less common but are also associated with cerebellar disease.

(2) Ocular flutter – these horizontal movements are like those seen in ocular dysmetria except they occur spontaneously in the primary position. If these movements have a vertical or torsional component the abnormality is termed opsoclonus or saccadomania. The most common cause for these abnormalities is non-specific encephalitis with associated cerebellar and long tract signs. However, in otherwise well children neuroblastoma should be suspected until proven otherwise.

(3) Square wave jerks – are subtle non-rhythmic breaks in fixation which are followed by a single movement of refoveation.

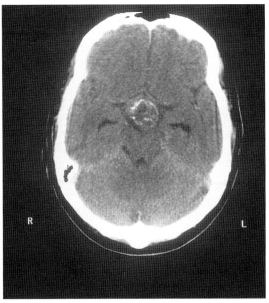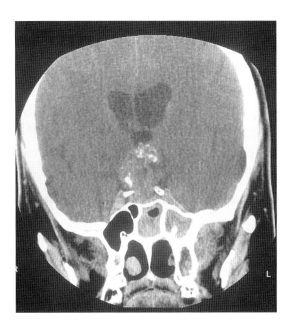

Fig. 9.5a

Accurate definition of masses involving the sella turcica and suprasellar region is of paramount importance as it will determine whether treatment should be surgical or non-surgical. It will also determine whether surgery is performed via a trans-sphenoidal or an intracranial approach.

Q: *Describe this CT scan. What is the diagnosis? (see Fig 9.4a)*

A: There is a relatively well-circumscribed cystic lesion arising from the suprasellar space. Punctate areas of calcification are visible within the walls and substance of the lesion. The third ventricle is dilated indicating a degree of hydrocephalus. This is an example of a craniopharyngioma.

The following radiological features are typical of craniopharyngiomas:

(1) Calcification – is found in 64% of craniopharyngiomas but it is not pathognomonic as calcification may be present in other sellar lesions such as sphenoidal masses (56%) and aneurysms (26%). Calcification is rarely seen in macroadenomas (5%) or sellar meningiomas (13%).

(2) Cystic change on MRI is another characteristic feature occurring in approximately 80% of craniopharyngiomas. Less marked cystic change secondary to necrosis may occasionally be a feature of macroadenomas (18%).

Craniopharyngiomas arise from the pituitary stalk and may present at any time from the neonatal period to the eighth decade. They are the most common non-glial intracranial neoplasm occurring in the first two decades. Chiasmal compression from behind and above is typical often causing profound visual impairment. Children tend to present with hypothalmic–pituitary disturbance (e.g. growth failure, retarded sexual development, infantilism, obesity and diabetes insipidus), hydrocephalus (sec-

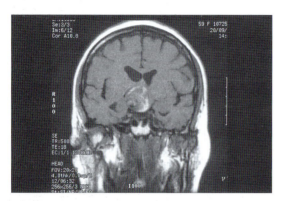

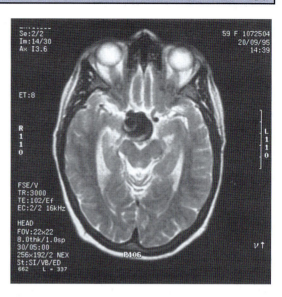

Fig. 9.5b

ondary to compression of the third ventricle), see-saw nystagmus (a pendular nystagmus comprising conjugate rotatory and disconjugate vertical components – this results in one eye which supraducts and intorts while the other infraducts and excyclotorts) or a squint. Visual impairment is not usually appreciated until the above features have prompted a referral. The presenting complaint in adults is progressive visual deterioration, which may be accompanied by a deterioration in the patient's mental state or signs of hypothalmic-pituitary dysfunction, e.g. impotence, decreased libido or galactorrhoea. Tumours are usually treated surgically with or without radiotherapy. Visual field improvement can be expected in approximately 60% of cases postoperatively.

Q: *Describe the MRI of this 75-year-old woman who presented with headaches and bilateral visual loss. (see Fig. 9.4b)*

A: This is another example of a well-circumscribed suprasellar lesion with a heterogeneous appearance. This lesion is an intracavernous carotid artery aneurysm. The hyperintense areas on T_1-weighted scans represent subacute thrombosis or flow-related enhancement. The hypointense areas on T_2-weighted scans signify intracellular deoxyhaemoglobin or methaemaglobin, calcification or flow voids.

Q: *These are the MR scans of a 28-year-old woman who presented with a 6-month history of headaches. What is the diagnosis? (see 9.4c)*

A: There is a mass filling the pituitary fossa that abuts the internal carotid arteries but does not encase them. It does not affect the chiasm. This is a typical pituitary macroadenoma. The characteristic radiological features of pituitary macroadenomas are:

(1) Sellar enlargement and erosion (94–100%). This is a non-specific sign as it is present in 50% of non-adenomatous masses. However, if it is absent the lesion is very unlikely to be a macroadenoma.

(2) Multilobulated upper tumour margin (60%).

(3) Cavernous sinus invasion, with encasement of the carotid arteries. This is usually unilateral and may be confused with intracavernous carotid artery aneurysms. Macroadenomas have a rather non-specific MR appearance, typically showing mild heterogeneous enhancement.

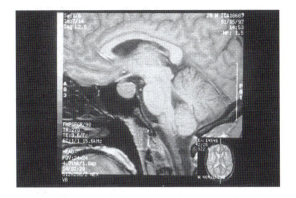

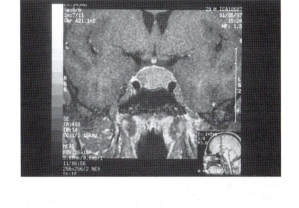

Fig. 9.5c

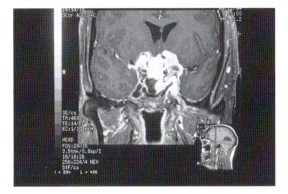

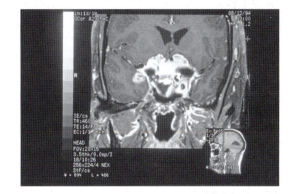

Fig. 9.5d

Q: *What are the radiological features that will distinguish a meningioma from a pituitary macroadenoma?*

A: Suprasellar and intrasellar meningiomas may arise from the diaphragma, tuberculum and dorsum sellae. These tumours typically exhibit dense homogeneous enhancement on MR (Fig. 9.4d – sellar meningioma that has invaded both cavernous sinuses). Although homogeneous signal intensity may be a feature in one third of macroadenomas and sphenoid tumours, it is never a feature of craniopharyngiomas or aneurysms. Obtuse dural margins involving the dorsum or tuberculum sellae are present in almost 70% of cases, as is dural tail enhancement. The latter is not a feature of macroaneurysms, but may be present in metastatic disease, sphenoidal tumours and lymphoma. Hyperostosis is found in one-third of sellar meningiomas; this is never a feature of macroadenomas, but may occasionally be confused with calcification in craniopharyngiomas. (see Fig. 9.4d)

Recommended reading

Donavon, J. L. and Nesbit, G. M. (1996) Distinction of masses involving the sella and suprasellar space: specificity of imaging features. *Am. J. Radiology*, **167**, 597–603.

9.6

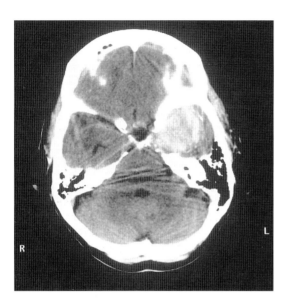
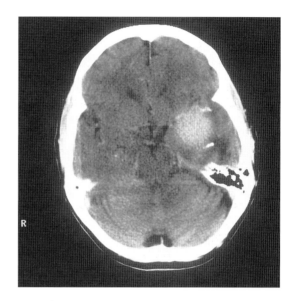

Fig. 9.6

Q: *This 58-year-old lady presented with a 5-year history of painless proptosis of her left eye. Describe these CT scans. What is the most likely diagnosis? (see Fig. 9.6)*

A: There is a marked hyperostosis of the entire left sphenoid ridge extending to involve the suprasellar area. There is also an associated well-defined and relatively homogeneous soft tissue mass that extends into the middle cranial fossa. These are the radiological appearances of a sphenoid ridge meningioma.

Intracranial meningiomas constitute 15% of adult intracranial tumours, sphenoid ridge meningiomas accounting for 18% of all intracranial meningiomas. Intracranial meningiomas occur three times more frequently in women than in men, the peak incidence being in the fifth decade

Q: *What are the ocular signs and symptoms of sphenoid ridge meningiomas?*

A: Tumours arising from the middle third of the sphenoid ridge will affect the neurovascular

structures passing through the optic canal and superior orbital fissure relatively early in the course of their development.

(1) Compression of the optic nerve by the tumour or by hyperostosis in the optic canal will result in visual loss that is slowly progressive in 90% of cases. Visual deterioration may be slow but intermittent in character ('stuttering' visual loss) and in 10% of cases acute visual loss will occur. Visual loss is bilateral in 50% of cases.

(2) The more medial parasellar tumours will affect adjacent vessels and the cavernous sinus early, causing diplopia secondary to cranial nerve involvement and chemosis and oedema secondary to venous obstruction.

(3) Tumours of the olfactory groove and lateral third of the sphenoid ridge tend to be larger before causing symptoms related to raised intracranial pressure.

(4) Proptosis, which may be axial or non-axial, and fullness of the temporalis fossa are

other common features of sphenoid ridge meningiomas. Old photographs are often invaluable when assessing expansion of the temporalis fossa or orbital displacement.

Q: *What treatment options are available in the management of sphenoid meningiomas?*

A: Treatment may not be required in the elderly patient or when the symptoms are minor and slowly progressive. However, in younger patients with progressive symptoms there are at present two main treatment modalities:

(1) Surgical resection – complete resection of intracranial meningiomas is often imposs- ible and is frequently associated with a high morbidity. This is due to the proximity of the tumour to the superior orbital fissure and the temporal and frontal lobes. If surgery is contemplated for slow growing tumours in the elderly patient the aim is usually to 'camouflage' the proptosis and to prevent corneal exposure.
(2) Radiotherapy – high doses of between 50 and 100 Gy are needed to treat these slowly dividing tumours. Complications of such treatment includes:
  (a) Radiation induced optic neuropathy.

(b) Malignant transformation in the meningioma.
(c) Formation of new tumours, e.g. menin- giomas or sarcomas.

The link between meningiomas and female hor- mones has been confirmed by the isolation of progesterone receptors in up to 70% of these tumours.

There have been several trials looking at the effect of progesterone antagonists on meningio- mas.

(1) Treatment with medroxyprogesterone acet- ate reduces progesterone receptor activity in meningiomas, but the agonist megestrol had little effect on tumour growth.
(2) Mifepristone has been shown to produce a subjective and/or an objective improvement (e.g. reduced tumour size on CT scanning). However, there was a high incidence of side effects such as nausea, fatigue, hot flushes and gynaecomastia due to the direct antag- onism of progesterone, and overactivity of the hypothalamic–pituitary–adrenal axis.

If the side effect profile of these drugs can be improved they may prove a useful adjunct to conventional therapy for large meningiomas.

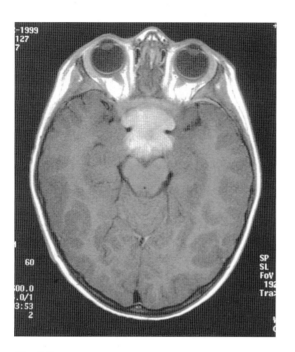

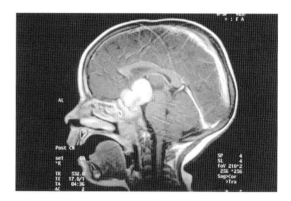

Fig. 9.7a

Q: *Describe these MRI appearances seen in an 8-year-old boy. What is the diagnosis? (see Fig. 9.7a)*

A: There is a large tumour of the optic chiasm elevating the floor of the fourth ventricle and displacing the midbrain posteriorly. These features are consistent with a pilocytic astrocytoma.

Although CT scan appearances are usually diagnostic MRI is the modality of choice for evaluation and follow-up of anterior visual pathway gliomas. MRI is especially useful when chiasmal involvement is suspected, as it has superior definition in distinguishing involved from uninvolved tissue. Typical radiological features of optic nerve gliomas include: a fusiform optic nerve swelling with smooth intact dural margins, anterior kinks adjacent to the globe, low-density cystic areas and no calcification.

Suprasellar extension and involvement of the optic tracts may also be seen in larger tumours.

Q: *What are the clinical features of optic nerve gliomas?*

A: Optic nerve gliomas are predominantly tumours of childhood, 75% of which present in the first decade of life (mean 8.8 years). The extent of visual pathway involvement is variable:

- 43% involve the chiasm.
- 22% are unilateral and limited to orbital portion of the optic nerve.
- 16% are diffuse with extrachiasmal involvement.
- 11% involve the optic nerve up to but not including the chiasm.
- 8% are diffuse but limited to optic nerve.

Neurofibromatosis type 1 is the underlying

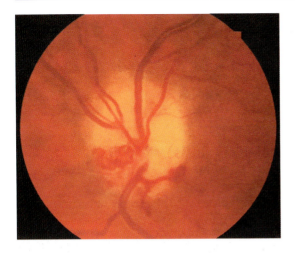

Fig. 9.7b

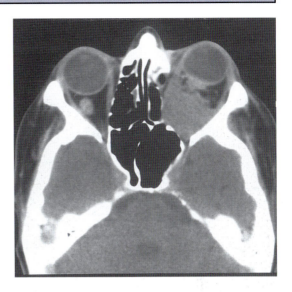

Fig. 9.7c

diagnosis in approximately 33–50% of cases. The overall prevalence of optic nerve glioma in neurofibromatosis type 1 (NF1) is approximately 20%.

Children present with axial proptosis (which may be of sudden onset), visual loss (with or without strabismus) or limitation of elevation. See-saw nystagmus may herald chiasmal involvement. The optic disc is usually pale but may be swollen and optociliary shunts have been reported. Visual field defects are invariably present. However, many series have shown these tumours to be silent in as many as 10% of patients with NF1.

Optic nerve gliomas are low-grade pilocytic astrocytomas. The vast majority have little potential for growth, although slow progression may be seen with serial MRIs. However, a more aggressive variant of optic nerve glioma with rapid growth is well reported.

Q: *What lesions may cause an enlargement of the optic nerve(s) in adults?*

A: The most common cause of an enlarged optic nerve in adults is an optic nerve meningioma. Like sphenoid ridge meningiomas they are more common in women (2 : 1 ratio), the majority occur between the third and sixth decades. Clinically they are characterised by a slowly developing compressive optic neuropathy; transient visual obscurations, mild dyschromatopsia, and an enlarged blindspot are typical early features. The development of proptosis (2–6 mm), progressive visual field loss and disc swelling with dilatation of the papillary vessels accompany enlargement of the tumour. Progressive disc gliosis and optociliary shunt vessels (Fig. 9.7b) are signs of marked optic nerve and vascular compromise respectively.

CT scans usually demonstrate one of three radiological patterns, diffuse thickening, fusiform swelling or globular enlargement (Fig. 9.7c).

In Fig. 9.7c the large posterior globular meningioma is causing proptosis of the left globe and there is a smaller nodular meningioma of the right optic nerve. This patient had NF2.

Meningiomas unlike gliomas do not cause kinking of the optic nerve and their nodular surface is in contrast to the smooth well-defined margins of optic nerve gliomas. Another characteristic feature is 'railroad tracking' caused by calcification in a subgroup of meningiomas (Fig. 9.7d).

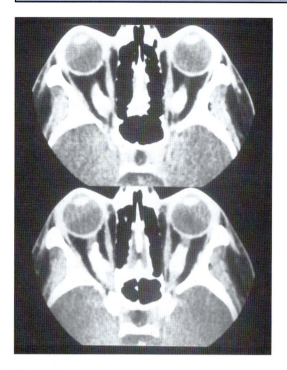

Fig. 9.7d

Tubular enlargement of the optic nerve may also be seen in the following conditions:

(1) Leukaemic infiltration.
(2) Optic neuritis.
(3) Papilloedema.
(4) Idiopathic orbital inflammation.

Recommended reading

Dutton, J. J. (1992) Optic nerve sheath meningiomas. *Surv. Ophthalmol.*, **37**, 167–183.
Dutton, J. J. (1994) Gliomas of the anterior visual pathway. *Surv. Ophthalmol.*, **38**, 427–452.

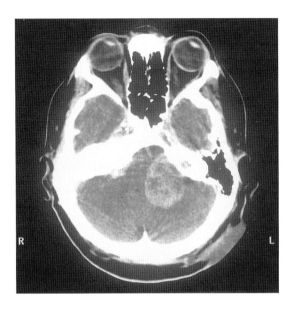

Fig. 9.8

Q: *How does an acoustic neuroma differ from a neurofibroma histologically?*

A:

(1) Neurofibromas are diffuse irregular proliferations of peripheral nerve sheath elements. The tumours are composed of elongated cells with basophilic nuclei and fine collagen fibres that have a 'maidenhair' appearance.

(2) Acoustic neuromas are neurilemmomas or schwannomas and as their name suggests they are composed of neoplastic Schwann cells. The spindled Schwann nuclei tend to form palisades, when this arrangement produces a compact texture it is known as the Antoni type A pattern. If the texture is loose and there are areas of necrosis this is called the Antoni type B pattern.

Q: *What is the diagnosis? Why may this patient present with a painless corneal ulcer? (see Fig. 9.8)*

A: There are bilateral masses in the cerebello-pontine angles. This CT scan appearance is typical of acoustic neuromas. These tumours arise from the VIIIth cranial nerve in the cerebello-pontine angle, where it lies in close proximity to the Vth, VIth and VIIth cranial nerves. Bilateral acoustic neuromas are characteristic of neurofibromatosis type 2.

The first structure to be damaged by an expanding acoustic neuroma is often the trigeminal nerve resulting in reduced corneal sensation. Corneal anaesthesia predisposes the cornea to a neurotrophic keratitis. Corneal sensation should always be assessed in patients presenting with ataxia, hearing loss or facial weakness, in whom the diagnosis of an acoustic neuroma is being considered.

Q: *Bilateral acoustic neuromas are a hallmark of NF2, what are the other features of this condition that distinguish it from NF1?*

A: The following features are typical of NF2:

(1) Cutaneous schwannomas.
(2) Spinal schwannomas.
(3) Absence of Lisch nodules and comparatively few café au lait spots.
(4) Juvenile cataracts (posterior subcapsular).
(5) Meningiomas tend to occur more frequently in patients with NF2.

Q: *How does the inheritance of NF1 differ from that of NF2?*

A: NF1 is inherited in an autosomal dominant pattern although 30 % of all cases are thought to be due to new mutations. The gene which is located on the long arm of chromosome 17 is

100% penetrant; however, expressivity is extremely variable. NF1 is the most common form of neurofibromatosis and has a frequency of approximately 1/3000.

NF2 is a much rarer condition with an incidence of 1/33 000–40 000. It too is transmitted as an autosomal dominant trait with variable expressivity (50% of all cases are spontaneous mutations). The NF2 gene is located on chromosome 22.

Q: *What type of gene is the NF1 gene?*

A: The NF1 gene has been cloned and characterised and there is increasing evidence that it acts as a tumour suppressor gene. A large segment of the gene codes for a protein which bears a close resemblance to the GTPase Activating Protein (GAP). This protein is thought to interact with the *ras* oncogene and act as a 'growth regulator'. The formation of tumours in NF1 is due to a combination of acquired mutations within the NF1 gene and other oncogenes or suppressor genes.

9.9

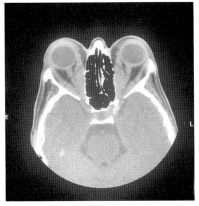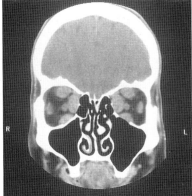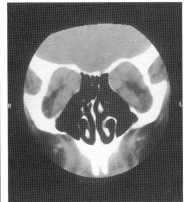

Fig. 9.9a

Q: *Describe these orbital CT scans. What is the differential diagnosis? (see Fig. 9.9a)*

A: These transverse and coronal orbital CT scans demonstrate gross enlargement of all the rectus muscles, especially the medial recti (note the enlargement involves the muscle belly behind the posterior margin of the globe). This has resulted in bilateral symmetrical proptosis and crowding at the orbital apices. The paranasal sinuses are clear and the superior ophthalmic veins visible on the transverse scans are of normal calibre.

These are the typical radiological appearances of advanced thyroid eye disease. Thyroid eye disease is the most common cause of unilateral or bilateral proptosis in an adult. Isolated muscles may be enlarged but more commonly there is involvement of two or more rectus muscles, the inferior and medial recti are most commonly affected. The radiological appearances are symmetrical in 60–70% of patients. Patients who demonstrate crowding at the orbital apices are at high risk of developing compressive optic neuropathy.

The differential diagnosis should include the following conditions:

(1) Idiopathic orbital inflammation – formerly termed orbital pseudotumour, this may present as an isolated myositis or with more global extraocular muscle involvement. It tends to be unilateral and is distinguished from dysthyroid disease radiologically by the involvement of the muscle tendons with fusiform enlargement of the entire muscle. There may also be local scleral and Tenon's capsule swelling.
(2) Orbital lymphoma – enlargement of muscles alone is rare. The presence of a poorly circumscribed diffuse lesion is more suggestive of lymphoma.
(3) Carotid-cavernous sinus fistulae – unilateral moderate enlargement of the extraocular muscles and dilation of the superior ophthalmic vein are the characteristic radiological features of this rare condition.

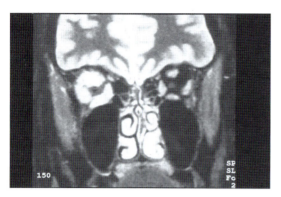

Fig. 9.9b

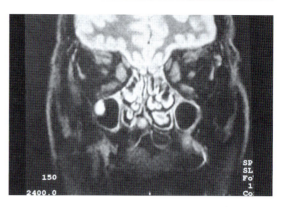

Fig. 9.9c

Q: *What advantages does MRI have over CT in the investigation and management of thyroid eye disease?*

A: MRI has a number advantages over CT in the assessment of thyroid eye disease. There is excellent soft tissue definition, no ionising radiation is used and no patient repositioning is required to take scans in different planes. Although CT provides accurate information regarding muscle size and crowding at the orbital apex it does not differentiate between muscles that are actively inflamed and those that have entered the fibrotic stage of the disease. The STIR (Short Tau Inversion Recovery) sequence suppresses the signal from orbital fat and enhances the signal from water containing tissues. Therefore actively inflamed muscles, which have a higher water content, will appear brighter relative to an adjacent uninvolved muscle such as temporalis (Fig. 9.9b). Fibrotic muscles, although equally enlarged, will have a less bright signal (Fig. 9.9c). Cine MRI techniques may also be used to demonstrate muscle elasticity, this is reduced in the burnt-out fibrotic stage of thyroid eye disease but is normal in actively inflamed muscles.

The ability to assess the activity of thyroid eye disease radiologically as well as clinically is particularly important if immunomodulatory therapy is being considered as this will only be of benefit in active disease. MRI is also helpful prior to strabismus surgery if there is any query

regarding inflammatory activity in the rectus muscles.

Q: Which patients with Graves' disease are at highest risk of developing compressive optic neuropathy?

A: The majority of patients with thyroid eye disease are young women, with the ratio female:male being 3.3:1. Patients with compressive optic neuropathy are older, are more frequently male (ratio female:male 1.6:1) and have a later onset of thyroid disease. There is also a higher incidence of diabetes mellitus (15% as opposed to 1.7% in those patients without optic nerve compromise). On examination these patients have more proptosis and a higher incidence of significant vertical deviation. Greater restriction of extraocular movements predisposes to more marked increases in intraocular pressure on upgaze.

Q: *How should patients with compressive optic neuropathy be managed?*

A: Compressive optic neuropathy is often insidious and may be masked by other symptoms such as diplopia. To avoid missing cases of optic nerve compression all patients with infiltrative thyroid eye disease should have a thorough assessment of optic nerve function including visual acuities, colour vision, disc examination and visual field assessment at each clinic visit. It should be noted that optic neuropathy often arises in patients with relatively little proptosis. This is because a rigid orbital septum restricts proptosis, thus allowing intraorbital pressure to rise.

Once compressive optic neuropathy has been diagnosed there are a number of treatment options. The treatment modality chosen depends on the severity of the eye disease, any complicating associated medical conditions and to an extent the previous experience of the ophthalmologist.

(1) Medical 'decompression' – in mild cases of optic nerve compression a short term course of prednisolone 40–50 mg o.d. may be effective. However a significant proportion of cases will not respond to this (or a higher dose) prednisolone regime alone. Over 50% of cases will relapse as treatment is curtailed. Oral prednisolone alone is rarely effective in severe cases of compressive optic neuropathy (Werner class 6b or c), such cases constitute an ophthalmological emergency and require rapid orbital decompression. This may be achieved by a series of pulsed intravenous methylprednisolone infusions (1 g over 1 h) separated by 48-h intervals; these infusions produce a rapid resolution of venous congestion within the orbit with a resultant decrease in intraorbital pressure. At the same time a prednisolone regime of 30–40 mg should be commenced plus a second line immunosuppressive agent such as cyclosporin A or azathioprine. These agents directed against the cell-mediated immune responses that drive thyroid eye disease, induce a prompt remission and enable patients to be maintained on relatively low doses of prednisolone so minimising the side effects of long-term therapy.

(2) Radiotherapy – a dose of 2000 cGy in 10 fractions over 12 days is a standard regime. Radiotherapy is most effective in producing a remission of soft tissue signs and orbital pain, with an improvement occurring in 70% of patients over a 2- to 4-week period. If it is to be used in cases of optic nerve compression it should be in conjunction with medical treatment because of its delayed onset of action. With modern delivery systems the risk of side effects such as radiation retinopathy and optic neuropathy are minimal, however coexistent microvascular disease, e.g. diabetes, is a relative contraindication to the use of radiotherapy.

(3) Surgical decompression – this should be limited to sight threatening cases which have failed to respond to medical therapy. Fortunately such cases are increasingly rare with the advent of combination immunosuppressive therapy and pulsed methylprednisolone. The key to successful decompression in cases of compressive optic neuropathy, regardless of the surgical approach, is removal of the apical portion of the orbital walls. Although rapid resolution of visual function may be achieved by decompression, with improvement in soft tissue signs, a significant number of patients will develop new diplopia. Patients may also experience worsening of pre-existing diplopia requiring strabismus surgery.

9.10

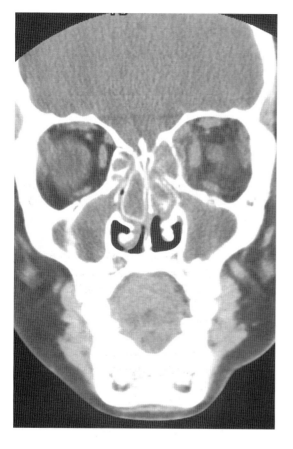 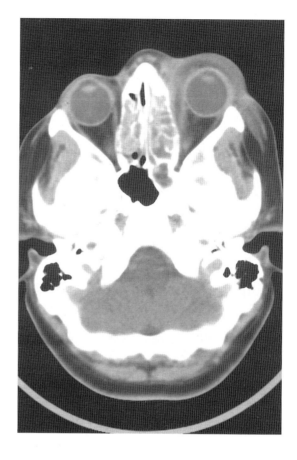

Fig. 9.10a

Q: *Describe the CT scan of this 35-year-old man who presented with a 3-day history of a red left eye associated with increasing lid swelling, ocular pain and fever. What is the likely diagnosis? (see Fig. 9.10a)*

A: This transverse CT scan demonstrates marked soft tissue swelling of the left lids and periorbital tissues. The medial and lateral recti and optic nerve are visible although the soft tissue involvement appears to extend posteriorly to involve the medial orbit. All the ethmoidal sinuses and both maxillary sinuses are opaque as is the left sphenoid sinus indicating widespread sinusitis.

These radiological features in conjunction with the history all point to a diagnosis of orbital cellulitis. In adults sinusitis (most commonly ethmoidal) is the cause of 58-85% of orbital cellulitis, 10–28% of cases have a cutaneous origin, the remaining cases are secondary to lacrimal infection, facial fractures or dental sources.

Q: *What are the complications of orbital cellulitis?*

A: Initial signs of progression include increasing pain, proptosis, chemosis, motility dysfunction, fever and malaise. Even with prompt and appropriate therapy, i.e. intravenous antibiotics, plus surgical drainage of the sinuses when indicated, the following complications may develop:

(1) Subperiosteal abscess formation – this may occur rapidly with motor and sensory signs out of proportion to the degree of inflammation. A marked non-axial proptosis associated with increased orbital tension and intraocular pressure, and decreased extraocular movement are typical of subperiosteal abscess formation. These abscesses are usually found on the medial wall of the orbit and are visible on CT scan as a homogeneous or heterogeneous fluid collection. As the collection increases in size the periosteum is displaced away from the orbital wall where it is not firmly adherent at the suture lines, producing a convex configuration.

(2) Orbital abscess formation – spread from a subperiosteal focus or progression of intraorbital cellulitis will lead to worsening of the inflammatory signs, proptosis and ophthalmoplegia. Signs of optic nerve compromise may develop rapidly, therefore all patients with orbital cellulitis should have their visual acuity, colour vision and pupillary reactions assessed at least every 4 h. Increasing malaise and fever are other signs of progression. Orbital abscesses are most commonly found in the retrobulbar space or superiorly, they are visible as rather ill-defined masses of lesions on CT scan.

(3) Cavernous sinus thrombosis – worsening of the inflammatory signs described above (which often become bilateral) accompanied by a varying level of consciousness, nausea and vomiting are suggestive of cavernous sinus thrombosis. In addition to the radiological signs described above there will be enlargement of the extraocular muscles and superior ophthalmic veins (typically bilateral). Even with appropriate antibiotic therapy cavernous sinus thrombosis has a 25% mortality.

(4) Ocular complications:
  (a) Exposure and neurotrophic keratitis.
  (b) Secondary glaucoma.
  (c) Septic uveitis, retinitis and in severe cases panophthalmitis.
  (d) Exudative retinal detachment and/or chorioretinal folds.
  (e) Compressive optic neuropathy.

Q: *How would your management of suspected orbital cellulitis differ if the patient was a poorly controlled diabetic with a history of recurrent ketoacidotic episodes?*

A: Signs and symptoms of orbital cellulitis in a brittle diabetic should be considered to be secondary to mucormycosis infection until proven otherwise. Rhino-orbito-cerebral mucormycosis is the most rapidly fatal fungal infection in man which until recently carried an almost 100% mortality rate. The classical presentation is that of a dehydrated diabetic patient in ketoacidosis with a blind immobile eye and a relative lack of inflammatory signs. Nasal stuffiness, epistaxis, rhinorrhoea with a granular or purulent discharge are other typical features. The fungus thrives in the glucose rich environment where it causes vascular occlusion with resultant tissue hypoxia. The following features help distinguish this condition from a pyogenic orbital cellulitis:

(1) Relatively mild proptosis and lid oedema.
(2) Paralytic ptosis and varying degrees of ophthalmoplegia secondary to orbital ischaemia (not orbital congestion as is the case in orbital cellulitis).
(3) Early onset of visual loss secondary to optic nerve ischaemia is the norm, unlike pyogenic cellulitis where visual loss is only seen in advanced cases.
(4) The classic black eschar involving the skin, palate or nasal mucosa. Initially it is only

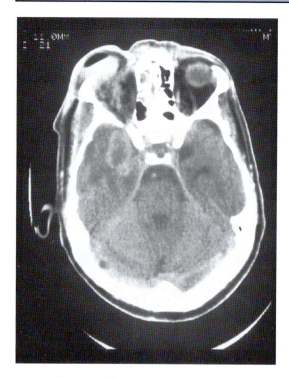

Fig. 9.10b

present in the minority of cases, but invariably develops as the infection progresses.

The critical factor in the successful management of orbital mucormycosis is early diagnosis based on the prompt recognition of the signs listed above in susceptible patients. Tissues should be obtained for microscopic examination, fungal culture and histopathology and any metabolic imbalance corrected. Wide local excision of involved tissue in combination with intravenous amphotericin B and irrigation of the tissues with amphotericin B is the currently recommended treatment. Liposomal amphotericin B should be considered in those patients with already compromised renal function. Hyperbaric oxygen therapy may also be of benefit although whether it should be used in all patients remains to be determined.

Figure 9.10b demonstrates a left middle cranial fossa abscess in a patient with advanced mucormycosis involving the left orbit.

Q: *What other conditions will predispose to mucormycosis infection?*

A: The following are also associated with a higher incidence of mucormycosis infection:

(1) Renal failure – 14% of patients in one large series were either in renal failure or had had renal transplantation.
(2) Desferrioxamine therapy – the iron chelate form feroxamine provides iron to Mucorales which is an important growth factor for the organism. Desferrioxamine has been shown to increase pathogenicity of Mucorales *in vitro*, as well as *in vivo*.
(3) Disseminated malignancy.
(4) Immunosuppressive therapy.
(5) Extensive burns.

Recommended reading

Yohai, R. A., Bullock, J. D., Aziz, A. A. and Markert R. J. (1994) Survival factors in rhino-orbital-cerebral mucormycosis. *Surv. Ophthalmol.*, **39**, 322.

9.11

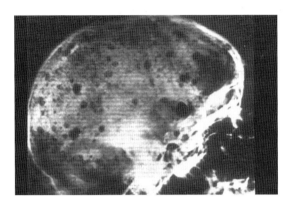

Fig. 9.11

Q: *Describe the skull X-ray of this 72-year-old man. What is the diagnosis? (see Fig. 9.11)*

A: There are numerous lytic lesions in the skull vault. These changes are pathognomonic of multiple myeloma. They arise as a result of increased osteoclastic bone resorption and inhibition of osteoblastic bone formation. The pronounced bone loss produced by this abnormal bone remodelling causes bone pain and predisposes to pathological fractures and hypercalcaemia.

Less numerous lytic skull lesions may be associated with bronchial carcinoma, breast carcinoma, thyroid carcinoma (rare) and renal carcinoma (rare).

Q: *What are the minimal diagnostic criteria for multiple myeloma? What ancillary investigations will help determine the extent of the disease?*

A: Myeloma is characterised by the classical triad of infiltration of the bone marrow by plasma cells, lytic bone lesions on skeletal radi-ology and the presence of M protein in the serum or urine or both.

The minimal diagnostic criteria for multiple myeloma are:

(1) More than 10% plasma cells in the bone marrow or plasmacytoma on biopsy.
(2) Clinical features of myeloma:
    (a) Bone pain and pathological fractures.
    (b) Anaemia and bone marrow failure.
    (c) Infection due to immune paresis and neutropaenia.
    (d) Renal impairment.
(3) At least one of the following:
    (a) Serum M band (IgG >30 g/l; IgA >20 g/l).
    (b) Urine M band (Bence–Jones protein-uria) – a urine sample should always be analysed for Bence–Jones proteins in cases of suspected myeloma as solitary free light chains are commonly unde-tected by routine serum electrophor-esis.
    (c) Osteolytic lesions on a skeletal survey.

Other investigations should include:

(4) Full blood count – look for evidence of:
    (a) Normochromic normocytic anaemia.
    (b) Neutropaenia.
    (c) Thrombocytopaenia may cause a bleeding diathesis.
(5) Erythrocyte sedimentation rate (ESR) – this is usually grossly elevated, i.e. >100 mm/h but may be normal in up to 10% of cases.
(6) Urea and electrolytes – the serum creatinine concentration is raised in 20% of cases at presentation. Renal failure may be second-ary to deposition of the protein in the renal tubules, hypercalcaemia, hyperuricaemia, or rarely associated amyloidosis. The 12-month survival in the presence of severe renal failure is <50%.

(7) Liver function tests – a raised alkaline phosphatase and a low serum albumin are poor prognostic signs.

Q: *Why may this patient present with a sudden unilateral loss of vision?*

A: Patients with multiple myeloma (especially IgG myelomas) may have symptoms of hyperviscosity. The most common ocular manifestation of this will be retinal venous occlusions. The possibility of a hyperviscosity syndrome should always be considered in patients with retinal venous occlusive disease, especially if there are no other risk factors present such as hypertension, diabetes or glaucoma. Heart failure, confusional states, coma, purpura and oral or nasal haemorrhage are other manifestations of hyperviscosity syndromes.

Q: *What are the causes of a monoclonal gammopathy other than multiple myeloma?*

A: Monoclonal gammopathy of undetermined significance is the most common cause of monoclonal gammopathy with a prevalence 20 times greater than that of multiple myeloma. The diagnosis is made when there is a serum M concentration of $<30\,g/l$ and there is no evidence of other causes of a monoclonal gammopathy such as multiple myeloma, Waldenström's macroglobulinaemia, amyloidosis or lymphoma. No treatment is required but follow up is necessary as 26% of these patients will eventually develop one of the conditions mentioned above.

Recommended reading

Knapp, A. J., Gartner, S. and Henkind, P. (1987) Multiple myeloma and its ocular manifestations. *Surv. Ophthalmol.*, **31**, 343–351.

Singer, C. R. J. (1997) Multiple myeloma and related conditions (Clinical review). *Br. Med. J.*, **314**, 960–963.

9.12

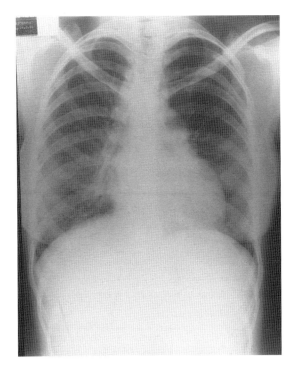

Fig. 9.12a

Q: *Describe the radiographic features of this chest X-ray. What is the differential diagnosis? (see Fig. 9.12)*

A: There is bilateral symmetrical enlargement of the hilar lymph nodes. The outer border of the shadow cast by the enlarged lymph nodes is clearly defined with multiple smooth contours. There are no other radiological changes of pulmonary disease.

The differential diagnosis should include:

(1) Sarcoidosis – the above are the classical features of bilateral hilar lymphadenopathy (BHL) associated with sarcoidosis. Rarely enlargement may be unilateral (right sided) or accompanied by calcification.

(2) Pulmonary tuberculosis – hilar or mediastinal lymphadenopathy may arise soon after primary infection as part of the primary complex. It is more commonly seen in children and tends to be unilateral. BHL as a feature of more extensive tuberculosis is more common in immigrants from Asia, Africa or the West Indies. The lymphadenopathy is not discrete, the enlarged nodes forming a large but ill-defined paramediastinal shadow and there may be associated pleural effusions or evidence of localised lung involvement.

(3) Hodgkin's disease and other lymphomas – the intrathoracic lymphadenopathy of Hodgkin's disease differs from that associated with sarcoidosis in a number of respects. Firstly, the lymphadenopathy tends to have a single contour (as opposed to multiple contours) and is usually asymmetrical. Secondly, the inferior part of the shadow is continuous with the heart shadow (in sarcoidosis there is a clear band between the inner border and the heart shadow).

(4) Metastatic carcinoma in hilar lymph nodes rarely mimics the symmetrical BHL of sarcoidosis.

(5) Coccidioidomycosis and histoplasmosis are other rare causes of hilar and mediastinal lymphadenopathy.

Q: *What is the natural history and prognosis of BHL secondary to sarcoidosis?*

A: BHL with or without clinical symptoms and signs of erythema nodosum or arthropathy is frequently the first manifestation of sarcoidosis. In a high proportion of patients BHL is detected on routine radiography and there will be no history of respiratory or systemic complaints. BHL resolves over a 1- to 2-year period with no additional pulmonary changes in approximately 60–70% of cases. Patients

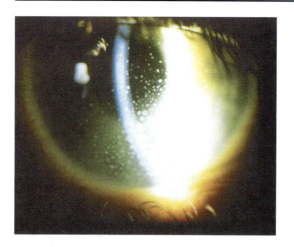

Fig. 9.12b

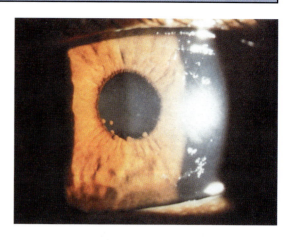

Fig. 9.12c

whose illness starts with erythema nodosum or febrile arthropathy have a better prognosis, with 85-90% attaining a normal chest radiograph. This figure is reduced to 48% for those who initially had constitutional or respiratory symptoms. These figures refer to a predominantly Caucasian population, in black patients presenting with BHL as few as 30% will attain complete resolution of radiological changes.

When BHL subsides spontaneously and completely without lung infiltration it is extremely rare for further manifestations of sarcoidosis to develop.

Q: *What are the clinical and radiological features of advanced pulmonary sarcoidosis?*

A: With increasing lung parenchymal involvement a restrictive airways disease causing exertional dyspnoea will develop. Pulmonary function tests will demonstrate a reduced total lung capacity, a decreased FEV1 and FVC, and a reduced gas transfer. This may eventually lead to pulmonary hypertension, cor pulmonale and death. Initially the chest X-ray will exhibit mottling in the mid-zones, this is followed by fine nodular shadows, and finally pulmonary line shadows and/or a honeycomb appearance indicative of pulmonary fibrosis may develop.

Q: *What is the relevance of BHL to the ophthalmologist?*

A: Acute anterior uveitis is the presenting feature of approximately 10% of cases of sarcoidosis. Uveitis (of any type) has been reported in 7–33% of patients with sarcoidosis at some point in their illness. However, the proportion of uveitis patients who were found to have sarcoidosis in several large ophthalmological series is less than 3%. The incidence of uveitis is highest in young women, who also invariably have BHL and/or erythema nodosum. Uveitis associated with BHL tends not to be granulomatous and is predominantly anterior. Although progression to a more insidious and granulomatous pattern, with more posterior uveal involvement, may occur as the disease progresses. Chronic granulomatous anterior uveitis tends to affect older patients with chronic lung fibrosis, it is characterised by mutton fat keratic precipitates (Fig. 9.12b) and Koeppe nodules (Fig. 9.12c).

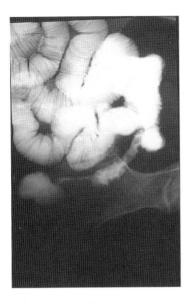

Fig. 9.13a

Q: *This 32-year-old woman had a 5-year history of general ill-health, intermittent abdominal pain and chronic diarrhoea. Describe this radiological investigation. What is the most likely diagnosis? (see Fig. 9.13a)*

A: This small-bowel barium follow-through demonstrates several of the cardinal radiological signs of Crohn's disease of the terminal ileum. There is a long area of narrowing (string sign) and deep ulceration with a characteristic 'rose-thorn' appearance, flanked by normal bowel (skip lesions).

Q: *What other small intestinal conditions should be considered in the differential diagnosis of Crohn's disease?*

A: The following conditions of the small intestine may mimic Crohn's disease:

(1) Ileocaecal tuberculosis – radiologically this may be identical to Crohn's disease, however the presence of longitudinal ulceration seen in tuberculous disease is a distinguishing feature. Ileocaecal tuberculosis should be considered in all patients with chronic diarrhoea and malabsorption especially those of Asian or African origin.

(2) Small bowel lymphomas – the presence of large focal ulceration is more typical of lymphoma.

(3) *Yersinia* enterocolitis – early disease confined to the terminal ileum may initially be confused with this transient condition. *Yersinia* enterocolitis never results in stricture or fistula formation.

(4) Small bowel ischaemia – the sudden onset and rapid resolution or perforation help to differentiate this condition from Crohn's disease.

(5) Carcinoid tumours – these may occasional cause fibrosis which mimics Crohn's disease.

Q: *What are the extra-intestinal features of Crohn's disease?*

A: Extra-intestinal manifestations of Crohn's disease include:

(1) Hepatic disease – this may range from minor abnormalities of liver function to established cirrhosis, pericholangitis, chronic active hepatitis, amyloidosis, gallstones and carcinoma of the biliary tree.

(2) Dermatological manifestations – erythema nodosum may precede, coincide with or follow the development of bowel symptoms. It is reported in between 0.5 and 9.0% of patients with Crohn's disease. Pyoderma gangrenosum is characterised by a painful necrotic ulcer with an advancing rolled or undermined border and a pustular centre. It is most commonly found over the shins and may also be associated with other gastrointestinal

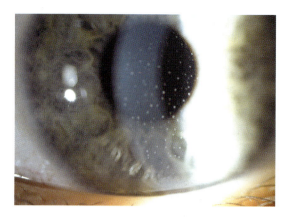

Fig. 9.13b

diseases including ulcerative colitis, diverticulosis and chronic active hepatitis.

(3) Articular manifestations – there are two types of arthritis associated with inflammatory bowel disease: enteropathic arthritis and sacroileitis or ankylosing spondylitis. The former is an inflammatory synovitis limited to a few large joints, radiological changes are minimal and permanent joint disease is rare. Improvement tends to follow treatment of the inflammatory bowel disease. Sacroileitis is frequently silent with the diagnosis being made on radiological grounds. Fewer patients with ankylosing spondylitis associated with inflammatory bowel disease are HLA B27-positive compared with sporadic cases (35 versus 90%). Spondylitis is slowly progressive and does not correlate with the activity of the inflammatory bowel disease.

(4) Ocular disease – uveitis has been reported as a complication in 4% of patients with inflammatory bowel disease, although there may be a higher incidence in Crohn's disease localised to the large bowel. The majority of patients with uveitis are HLA B27-positive and have a non-granulomatous anterior uveitis (Fig. 9.13b), which responds rapidly to topical steroid therapy. Episcleritis although less common than uveitis is a well recognised ocular manifestation of inflammatory bowel disease.

(5) Haematological disease – a broad spectrum of haematological abnormalities have been described in association with inflammatory bowel disease ranging from nutritional anaemias to acute myeloid leukaemia. Arterial and venous thrombosis secondary to hypercoagulable states are also well described.

Q: *What other conditions may present with gastrointestinal upset and ocular infection/inflammation?*

A:

(1) Ulcerative colitis – the ocular manifestations are identical to those of Crohn's disease.

(2) Reiter's syndrome – this consists of the triad of a seronegative reactive arthritis, a non-specific urethritis and conjunctivitis. Iritis occurs in approximately 20% of patients with the first attack of Reiter's syndrome. Approximately 80% of patients are HLA-B27-positive. However, it may also be precipitated by gastrointestinal infections such as *Shigella, Yersinia, Salmonella* or *Campylobacter*.

(3) Behçet's disease may occasionally cause an acute colitis (that may mimic Crohn's colitis) in association with the more typical spectrum of ocular inflammation, e.g. hypopyon uveitis and retinal vasculitis (see Question 1.20).

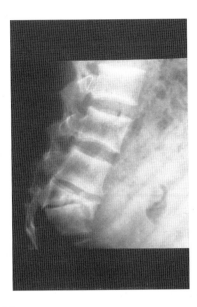

Fig. 9.14a

Q: *What is the diagnosis and underlying aetiology? What is the relevance of this condition to the ophthalmologist? (see Fig. 9.14a)*

A: This lateral thoracic/lumbar spine X-ray depicts a crush fracture of the T10 vertebra.

The relatively radiolucent adjacent vertebral bodies are indicative of marked osteoporosis, which is the underlying pathology in this crush fracture.

Osteoporosis is of particular relevance to the ophthalmologist as it is one of the major complications of corticosteroid therapy. Epidemiological data suggest that corticosteroid treatment doubles the risk of fractures of the hip and distal radius and at least quadruples the risk of vertebral fracture.

The ophthalmologist is frequently involved in the management of conditions that require prolonged corticosteroid therapy such as:

(1) Giant cell arteritis.
(2) Thyroid eye disease.
(3) Posterior uveitis/retinal vasculitis.
(4) Scleritis.

In a significant proportion of these conditions the patient is a post-menopausal woman.

Q: *What precautions should the clinician take before commencing a patient on a course of corticosteroids?*

A: Prior to commencing any patient on oral corticosteroids, irrespective of their dose or duration, the clinician should consider the following:

(1) Does the patient have any of the following strong risk factors for osteoporosis?
    (a) Premature menopause (<45 years).
    (b) Personal or family history of low-trauma fractures.
    (c) History of amenorrhoea.
    (d) Slender build (bone mass index <20 kg/m^2).
(2) Advise the patient of the risk of osteoporosis.
(3) Recommend lifestyle changes, such as not smoking, not drinking alcohol to excess, taking regular exercise and taking measures to avoid falls.
(4) Recommend calcium and vitamin D supplementation if deficient in the normal diet or in high-risk patient groups such as house-bound or elderly patients.
(5) If taking hormone replacement therapy, encourage to continue treatment.

Q: *What investigations are appropriate in the case of an osteoporotic fracture?*

A: The following diagnostic test should be considered to exclude other secondary causes of osteoporosis such as myeloma, endocrinopathies, other metabolic bone diseases and premature hypogonadism.

(1) FBC and ESR.
(2) Serum calcium and alkaline phosphatase.

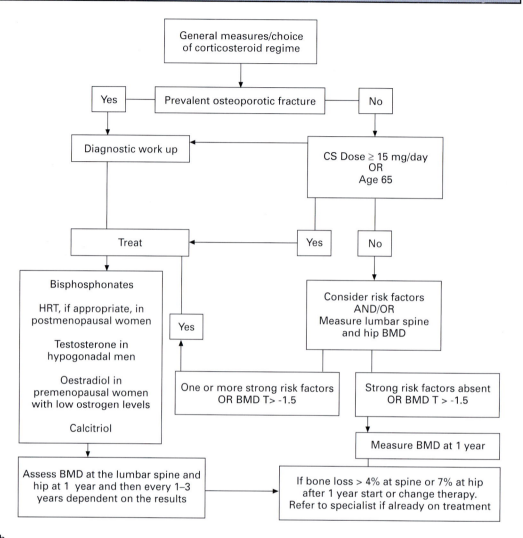

Fig. 9.14b

(3) Protein electrophoresis.
(4) Total testosterone in men and oestradiol in amenorrhoeic premenopausal women.
(5) Thyroid function tests.

Q: *Which patients taking oral corticosteroids should be monitored for osteoporosis? What are the indications for prophylactic treatment? What are these treatment options?*

A: The National Osteoporosis Society (NOS) guidelines recommend that any adult patient about to commence or currently being pre-scribed an oral dose of 7.5 mg/day or more of prednisolone (or equivalent dose of another corticosteroid) for six months or more, should be considered to be at risk of developing osteo-porosis and monitored appropriately. Studies indicate that at present only a small proportion (8–14%) of patients treated with corticosteroids are co-prescribed therapy to prevent bone loss. To address this problem the NOS have devised an algorithm for the prevention and manage-ment of corticosteroid induced osteoporosis (Fig. 9.14b).

Bone mineral density (BMD) can be measured with dual X-ray absorptiometry. BMD measurements are conventionally expressed as standard deviation scores. The *T* score indicates the difference between the patient's bone density and the ideal peak bone mass achieved by a young adult. The critical *T* score value of below −1.5 suggested by the NOS is consistent with the proposed European regulatory guidelines.

Bisphosphonates are the first option for treatment especially in those who are eugonadal or who are unwilling or unable to take hormone replacement therapy. At present the bisphosphonate etidronate is the only licensed preparation for the prevention or treatment of corticosteroid induced osteoporosis. Calcitriol has been shown to be an effective preventative therapy but the evidence for it as a treatment option is less convincing. The evidence that replacing low hormone levels alone prevent corticosteroid induced osteoporosis is limited.

Recommended reading

Lips, P. (1999) Prevention of corticosteroid induced osteoporosis [Editorial]. *Br. Med. J.*, **318**, 1366–1367.

National Osteoporosis Society (1998) *Guidance on the Management of Corticosteroid Induced Osteoporosis*. National Osteoporosis Society, Bath.

10.1

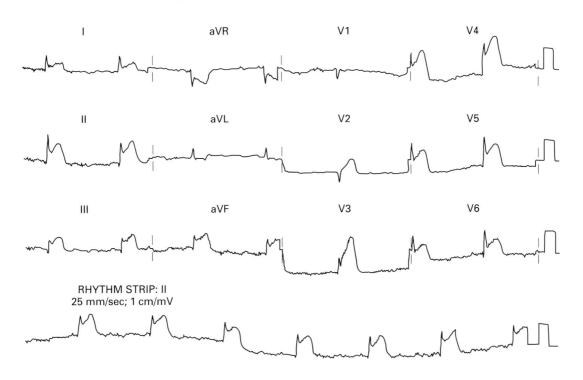

I aVR V1 V4

II aVL V2 V5

III aVF V3 V6

RHYTHM STRIP: II
25 mm/sec; 1 cm/mV

Fig. 10.1

Q: *Describe this ECG. What is the diagnosis? (see Fig. 10.1)*

A: There is marked ST elevation in leads II, III, AVF and V$_3$ to V$_6$. The ST segments are also moderately elevated in leads I and V$_2$. There is no evidence of T wave inversion in any leads. These changes are indicative of an acute inferior myocardial infarction.

Q: *How would the following influence your decision to commence thrombolytic treatment: (1) a history of proliferative diabetic retinopathy and (2) routine cataract surgery 3 days prior to the infarction?*

A: The benefits of thrombolysis in patients with acute myocardial infarction are well documented; in a published overview fibrinolytic therapy typically avoided 20–30 deaths per 1000 patients treated and was associated with only approximately four extra strokes per thousand during days 0–1. Two of these strokes were associated with early death and were already accounted for in the overall mortality reduction.

Diabetics are at above-average risk of death following myocardial infarction and the benefit of fibrinolytic therapy was if anything slightly greater in diabetic patients.

The ISIS-3, GISSI-2 and GUSTO studies, which included over 70 000 patients (11–15% of whom were diabetic), did not report any ocular complications following thrombolytic therapy. In fact there is only a single reported case of a vitreous haemorrhage in an eye with known proliferative retinopathy reported in the literature. Ocular haemorrhagic complications including subconjunctival haemorrhages, haemorrhagic choroidal detachments (associated with pre-existing telangiectasia) and vitreous haemorrhages have been reported in non-diabetic patients receiving thrombolytic therapy. In none of the above patients was there any permanent visual deficit following the haemorrhagic episode.

In view of the above evidence, although diabetic retinopathy is listed as a relative contraindication to thrombolysis it should not be withheld from diabetic patients with retinopathy. By the same token the presence of other retinal conditions including hypertensive retinopathy grades III–IV, Coats' disease and proliferative sickle cell retinopathy should not deter physicians from giving thrombolytic therapy.

The risk of haemorrhagic complications following uncomplicated cataract surgery (especially if the incision is corneal) is minimal, although a total hyphaema following thrombolytic therapy 8 days after extracapsular cataract extraction has been reported. As in the cases mentioned above, the haemorrhage in this case resolved speedily (within 4 days). Recent cataract surgery would therefore not appear to be a contraindication for thrombolytic therapy.

Recommended reading

Fibrinolytic Therapy Trialists (FTT) Collaborative Group (1994) Indications for fibrinolytic therapy in suspected acute myocardial infarction: collaborative overview of early mortality and major morbidity results form all randomised trials of more than 1000 patients. *Lancet*, **343**, 311–322.

Gruppo Italiano per lo Studio della Streptochinasi nell'Infarto miocardico (1990) GISSI-2: a factorial randomised trial of alteplase versus streptokinase and heparin versus no heparin among 12 490 patients with acute myocardial infarction. *Lancet*, **336**, 6571.

ISIS-3 (Third International Study of Infarct Survival) Collaborative Group (1993) ISIS-3: a randomised trial of streptokinase vs tissue plasminogen activator vs anistreplase and of aspirin plus heparin vs aspirin alone among 41 299 cases of suspected acute myocardial infarction. *Lancet*, **339**, 753–770.

The GUSTO Investigators (1993) An international randomised trial comparing four thrombolytic strategies for acute myocardial infarction. *N. Engl. J. Med.*, **329**, 673–682.

10.2

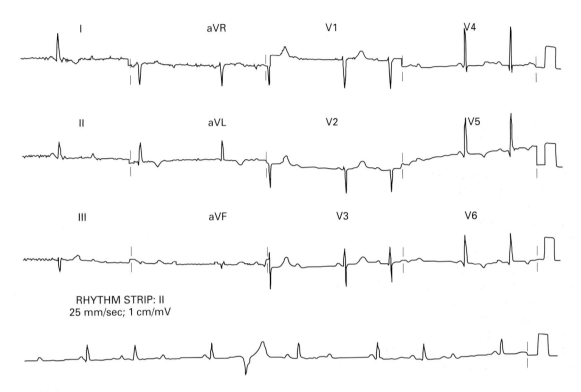

I aVR V1 V4

II aVL V2 V5

III aVF V3 V6

RHYTHM STRIP: II
25 mm/sec; 1 cm/mV

Fig. 10.2

Q: *Describe the ECG of this asymptomatic 65-year-old man. What ophthalmic conditions may be associated with this cardiac arrhythmia? (see Fig. 10.2)*

A: The rhythm strip demonstrates two normal P waves and QRS complexes followed by a solitary P wave, this pattern is then repeated. There is also an isolated ventricular ectopic. As there is an increase in the PR interval before the failure of conduction this is an example of a Mobitz Type I second-degree atrioventricular block (2:1). A Mobitz Type II second-degree atrioventricular block is characterised by a constant PR interval. This condition is commonly associated with distal conducting system disease, resulting in the presence of bundle branch block. There is also a high risk of progression to complete atrioventricular block.

Cardiac conduction defects including atrioventricular block may be found in a number of conditions with well recognised ocular manifestations.

(1) Myotonic dystrophy (see Question 5.8) – presenile cataract and symmetrical ptosis are almost universal ocular manifestations of this hereditary myopathy. Ophthalmologists should be aware that cardiac conduction defects, including AV block, are associated with myotonic dystrophy. A preoperative ECG is therefore mandatory if general anaesthesia is being considered for cataract surgery.

(2) Chronic progressive external ophthalmoplegia (see Question 3.7) – the Kearns–Sayer variant is associated with a pigmentary retinopathy and cardiac conduction defects.

(3) Glaucoma – β-blockers are known to cause AV block. The administration of intravenous verapamil to a patient taking β-blockers is particularly hazardous.

(4) Lyme disease – uveitis ranging from a mild iritis to a panophthalmitis is a feature of stage II Lyme disease. Approximately 10% of patients with stage II Lyme disease will develop myocarditis or heart block.

Q: *What other conditions may cause AV block?*

A: The following conditions may also cause AV block:

(1) Drugs – digoxin, verapamil, class I antiarrhythmics.

(2) Idiopathic conducting system fibrosis.

(3) Acute myocardial ischaemia or infarction.

(4) Infiltration – calcific aortic stenosis, sarcoid, scleroderma and syphilis.

(5) Infection – diphtheria, rheumatic fever and endocarditis.

(6) Vagal – athletic heart, carotid sinus and vasovagal syndrome.

10.3

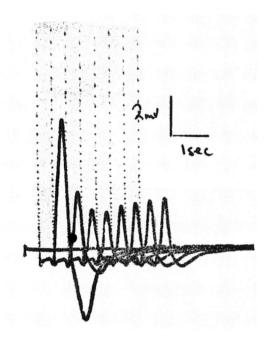

Fig. 10.3

Q: *Describe this repetitive nerve stimulation (RNS) EMG recording. What is the underlying condition? (see Fig. 10.3)*

A: RNS utilises an EMG to measure action potentials evoked by repetitive slow (25 Hz) supramaximal nerve stimulation. This produces no change in the amplitude of response in normal individuals. The RNS recording exhibits the characteristic decrement in the amplitude of the action potential seen in myasthenia gravis, which plateaus off by the fourth or fifth response.

Q: *What clinical features will distinguish between myasthenia gravis and Eaton–Lambert syndrome?*

A: Myasthenia gravis is characterised by muscle weakness that is exacerbated by exercise, i.e. the muscles exhibit fatiguability. The most

commonly involved muscles are the proximal limb, ocular and bulbar muscles. The muscle weakness in the Eaton–Lambert syndrome is caused by defective release of acetylcholine at the neuromuscular junction and actually improves with exercise. The proximal limb musculature is primarily affected, but ocular and bulbar involvement is rare. The RWS recording in Eton–Lambert syndrome shows the opposite pattern with an initially low amplitude action potential increasing steadily with motor nerve stimulation. The Eaton–Lambert syndrome is a rare non-metastatic manifestation of malignancy (60% are related to an oat-cell carcinoma).

Q: *What other investigations are indicated in cases of suspected myasthenia gravis?*

A: The tensilon test (see Question 3.6) and RNS although readily available are the least specific and least sensitive tests for suspected myasthenia gravis. Supplementary investigations include:

(1) Anti- acetylcholine receptor (AChR) antibody is specific to myasthenia gravis, and with newer assays it is found to be elevated in over 95% of patients with generalised myasthenia and in 60% of patients with ocular myasthenia. Although it is well documented that the extent of the acetylcholine receptor loss tends to parallel the severity of myasthenia, there is considerable debate as to whether actual antibody titres correlate with disease severity.
(2) Anti-striated muscle antibody is present in only 30% of myasthenic patients. However, titres are elevated in 90% of patients with a thymoma.
(3) Single-fibre electromyography (SFEMG) is more sensitive (88–92%) than RNS in the detection of myasthenia gravis. It may be helpful in patients with negative anti-AChR

antibody assays, an equivocal RNS or in those with mild myasthenia. The disadvantages are that it is a long and technically difficult test, which is not specific to myasthenia and is highly operator dependent.

(4) Mediastinal contrast enhanced CT or MRI to rule out thymomas which are present in 12% of myasthenic patients.

(5) Ancillary investigations to detect concurrent conditions:

(a) Thyroid function tests and antithyroid antibodies.
(b) Antinuclear antibodies and rheumatoid factor.

Recommended reading

Drachman, D. B. (1994) Myasthenia gravis [Review]. *N. Engl. J. Med.*, **330**, 1797–1810.

Kessey, J. C. (1989) Electrodiagnostic approach to defects of neuromuscular transmission. *Muscle Nerve*, **12**, 613.

10.4

Q: *The upper waveforms are an example of pattern reversal visually evoked potentials (VEP) in a control patient. What does the VEP represent? How is it measured, and what are the clinically important components of its waveform? (see Fig. 10.4a)*

A: The VEP is a measure of the response of the occipital cortex to visual stimulation. It is extracted, using scalp electrodes, from the background electroencephalographic activity by the computerised averaging of the responses to repeated stimuli. A reversing checkerboard pattern is the usual stimulus, although a diffuse flash may also be used. The VEP contains a prominent positive component at approximately 100 ms (the P_{100} component), the latency of this component is the most frequently used measure, although amplitude may also be relevant.

Q: *Waveforms A, B and C were recorded from three patients with acute unilateral visual loss. The dotted line represents two standard deviations from the mean P_{100} value taken from a group of control patients. Describe the pattern reversal VEPs for each patient. What is the likely diagnosis in each case?*

A:

- Waveform A – the VEP of the right eye is of normal latency and amplitude, the amplitude of the left VEP is normal but the latency is significantly prolonged (126 ms). Increased VEP latency although not pathognomonic, is very suggestive of demyelination. Approximately 90% of patients with definite multiple sclerosis will have VEP latencies greater than two standard deviations longer than those of control patients (mean delay 30–40 ms). Ischaemic optic neuropathies and other causes of optic atrophy may be associated with a slightly increased VEP latency in the order of

15–25 ms. The increased latency is thought to reflect a reduced conduction velocity in damaged visual pathway fibres, although delay at a retinal or cortical level may account for some of this prolongation. The visual acuities in this patient were RE 6/6, LE 6/12, there was reduced colour vision in the left eye, a left relative afferent pupillary defect but no disc swelling. The pattern reversal VEP supported the clinical diagnosis of a left retrobulbar optic neuritis.

- Waveform B – the VEP of the right eye is of normal latency and amplitude, the amplitude of the left VEP is reduced and the latency significantly prolonged (130 ms). The increased latency is again suggestive of demyelination. The VEP amplitude in demyelinating optic neuritis is normal or slightly reduced in the majority of cases, although extinguished VEPs have been reported in the acute phase of demyelinating optic neuritis. The reduced amplitude is secondary to a complete conduction block in damaged visual pathway fibres. On examination visual acuities were RE 6/6 and LE 6/36, no Ishihara colour plates were recognised by the left eye, there was a left relative afferent pupillary defect, and the left optic nerve head was swollen.

- Waveform C – the left VEP is almost flat and it could be argued that the latency of the small P wave is prolonged. Although the amplitude of the right VEP is normal the latency is prolonged (120 ms). A flat VEP is typical of ischaemic optic neuropathy and Leber's optic atrophy, but as mentioned above, may also be a feature of demyelinating optic neuritis.

This 40-year-old woman presented with a 1-week history of visual loss in her left eye. On examination visual acuities were RE 6/6 and LE 6/60, the colour vision in the asymptomatic right eye was reduced, the

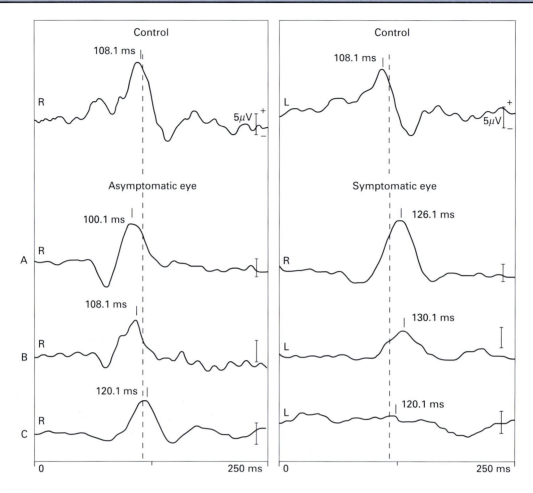

Fig. 10.4a

left disc was not swollen but there was a degree of right disc pallor. The clues to the underlying pathology in this case are the increased VEP latency, reduced colour vision and disc pallor of the asymptomatic right eye. These findings suggest a previous 'silent' episode of demyelinating optic neuritis in the right eye, making demyelination the most likely cause of the acute pathology in the left eye.

Q: *This 35-year-old man presented with sudden unilateral visual loss. On examination his visual acuities were RE 6/60 and LE 6/6, colour vision was reduced in the right eye, and*

there was a right relative afferent pupillary defect and a mild degree of right disc swelling. The left VEP was of normal amplitude and latency. Comment on the pattern reversal VEP of his right eye. What is the likely diagnosis? (see Fig. 10.4b)

A: The right VEP amplitude is markedly reduced but the latency is not prolonged. From the history and examination demyelinating optic neuritis would be the most likely diagnosis, however, the normal VEP latency rules this out. The second most common cause of unilateral visual loss associated with disc swel-

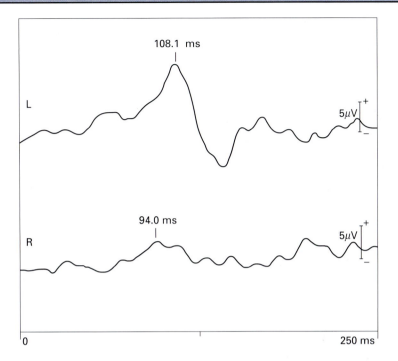

Fig. 10.4b

ling in a young man is Leber's optic neuropathy (see Question 3.7). The visual acuity in the right eye remained at 6/60, 6 weeks after his initial presentation he experienced a sudden deteriora-tion in the vision of his left eye associated with disc swelling and a similar VEP, so confirming the diagnosis of Leber's optic neuropathy.

10.5

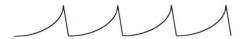

Fig. 10.5a

Q: *A 25-year-old woman with a history of dizzy spells and headaches was referred for a neurological opinion. Her visual acuities were 6/12 in both eyes. On examination the only feature of note was nystagmus, the waveform of which is illustrated above. What is the significance of this nystagmus waveform?*

A: The most significant feature of this waveform is the accelerating slow phase component. This waveform is typical of congenital idiopathic nystagmus (CIN) and sensory nystagmus (SN). SN maybe secondary to conditions such as albinism, aniridia, congenital stationary night blindness and other retinal dystrophies. All other forms of nystagmus have an exponentially decreasing slow phase velocity. The importance of distinguishing between CIN/SN and neurological nystagmus is that unnecessary neurological investigations may be avoided.

Q: *What clinical features of CIN will distinguish it from neurological nystagmus?*

A: The first step in evaluating any patient with nystagmus is to take a history:

(1) Is there a previous history of 'jumping eyes', 'dancing eyes' or 'wobbly eyes'? Remember that congenital nystagmus may wax and wane throughout life, but is almost always present before the age of 6 months.

(2) Is there a family history of nystagmus and associated conditions?
(3) Did the patient ever have patching treatment or wear glasses as a child?
(4) Is there a history of an infantile convergent squint?
(5) Is the nystagmus secondary to poor vision (i.e. SN)?
(6) Is oscillopsia present (illusion of environmental movement)? Patients with congenital nystagmus do not experience oscillopsia.

The clinical characteristics of congenital nystagmus include the following:

(1) It is uniplanar, i.e. the plane of the nystagmus (usually horizontal) remains unchanged in all positions of gaze, including vertical gaze. Only peripheral vestibular nystagmus and periodic alternating nystagmus are also uniplanar.
(2) The amplitude of the nystagmus is similar in both eyes.
(3) It is binocular and conjugate.
(4) It is dampened by convergence and exacerbated by fixation effort.
(5) There may be a 'null point' where the nystagmus is least marked and the patient may adopt a compensatory head posture to place the 'null point' in the primary position.
(6) There may be a superimposed latent nystagmus.
(7) There may be inversion of the optokinetic reflex.

The character of any form of nystagmus may be accurately documented using the following scheme (Fig. 10.5b).

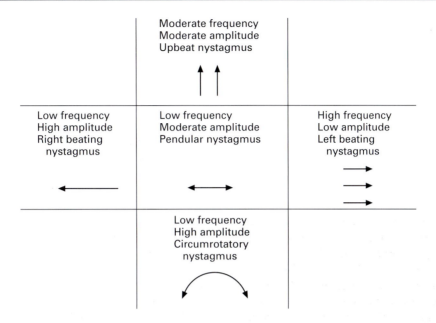

Fig. 10.5b

Index